Magnesium and Its Importance for Human Health and Disease Management

Magnesium and Its Importance for Human Health and Disease Management

Editor: Chester Cooke

AMERICAN
MEDICAL PUBLISHERS
www.americanmedicalpublishers.com

AMERICAN
MEDICAL PUBLISHERS
www.americanmedicalpublishers.com

Cataloging-in-Publication Data

Magnesium and its importance for human health and disease management / edited by Chester Cooke.
   p. cm.
Includes bibliographical references and index.
ISBN 978-1-63927-713-1
1. Magnesium--Physiological effect. 2. Magnesium in the body. 3. Magnesium--Health aspects.
4. Magnesium--Therapeutic use. 5. Magnesium deficiency diseases. 6. Magnesium--Metabolism--Disorders.
7. Magnesium--Metabolism. I. Cooke, Chester.
RC627.M3 M34 2023
613.285 2--dc23

American Medical Publishers,
41 Flatbush Avenue,
1st Floor, New York,
NY 11217, USA

ISBN 978-1-63927-713-1 (Hardback)

Contents

Preface

Magnesium is a mineral present in a range of foods. It plays a significant role in facilitating a wide range of chemical reactions in the body, like regulation of blood sugar, supporting the functioning of nerves and muscles, building strong bones, and regulation of blood pressure. Magnesium helps in steady functioning of the heart and facilitates contraction of the muscles by acting as an electrical conductor. It is a major nutrient which helps in the smooth functioning of various body parts like nerves, heart, bones, etc. Magnesium can be found in foods like whole grains, legumes, seeds, nuts and green leafy vegetables. The consumption of magnesium in enough amounts can help in the prevention and treatment of diseases, like migraine, Alzheimer's disease, cardiovascular disease and type 2 diabetes. The early symptoms of magnesium deficiency include weakness, loss of appetite, fatigue, nausea and vomiting. This book unravels the recent studies on the importance of magnesium for human health and disease management. It will serve as a reference to a broad spectrum of readers.

All of the data presented henceforth, was collaborated in the wake of recent advancements in the field. The aim of this book is to present the diversified developments from across the globe in a comprehensible manner. The opinions expressed in each chapter belong solely to the contributing authors. Their interpretations of the topics are the integral part of this book, which I have carefully compiled for a better understanding of the readers.

At the end, I would like to thank all those who dedicated their time and efforts for the successful completion of this book. I also wish to convey my gratitude towards my friends and family who supported me at every step.

Editor

Magnesium Deficiency Questionnaire: A New Non-Invasive Magnesium Deficiency Screening Tool Developed Using Real-World Data from Four Observational Studies

Svetlana Orlova [1], Galina Dikke [2], Gisele Pickering [3], Sofya Konchits [4], Kirill Starostin [4],*[iD] and Alina Bevz [4]

[1] Department of Dietetics and Clinical Nutritiology of Continuing Medical Education, Medical Institute, RUDN University, 119571 Moscow, Russia; rudn_nutr@mail.ru

[2] Department of Obstetrics and Gynecology with a Course of Reproductive Medicine, The Academy of Medical Education F.I. Inozemtsev, 190013 Saint-Petersburg, Russia; galadikke@yandex.ru

[3] Department of Clinical Pharmacology, University Hospital and Inserm 1107 Fundamental and Clinical Pharmacology of Pain, Medical Faculty, F-63000 Clermont-Ferrand, France; gisele.pickering@uca.fr

[4] Medical Affairs, Sanofi, 125009 Moscow, Russia; sofya.konchits@sanofi.com (S.K.); alina.bevz@sanofi.com (A.B.)

* Correspondence: kirill.starostin@sanofi.com

Abstract: Due to the high estimated prevalence of magnesium deficiency, there is a need for a rapid, non-invasive assessment tool that could be used by patients and clinicians to confirm suspected hypomagnesemia and substantiate laboratory testing. This study analyzed data from four large observational studies of hypomagnesemia in pregnant women and women with hormone-related conditions across Russia. Hypomagnesemia was assessed using a 62-item magnesium deficiency questionnaire (MDQ-62) and a serum test. The diagnostic utility (sensitivity/specificity) of MDQ-62 was analyzed using area under the receiver operating characteristic curve (AUROC). A logistic regression model was applied to develop a shorter, optimized version of MDQ-62. A total of 765 pregnant women and 8836 women with hormone-related conditions were included in the analysis. The diagnostic performance of MDQ-62 was "fair" (AUROC = 0.7–0.8) for women with hormone-related conditions and "poor" for pregnant women (AUROC = 0.6–0.7). The optimized MDQ-23 (23 questions) and MDQ-10 (10 questions) had similar AUROC values; for all versions of the questionnaire, there was a significant negative correlation between score and changes in total serum magnesium levels ($p < 0.0001$ for all comparisons; correlation coefficients ranged from −0.1667 to −0.2716). This analysis confirmed the value of MDQ in identifying women at risk of hypomagnesemia.

Keywords: hypomagnesemia; magnesium deficiency questionnaire; pregnancy; hormone-related conditions

1. Introduction

Magnesium deficiency and low magnesium intake are associated with altered levels of other electrolytes, cardiovascular events, various metabolic and neuromuscular conditions, type II diabetes mellitus, and depression [1]. Studies of various populations showed that 15–42% of apparently healthy adults have subnormal serum magnesium levels; magnesium deficiency is more frequent in women than in men, and the proportions are much higher in post-menopausal women and in individuals with obesity or type 2 diabetes [1,2].

Despite its implications in clinical practice, diagnosing magnesium deficiency still presents a challenge. To date, there is no gold standard for how to determine magnesium levels. Most of the magnesium tests used in research, such as 24-hour urine magnesium load test, muscle and bone concentration measurements, nuclear magnetic resonance imaging, and isotope studies, are considered impractical in the clinic [3]. The measurement of total magnesium concentration in serum using spectrophotometry with titan yellow or xylidyl blue is the most practical and reliable approach; however, there is an argument that the results can only serve as an approximation of magnesium concentrations in tissues [1–3]. The optimal cut-off serum concentration that indicates magnesium deficiency is also a matter of ongoing debate. In Russia and other countries, the most commonly used lower reference limit is 0.66 mmol/L [4]. However, the largest historical study in the US identified 0.75 mmol/L as the reference limit, and recent publications suggest that the cut-off should be set at 0.8 mmol/L [2,3,5].

Only about 0.8% of total body magnesium is present in blood, with the rest stored in soft tissue (19%), muscle (27%), and bone (53%), meaning that magnesium deficiency can be present even when serum magnesium levels are in the normal range [1,3,6–8]. Conversely, a low serum magnesium level is a clear indication of overall magnesium deficiency. However, due to the lack of specific symptoms, magnesium deficiency is rarely suspected in the clinic, and furthermore, serum levels or other tests (e.g., magnesium level in red blood cells) may not be reimbursed [3]. For these reasons, in many countries including Russia, magnesium tests are rarely reimbursed by insurance companies, emphasizing the need for a simple, reliable, and affordable screening tool to help identify magnesium deficiency.

Magnesium deficiency can be suspected and diagnosed with the help of the 'magnesium deficiency questionnaire' (MDQ-62), consisting of 62 questions that can be grouped into 5 general categories: wellbeing, lifestyle, pregnancy, disease, and medication [9]. Although MDQ-62 may help identify non-specific symptoms frequently accompanying magnesium deficiency, the questionnaire is cumbersome and time-consuming, and several questions are very similar. It is currently unclear to what extent MDQ-62 scores correlate with total magnesium serum concentration and whether it can be a reliable surrogate for laboratory values.

Four large observational studies conducted between 2012 and 2016 across multiple regions and cities in the Russian Federation assessed the prevalence and clinical management of magnesium deficiency in pregnant women (MAGIC, MAGIC2) and in women with hormone-related conditions (MAGYN, MAGYN2) using MDQ-62 and laboratory tests [10–13]. Here, we report the results of a secondary analysis using pooled data from these studies, designed to describe the prevalence of magnesium deficiency in these populations and to identify associated risk factors and comorbidities. Another key objective of this analysis was to develop shorter, optimized versions of the questionnaire that would offer the same level of accuracy in identifying suspected hypomagnesemia.

2. Materials and Methods

This manuscript summarizes a part of the secondary analysis of pooled data collected in four observational studies of magnesium deficiency in pregnant women and women with hormone-related conditions: MAGIC (DIREGL06157), MAGIC2 (DIREGL06468), MAGYN (MAGNEL06863), and MAGYN2 (MAGNEL07741) [10–13].

MAGIC and MAGIC2 enrolled pregnant women ($N = 1130$ and $N = 2117$, respectively) during routine visits to maternity welfare centers. Women were included in the studies if they were >18 years of age, were pregnant, and had suspected magnesium deficiency (fatigue, muscle cramps, etc.). The study excluded women who reported other known or obvious reasons for magnesium deficiency beside pregnancy [11,13]. MAGYN and MAGYN2 studies enrolled women with hormone-related conditions ($N = 9168$ and $N = 11,424$, respectively) attending outpatient clinics. Women were included if they were 18–60 years of age and used hormonal contraception or hormone replacement therapy (HRT) or had one of the following conditions: premenstrual syndrome (PMS), climacteric syndrome without HRT, osteoporosis, or other hormonal conditions (including endometriosis, polycystic ovarian disease, uterine leiomyoma, algodysmenorrhea, endometrial hyperplastic processes). Women were excluded if they had severe conditions potentially hindering their participation in the study or were receiving magnesium supplementation at baseline [10,12].

The present analysis included all patients who fulfilled the inclusion/exclusion criteria in the studies (Figure 1). Patients with missing data, contradictory/inconsistent data, or outlier data were excluded from the analysis (exclusion was performed separately for each variable of interest). Pooled databases were created for patient populations of "pregnant women" (MAGIC and MAGIC2) and 'women with hormone-related conditions' (MAGYN and MAGYN2).

Figure 1. Study population: **(a)** Pregnant women cohort; **(b)** Women with hormone-related conditions cohort.

2.1. Study Visits and Treatment

MAGIC, MAGIC2, MAGYN, and MAGYN2 were observational studies; during these studies, all treatment decisions were made by the treating physicians.

Epidemiological data were collected at baseline (Visit 1) for all participants. Patients with low serum magnesium at this visit or with suspected deficiency based on MDQ-62 attended Visit 2 and underwent a second assessment of serum magnesium. Visit 2 was scheduled by the treating physicians according to their standard practice; in MAGYN and MAGYN2, it occurred approximately 4 weeks after Visit 1.

The analysis of the effectiveness of magnesium supplementation included participants who had mild hypomagnesemia at Visit 1 (serum levels above 0.5 mmol/L but below 0.66 mmol/L or 0.8 mmol/L, depending on the specific cut-off used) and who were prescribed a combination of magnesium and vitamin B6, Magne B6® or Magne B6 Forte® (Sanofi), for approximately 4 weeks. Patients who received other types of magnesium supplementation were excluded from the analysis.

2.2. Study Objectives and Endpoints

The objectives of this secondary analysis were (1) to assess the sensitivity and specificity of MDQ-62; (2) to develop a shortened version of MDQ using regression modelling; (3) to assess the sensitivity and specificity of this new shortened version of MDQ, and (4) to analyze the ability of MDQ and shortened MDQ to reflect dynamic changes in serum magnesium level.

The following research questions were assessed.

Question 1: What are the sensitivity and specificity of MDQ-62 when detecting hypomagnesemia in women with hormone-related conditions, using serum magnesium level cut-offs of 0.66 mmol/L or 0.8 mmol/L?

Question 2: What are the sensitivity and specificity of MDQ-62 when detecting hypomagnesemia in pregnant women, using serum magnesium level cut-offs of 0.66 mmol/L or 0.8 mmol/L?

Question 3: Can the number of questions in MDQ be reduced without a loss of diagnostic quality?

Question 4: Is it possible to detect changes in the serum magnesium level using MDQ-62 or shortened MDQ?

2.3. Questionnaires

The MDQ-62, consisting of 62 questions, was developed previously and adapted for use in the Russian Federation [9,11]. Each question contributed 2–5 points to the overall score. A score of 51 points or more was used as an indication that magnesium deficiency was 'highly probable', whereas a score of 30–50 points was interpreted as 'likely' magnesium deficiency [9,11].

To optimize the questionnaire, each of 62 questions was tested for contribution to the total MDQ score as well as for association with the magnesium level using the population of women with hormone-related conditions as the training sample (see Statistical analysis for further details). Questions independently associated with hypomagnesemia were selected and assembled in the modified MDQ. The modified shortened MDQ was tested on the pregnant women cohort (testing sample).

The diagnostic performance of MDQ-62 and modified MDQ was analyzed in women who had serum magnesium level data and questionnaire data at Visit 1.

2.4. Statistical Analysis

The sensitivity and specificity of MDQ-62 were analyzed using area under the receiver operating characteristic curve (AUROC), MDQ cut-off, positive and negative predictive values, and the likelihood ratio. Statistical significance of AUROC was analyzed using a Mann–Whitney test.

For the development of the modified MDQ, stepwise multiple regression was applied to obtain a shortened version of the questionnaire. All 62 questions of MDQ-62 were included and excluded into the testing empty model step by step, using a bidirectional stepwise selection approach and assessing explanatory capabilities each time after inclusion or exclusion of a variable with the following parameters or variable to select and to keep: stepwise slEntry = 0.00001, slStay = 0.1, accordingly (software SAS version 9.4, SAS Institute Inc., Cary, NC, USA). The model was developed for both cut-offs, <0.66 mmol/L and <0.8 mmol/L. The quality of the final model was also analyzed and compared with the quality of the initial model.

Optimization was considered to be achieved for the modified MDQ if it consisted of a smaller number of questions than MDQ-62, if its sensitivity was equal or higher than that of MDQ-62, and if the difference in specificity between MDQ-62 and the modified MDQ was equal to or lower than 20%. Alternatively, optimization was considered to be achieved if the modified MDQ consisted of 15 questions, and if the difference in specificity between MDQ-62 and the modified MDQ was equal to or lower than 10%.

The training sample consisted of the cohort of women with hormone-related conditions, and the test sample consisted of the pregnant women cohort.

The sensitivity and specificity of the modified MDQs were analyzed using the same approach as for MDQ-62.

Correlation coefficients (r) were calculated based on changes from baseline to week 4 in terms of MDQ-62/modified MDQ scores and serum magnesium concentration and analyzed as continuous or dichotomous variables (hypomagnesemia: yes/no). Sensitivity and specificity were estimated using standard formulae [14]. The absolute magnesium concentration was defined as reference.

The study group characteristics (such as demographics) were analyzed using descriptive statistics, and differences were analyzed using the chi square test, unpaired t-test, and non-parametric tests. Statistical significance threshold was set at $p < 0.05$.

3. Results

3.1. Study Population

A flow chart of the study population is presented in Figure 1 (duplicated records, subjects without serum magnesium test, and subjects <18 years old were excluded from the analysis). In total, 983 participants in the "pregnant women" cohort and 9444 participants in the "women with hormone-related conditions" cohort were eligible for analysis. Participants in the "pregnant women" cohort had a median age of 28.0 years (range 18–52 years) and a mean (SD) serum magnesium level of 0.714 (0.125) mmol/L (range 0.12–1.92 mmol/L). Participants in the "women with hormone-related conditions" cohort had a median age of 44.0 years (range 18–60 years) and a mean (SD) serum magnesium level of 0.776 (0.198) mmol/L (range 0.08–4.08 mmol/L).

The prevalence of magnesium deficiency assessed by serum levels in pregnant women was 34.0%/78.9% when using 0.66/0.8 mmol/L, respectively, as the cut-off. In women with hormone-related conditions, the prevalence was 24.1%/54.8% when using 0.66/0.8 mmol/L, respectively, as the cut-off (Figure 1). After taking magnesium supplements for four weeks, a large proportion of women in both cohorts was able to achieve a magnesium level above the target cut-offs (Figure 2).

Figure 2. Prevalence and clinical management of magnesium deficiency: (**a**) Proportion of women with magnesium deficiency at Visit 1; (**b**) Proportion of women achieving the target level after four weeks of magnesium supplementation. [a] Includes women who had a magnesium serum level below the corresponding target at baseline.

3.2. Diagnostic Performance of MDQ-62

The diagnostic performance of MDQ was examined separately in pregnant women and in women with hormone-related conditions using two different cut-offs of magnesium serum levels: 0.8 mmol/L and 0.66 mmol/L. The analysis included 765 pregnant women and 8836 women with hormone-related conditions who both had the results of total serum magnesium test and had filled the MDQ-62 at Visit 1.

In pregnant women, using the cut-off of 0.8 mmol/L, AUROC for MDQ-62 was 0.6301 (standard error [SE] = 0.0251; 95% confidence interval [CI]: 0.5810–0.6792; $p < 0.0001$); using the cut-off of 0.66 mmol/L, AUROC for MDQ-62 was 0.6446 (SE = 0.0210; 95% CI: 0.6036–0.6857; $p < 0.0001$).

The positive predictive value of MDQ-62 was slightly better with the cut-off 0.66 mmol/L than that obtained with the cut-off of 0.8 mmol/L (Supplementary Tables S1 and S2).

In women with hormone-related conditions, using the cut-off of 0.8 mmol/L, AUROC for MDQ-62 was 0.7893 (SE = 0.0049; 95% CI: 0.7797–0.7990; $p < 0.0001$); using the cut-off of 0.66 mmol/L, AUROC for MDQ-62 was 0.7412 (SE = 0.0057; 95% CI: 0.7300–0.7524; $p < 0.0001$) (Figure 3). For this group, the positive predictive value was slightly worse with the cut-off of 0.66 mmol/L compared to that with the cut-off of 0.8 mmol/L (Supplementary Tables S1 and S2).

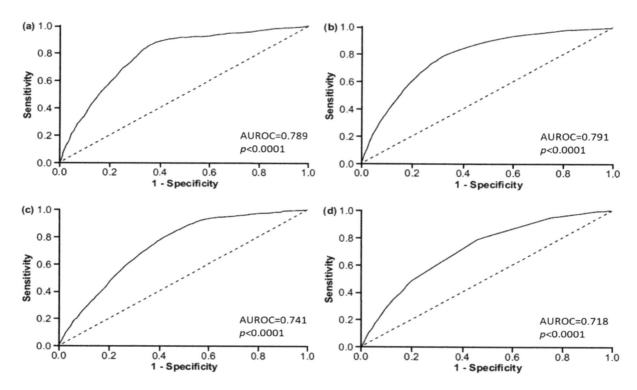

Figure 3. AUROC curves showing the questionnaires' ability to predict hypomagnesemia in women with hormone-related conditions for: (**a**) MDQ-62 using the cut-off <0.8 mmol/L; (**b**) MDQ-62 using the cut-off <0.66 mmol/L; (**c**) MDQ-23using the cut-off <0.8 mmol/L; (**d**) MDQ-10 using the cut-off <0.66 mmol/L. AUROC, area under the receiver operating characteristic; MDQ, magnesium deficiency questionnaire; The presented p values are related to ROC curves implying the H0 hypothesis: AUC = 0.5.

In all analyses, an MDQ-62 cut-off ≥51 points provided better specificity, worse sensitivity, better positive likelihood ratio, and worse negative likelihood ratio compared with an MDQ-62 cut-off ≥30. Formally, based on the previously published rough classification system, MDQ-62 had a "poor" (AUROC 0.6–0.7) diagnostic value in pregnant women and a "fair" (AUROC 0.7–0.8) diagnostic value in women with hormone-related conditions [15].

3.3. Development of Modified MDQs

Each of the 62 MDQ questions was tested for contribution to the total MDQ score as well as for association with the serum magnesium level in women with hormone-related conditions (training sample), using both cut-offs of <0.8 mmol/L and <0.66 mmol/L. For each of the cut-offs, a modified MDQ was developed that contained questions that showed statistically significant correlation with hypomagnesemia defined as the corresponding cut-off (Supplementary Table S3).

MDQ-23 contained 23 questions that showed a significant correlation with hypomagnesemia defined as <0.8 mmol/L (Supplementary Table S3); its total score range was 0–41, and the optimal cut-off value was >9. MDQ-10 contained 10 questions that showed a significant correlation with hypomagnesemia defined as <0.66 mmol/L (Supplementary Table S4); its total score range was 0–31, and the optimal cut-off value was >5.

The diagnostic performance of the modified MDQs to detect hypomagnesemia at the corresponding cut-offs was tested on the data from pregnant women with symptoms of magnesium deficiency (testing sample).

3.4. Diagnostic Performance of MDQ-23 and MDQ-10

The diagnostic performance of MDQ-23 was compared with that of MDQ-62 using the total serum magnesium level cut-off of 0.8 mmol/L (Table 1; Figure 3). MDQ-23 had similar AUROC, higher sensitivity, and lower specificity than MDQ-62 at cut-off ≥30; the 95% CIs overlapped, suggesting that the slight differences were not statistically significant.

Table 1. Diagnostic performance of MDQ-23 compared with that of MDQ-62 using a serum magnesium level cut-off of 0.8 mmol/L.

	MDQ-62 Score ≥ 30		MDQ-62 Score ≥ 51		MDQ-23 Score> 9	
	Value	95% CI	Value	95% CI	Value	95% CI
Training Sample: Women with Hormone-Related Conditions						
Sensitivity	0.884	0.874–0.893	0.248	0.236–0.260	0.888	0.879–0.897
Specificity	0.616	0.601–0.631	0.938	0.930–0.945	0.524	0.508–0.539
AUROC	0.789	0.780–0.799	0.789	0.780–0.799	0.791	0.781–0.800
p value	<0.001				<0.001	
Testing Sample: Pregnant Women with Symptoms of Magnesium Deficiency						
Sensitivity	0.845	0.815–0.872	0.283	0.248–0.320	0.864	0.835–0.890
Specificity	0.235	0.165–0.316	0.864	0.793–0.917	0.197	0.133–0.275
AUROC	0.630	0.581–0.679	0.630	0.581–0.679	0.610	0.560–0.659

CI, confidence interval; the presented p values are related to ROC curves implying the H0 hypothesis: AUC = 0.5.

The diagnostic performance of MDQ-10 was compared with that of MDQ-62 using the total serum magnesium level cut-off of 0.66 mmol/L (Table 2; Figure 3). MDQ-10 had a similar AUROC to that of MDQ-62 at score cut-off ≥30 and a higher sensitivity than MDQ-62 in the training sample, but a slightly lower sensitivity in the testing sample and a lower specificity in both samples; the 95% CIs overlapped, suggesting that the detected differences were not statistically significant.

Table 2. Diagnostic performance of MDQ-10 compared with that of MDQ-62 using a serum magnesium level cut-off of 0.66 mmol/L.

	MDQ-62 Score ≥ 30		MDQ-62 Score ≥ 51		MDQ-10 Score> 5	
	Value	95% CI	Value	95% CI	Value	95% CI
Training Sample: Women with Hormone-Related Conditions						
Sensitivity	0.927	0.915–0.938	0.310	0.290–0.331	0.940	0.929–0.950
Specificity	0.427	0.415–0.439	0.881	0.873–0.889	0.260	0.250–0.271
AUROC	0.741	0.730–0.752	0.741	0.730–0.752	0.718	0.706–0.730
p value	<0.001				<0.001	
Testing Sample: Pregnant Women with Symptoms of Magnesium Deficiency						
Sensitivity	0.887	0.843–0.922	0.358	0.301–0.418	0.869	0.823–0.906
Specificity	0.200	0.165–0.238	0.798	0.760–0.833	0.171	0.139–0.207
AUROC	0.645	0.604–0.686	0.645	0.604–0.686	0.610	0.568–0.652

The presented p values are related to ROC curves implying the H0 hypothesis: AUC = 0.5.

The ability of MDQ-23 and MDQ-10 to detect changes in total serum magnesium level was determined by estimating the correlation between serum magnesium level change and questionnaire score change from Visit 1 to Visit 2. In total, 765 pregnant women and 933 women with hormone-related conditions were included in the analysis (Table 3). In both datasets, statistically significant negative correlations were observed ($p < 0.0001$); however, the correlation coefficients were low (ranging from -0.1667 to -0.2716). For all tested questionnaires, the correlation coefficients were higher for women with hormone-related conditions than for pregnant women.

Table 3. Correlation between changes from Visit 1 to Visit 2 for total serum magnesium level and for initial (MDQ-62) and modified (MDQ-23 and MDQ-10) questionnaire scores.

| | Women with Hormone-Related Conditions ($N = 933$) | | Pregnant Women with Symptoms of Magnesium Deficiency ($N = 765$) | |
	r	p Value	r	p Value
MDQ-62	-0.2716	<0.0001	-0.2253	<0.0001
MDQ-23	-0.2890	<0.0001	-0.1729	<0.0001
MDQ-10	-0.2072	<0.0001	-0.1667	<0.0001

r, Pearson correlation coefficient. The presented p values are related to the Pearson correlation coefficient implying the H0 hypothesis: r = 0.

4. Discussion

This study is one of the largest and the most comprehensive real-world studies of magnesium deficiency in women. The study population consisted of pregnant women and women with hormone-related conditions from multiple cities and regions of the Russian Federation, providing a wide geographical coverage and a large sample size (a total of 10,427 women).

Among various magnesium tests, total serum concentration is considered to be the most practical for use in the clinic; however, the prevalence of magnesium deficiency may be underestimated if only blood levels are used [1–3,8]. Because of these considerations and the lack of clinical symptoms that specifically indicate magnesium deficiency, serum magnesium tests are rarely ordered and often not reimbursed by insurance companies [3]. There is an unmet need for a non-invasive assessment method that could be used as a surrogate for a clinical diagnosis of magnesium deficiency and at the very least serve as the basis for more detailed laboratory investigations.

This study measured the predictive ability of an existing non-invasive magnesium deficiency screening tool (MDQ-62). It was classified as a "fairly predictive" diagnostic tool for women with hormone-related conditions based on the rough classification of AUROC values [16]; nevertheless, it provided a clinically useful estimate of the magnesium status that may help physicians to identify a possible magnesium deficiency and provide a basis for laboratory testing. This questionnaire may also be used by the general populations to raise or dispel a possible suspicion of magnesium deficiency. The study used the existing MDQ-62 [9] to develop two new short questionnaires (MDQ-23 at cut-off <0.8 mmol/L and MDQ-10 at cut-off <0.66 mmol/L) that have nearly the same diagnostic performance as the original MDQ-62 when assessing likely magnesium deficiency but contain fewer questions and are therefore less time-consuming and easier to administer in routine clinical practice (the initial MDQ-62 and the modified MDQ-23 and MDQ-10 questionnaires with individual questions' scores are presented below (Table 4).

Having a quick non-invasive cost-free method that could provide further evidence in cases of suspected magnesium deficiency would be very valuable for healthcare providers, especially where there are very few symptoms, and the need for serum testing is otherwise unclear. In this study, the initial long and cumbersome questionnaire was shortened by almost three-fold without losing sensitivity and with a minimal loss of specificity (less than 20%). Both MDQ-23 and MDQ-10 scores showed a statistically significant negative correlation with changes in serum magnesium levels, demonstrating their potential clinical utility in everyday practice as a tool to identify suspected cases of magnesium deficiency.

Table 4. Initial (MDQ-62) and modified (MDQ-23, MDQ-10) questionnaires with individual questions' scores.

Question Number in MDQ-62	Question	Question Score in MDQ-62	Question Score in MDQ-23	Question Score in MDQ-10
Q1	Excessive emotional stress	2	2	3
Q2	Irritable, or easily provoked to anger	3	2	3
Q3	Restless, or hyperactive	2	-	-
Q4	Easily startled by sound or light	4	-	-
Q5	Insomnia	2	1	3
Q6	Chronic headache or migraine	3	-	-
Q7	Convulsions	2	2	-
Q8	Tremor or shakiness in the hands	3	-	-
Q9	Fine, barely noticeable muscle twitching around your eyes, facial muscles, or other muscles of your body	3	1	-
Q10	Muscle spasms	3	-	-
Q11	Muscle spasms in hands or feet	3	2	-
Q12	Gag or choke from spasms in your esophagus (food tube)	4	2	-
Q13	Asthma, short breathing, rales	3	-	-
Q14	Emphysema, chronic bronchitis, or high respiratory rate (tachypnea)	2	-	-
Q15	Osteoporosis	5	-	-
Q16	Kidney stone disease (urolithiasis)	3	-	3
Q17	Chronic kidney disease	2	2	-
Q18	Diabetes	4	-	-
Q19	Hyperfunction of the thyroid or parathyroid gland	3	-	-
Q20	High blood pressure	3	-	-
Q21	Mitral valve prolapse ("floppy heart valve")	4	4	4
Q22	Tachycardia, irregular heartbeat, or arrhythmia	3	-	-
Q23	Chronic bowel disease, ulcerative colitis, Crohn's disease or irritable bowel syndrome	3	-	-
Q24	Frequent diarrhea or constipation	3	2	3
Q25	Suffer from premenstrual syndrome or menstrual cramps	3	-	-
Q26	Pregnant or recently pregnant	2	-	-
Q27	Take Digitalis (Digoxin)	3	-	-
Q28	Take any kind of diuretic	5	1	-
Q29	Recent radiation therapy or other type of radiation exposure	5	-	-
Q30	Have more than seven alcohol drinks weekly	4	1	-
Q31	Problems with excessive alcohol intake	3	-	-
Q32	Take more than three portions of caffeine-containing drinks daily	2	-	-
Q33	Consumption of sugar-containing products	2	-	-
Q34	Crave carbohydrates and/or chocolate	2	2	-
Q35	Crave salt and/or salt products	2	-	-
Q36	Eat a high-processed food/fast food diet	2	-	-
Q37	Eat a diet low in greens, leafy vegetables, seeds, and fresh fruit	2	1	-
Q38	Eat a low-protein diet	2	-	-
Q39	Presence of undigested food or fat in feces	2	-	-
Q40	High blood pressure or pre-eclampsia in previous pregnancy	4	-	-
Q41	Chronic fatigue	2	1	-
Q42	Muscle weakness	2	2	-
Q43	Feeling of cold hands and/or feet	2	-	-
Q44	Numbness in face, hands, or feet	2	-	-
Q45	Persistent tingling in the body	2	2	3
Q46	Feeling of chronic indifference or apathy	2	-	4
Q47	Poor memory	2	-	-
Q48	Loss of concentration	2	1	-
Q49	Anxiety	3	2	-
Q50	Chronic depression for no apparent reason	2	2	-
Q51	Feelings of disorientation as to time or place	2	-	-
Q52	Feeling depressed, lack of personal identity	2	-	-
Q53	Hallucinations	2	-	-
Q54	Feeling of persecution and hostility from others	2	-	-
Q55	Pale and puffy face or poor, bad complexion	2	-	-
Q56	Loss of considerable sexual energy or vitality	2	2	-

Table 4. *Cont.*

Question Number in MDQ-62	Question	Question Score in MDQ-62	Question Score in MDQ-23	Question Score in MDQ-10
Q57	Been told by your attending doctor that your blood calcium is low	2	-	3
Q58	Been told by your attending doctor that your blood potassium is low	3	-	-
Q59	Take calcium supplements regularly without magnesium	2	3	2
Q60	Take iron or zinc supplements regularly without magnesium	2	-	-
Q61	Chronic fluoride intake	2	-	-
Q62	Frequently use antibiotics, steroids, oral contraceptives, indomethacin, cisplatin, amphotericin B, cholestyramine, synthetic estrogens	3	1	-

The symptoms potentially related to magnesium deficiency and included into the MDQ-62 questionnaire are non-specific and may be related to a number of various medical disorders, for instance, B-vitamins deficiencies, low blood calcium, alcohol abuse [16]. Moreover, some of the medical conditions mentioned in the initial MDQ-62 questionnaire (for instance, diabetes) may contribute to some of these symptoms independently of the Mg status [9,17]. Knowing that we did not expect from the beginning a high specificity from the questionnaire based on subjective self-assessment and while establishing research questions, we consciously concentrated our efforts on keeping maximal sensitivity, setting it as a priority in questionnaire optimization. We chose this particular approach to develop a fast non-invasive screening tool to catch most true positive cases implying further laboratory diagnosis verification. The price in this case is usually false positive cases with symptoms/complaints related to other medical conditions and, therefore, a lower specificity of the questionnaire.

MDQ-23 and MDQ-10 showed a slightly worse performance in pregnant women than in women with hormone-related conditions, possibly because some symptoms or signs assessed in the questionnaire may be caused by pregnancy itself rather than by an underlying magnesium deficiency, for example, emotional stress, irritability, or frequent constipation. Another potential reason is that this study used the same questionnaire and cut-offs for pregnant women and women with hormone-related conditions; however, pregnancy may require a different questionnaire design and validation. Finally, pregnancy-related magnesium deficiency may be associated with specific enhanced needs of mother and child, and the natural course of hypomagnesemia may differ in this group of patients. Future studies in pregnant women would be useful to determine whether the questionnaire could be modified further to increase its sensitivity and specificity for this specific population.

The four observational studies (MAGIC, MAGIC2, MAGYN, and MAGYN2) and the analysis presented here were not designed to validate MDQ-62; therefore, it may not be possible to directly extrapolate the results obtained here to the general population without additional validation procedures. One should also bear in mind that the serum levels of magnesium may be misleading, as they do not always accurately reflect the levels in soft tissues and bones; on the other hand, magnesium deficiency can be asymptomatic. Consequently, MDQ and laboratory testing cannot fully replace each other in the assessment of the magnesium status, and the complementary use of both should be considered. It may be advisable to use them step by step, for example to use the questionnaire first to corroborate a suspected deficiency and then follow up with a serum magnesium test.

To our knowledge, MDQ-62 and the two shortened versions presented here are currently the only tools that can be used to assess magnesium deficiency in a non-invasive manner and at no cost. The main advantage of MDQ-23 and MDQ-10 is their relatively high sensitivity (0.8–0.9) in predicting magnesium serum levels <0.8 mmol/L (MDQ-23 score >9) or <0.66 mmol/L (MDQ-10 score >5). Using the modified questionnaires allows clinicians to identify those at a high risk of magnesium deficiency and to verify it further with blood test. The relatively low specificity and therefore potentially high false positive rate are not a major limitation for screening tests, as their main goal is not to miss true positive cases. We believe that MDQs could be very useful in the clinical practice as magnesium deficiency screening tools.

5. Conclusions

This analysis determined the sensitivity and specificity of MDQ-62 in identifying patients with suspected magnesium deficiency. Furthermore, we developed two shortened questionnaires (MDQ-23 and MDQ-10), which were non-inferior to MDQ-62. All versions of MDQ showed a better performance in women with hormone-related conditions than in pregnant women.

Table S1: Diagnostic utility of MDQ using a serum magnesium level cut-off of 0.8 mmol/L, Table S2: Diagnostic utility of MDQ using a serum magnesium level cut-off of 0.66 mmol/L, Table S3: Development of MDQ-23, Table S4: Development of MDQ-10.

Author Contributions: Conceptualization, K.S., A.B, and S.O.; methodology, K.S., S.K., G.D., G.P.; validation, S.O., G.D., K.S.; formal analysis, S.K.; investigation, K.S.; resources, A.B.; data curation, S.K.; writing—original draft preparation, K.S.; writing—review and editing, all authors.; supervision, G.P.; project administration, K.S.; funding acquisition, K.S., A.B. All authors have read and agreed to the published version of the manuscript.

Acknowledgments: The authors are grateful to the participants included in the studies, the investigators, coordinators, and the study teams. The authors thank Lionel Noah and Beatrice Bois de Fer of Consumer Healthcare, Sanofi, Paris, France, for critical review of the manuscript. The authors thank Atlant Clinical Ltd. Clinical Research Organization for their contribution to protocol development and conducting the analysis. Editorial support was provided by Olga Ucar and Mark Davies of inScience Communications, Springer Healthcare Ltd., UK, and was funded by Sanofi.

References

1. Workinger, J.L.; Doyle, R.P.; Bortz, J. Challenges in the diagnosis of magnesium status. *Nutrients* **2018**, *10*, 1201. [CrossRef] [PubMed]

2. Costello, R.B.; Elin, R.J.; Rosanoff, A.; Wallace, T.C.; Guerrero-Romero, F.; Hruby, A.; Lutsey, P.L.; Nielsen, F.H.; Rodriguez-Moran, M.; Song, Y.; et al. Perspective: The case for an evidence-based reference interval for serum magnesium: The time has come. *Adv. Nutr.* **2016**, *7*, 977–993. [CrossRef]

3. Elin, R.J. Assessment of magnesium status for diagnosis and therapy. *Magnes. Res.* **2010**, *23*, S194–S198. [CrossRef]

4. Bell, C. *Clinical Guide to Laboratory Tests*, 3rd ed.; Norbert, W.T., Ed.; Saunders, Elsevier: St. Louis, MO, USA, 2009.

5. Lowenstein, F.W.; Stanton, M.F. Serum magnesium levels in the United States, 1971–1974. *J. Am. Coll. Nutr.* **1986**, *5*, 399–414. [CrossRef]

6. Abbott, L.G.; Rude, R.K. Clinical manifestations of magnesium deficiency. *Miner. Electrolyte Metab.* **1993**, *19*, 314–322. [PubMed]

7. DiNicolantonio, J.J.; O'Keefe, J.H.; Wilson, W. Subclinical magnesium deficiency: A principal driver of cardiovascular disease and a public health crisis. *Open Heart* **2018**, *5*, e000668. [CrossRef]

8. Ismail, A.A.A.; Ismail, N.A. Magnesium: A mineral essential for health yet generally underestimated or even ignored. *J. Nutr. Food Sci.* **2016**, *6*. [CrossRef]

9. Slagle, P. Magnificent magnesium. In *The Way Up Newsletter*; The Way Up Ltd.: Rancho Mirage, CA, USA, 2001; Volume 30.

10. Makatsariya, A.D.; Dadak, C.; Bitsadze, V.O.; Solopova, A.G.; Khamani, N.M. Clinical features of patients with hormone-dependent conditions and magnesium deficiency. *Akusherstvo Ginekol.* **2017**, *5*, 124–131. [CrossRef]

11. Makatsariya, A.D.; Bitsadze, V.O.; Khizroeva, D.K.; Dzhobava, E.M. Prevalence of magnesium deficiency in pregnant women. *Vopr. Ginekol. Akusherstva Perinatol.* **2012**, *11*, 25–34.

12. Serov, V.N.; Baranov, I.I.; Blinov, D.V.; Zimovina, U.V.; Sandakova, E.A.; Ushakova, T.I. Results of evaluating Mg deficiency among female patients with hormone-related conditions. *Akusherstvo Ginekol.* **2015**, *6*, 91–97.

13. Serov, V.N.; Blinov, D.V.; Zimovina, U.V.; Dzhobava, E.M. Results of an investigation of the prevalence of magnesium deficiency in pregnant women. *Akusherstvo Ginekol.* **2014**, *6*, 33–40.

14.   Trevethan, R. Sensitivity, specificity, and predictive values: Foundations, pliabilities, and pitfalls in research and practice. *Front. Public Health* **2017**, *5*, 307. [CrossRef] [PubMed]
15.   Safari, S.; Baratloo, A.; Elfil, M.; Negida, A. Evidence based emergency medicine; Part 5 receiver operating curve and area under the curve. *Emergy (Tehran)* **2016**, *4*, 111–113.
16.   Shenkin, A. Micronutrients in health and disease. *Postgrad Med. J.* **2006**, *82*, 559–567. [CrossRef] [PubMed]
17.   Ramachandran, A. Know the signs and symptoms of diabetes. *Indian J. Med. Res.* **2014**, *5*, 579–581.

2

Higher Dietary Magnesium Intake and Higher Magnesium Status are Associated with Lower Prevalence of Coronary Heart Disease in Patients with Type 2 Diabetes

Christina M. Gant [1,2], Sabita S. Soedamah-Muthu [3,4], S. Heleen Binnenmars [2], Stephan J. L. Bakker [2], Gerjan Navis [2] and Gozewijn D. Laverman [1,*]

[1]   Department of Internal Medicine/Nephrology, ZGT Hospital, 7609 PP Almelo,
      The Netherlands; c.gant@zgt.nl
[2]   Department of Internal Medicine, Division of Nephrology, University of Groningen,
      University Medical Centre Groningen, 9713EZ Groningen, The Netherlands;
      s.h.binnenmars@umcg.nl (S.H.B.); s.j.l.bakker@umcg.nl (S.J.L.B.); g.j.navis@umcg.nl (G.N.)
[3]   Centre of Research on Psychology in Somatic Diseases (CORPS), Department of Medical and Clinical
      Psychology, Tilburg University, 5037 AB Tilburg, The Netherlands; S.S.Soedamah@uvt.nl
[4]   Institute for Food, Nutrition and Health, University of Reading, Reading RG1 5EX, UK
*   Correspondence: g.laverman@zgt.nl

Abstract: In type 2 diabetes mellitus (T2D), the handling of magnesium is disturbed. Magnesium deficiency may be associated with a higher risk of coronary heart disease (CHD). We investigated the associations between (1) dietary magnesium intake; (2) 24 h urinary magnesium excretion; and (3) plasma magnesium concentration with prevalent CHD in T2D patients. This cross-sectional analysis was performed on baseline data from the DIAbetes and LifEstyle Cohort Twente-1 (DIALECT-1, $n = 450$, age 63 ± 9 years, 57% men, and diabetes duration of 11 (7–18) years). Prevalence ratios (95% CI) of CHD by sex-specific quartiles of magnesium indicators, as well as by magnesium intake per dietary source, were determined using multivariable Cox proportional hazard models. CHD was present in 100 (22%) subjects. Adjusted CHD prevalence ratios for the highest compared to the lowest quartiles were 0.40 (0.20, 0.79) for magnesium intake, 0.63 (0.32, 1.26) for 24 h urinary magnesium excretion, and 0.62 (0.32, 1.20) for plasma magnesium concentration. For every 10 mg increase of magnesium intake from vegetables, the prevalence of CHD was, statistically non-significantly, lower (0.75 (0.52, 1.08)). In this T2D cohort, higher magnesium intake, higher 24 h urinary magnesium excretion, and higher plasma magnesium concentration are associated with a lower prevalence of CHD.

Keywords: coronary heart disease; diabetes mellitus type 2; dietary magnesium intake; urinary magnesium excretion; plasma magnesium concentration

1. Introduction

Coronary heart disease (CHD) is one of the most prevalent and high-impact complications related to type 2 diabetes mellitus (T2D) [1,2]. In the general population, magnesium (Mg) deficiency might be associated with a greater risk of CHD; however, data on the inverse associations between Mg status and intake and CHD are inconsistent [3–9]. In T2D, the prevalence of hypomagnesemia is increased 14–48%, compared with 3–15% in those without T2D [10,11]. This could partly be due to increased urinary Mg excretion caused by insulin resistance, and partly due to poor dietary Mg intake [10–13].

However, surprisingly few studies report on the association between Mg and CHD in patients with established T2D [14,15].

In the DIAbetes and LifEstyle Cohort Twente (DIALECT), we collected extensive data on dietary Mg intake, 24 h urinary Mg excretion, and plasma Mg concentration. We aimed to study the association between the parameters of Mg (i.e., dietary Mg intake, 24 h urinary Mg excretion, and serum Mg concentration) and CHD. When we found that dietary Mg intake was inversely associated with CHD risk, we also explored whether there was an association between Mg intake from specific dietary sources (i.e., cereals, potatoes, etc.) and CHD risk.

2. Materials and Methods

2.1. Study Design

This was a cross-sectional analysis performed in the DIAbetes and LifEstyle Cohort Twente-1 (DIALECT-1). The study population and study procedures have been described previously [16]. The study has been approved by the relevant institutional review boards (METC-Twente, NL57219.044.16; METC-Groningen, 1009.68020), is registered in the Netherlands Trial Register (NTR trial code 5855), and is performed according to the guidelines of good clinical practice and the declaration of Helsinki.

2.2. Participants

All patients with T2D treated in the outpatient clinic of our hospital, aged 18+ years, were eligible for the study. Exclusion criteria were inability to understand the informed consent procedure, insufficient command of the Dutch language, or dialysis dependency. The inclusion flowchart has been described previously [16]. In total, 1082 patients were eligible for the study, of which 470 agreed to participate. The most important reasons for non-participation were no interest in the trial ($n = 123$), inability due to co-morbidity ($n = 62$), and no transport options ($n = 58$). After the baseline visit, 20 patients were excluded due to the fact that their diabetes diagnosis changed from type 2 diabetes to type 1 diabetes. Therefore, a total of 450 patients with type 2 diabetes were included in DIALECT-1. Missing values for specific variables are listed in Table 1.

2.3. Study Procedures

Eligible patients with type 2 diabetes were selected from the electronic patient file. At the clinic, sociodemographic characteristics, medical history, lifestyle behaviors, and current medications were recorded and anthropometric dimension were measured. Blood pressure was measured in a supine position by an automated device (Dinamap®; GE Medical systems, Milwaukee, WI, USA) for 15 min with a one-minute interval. The mean systolic and diastolic pressure of the final three measurements was used for further analysis. Physical activity was assessed using the Short QUestionnaire to ASses Health enhancing physical activity (SQUASH) questionnaire, which was previously validated and is commonly used in the Netherlands for population research [17].

Blood was drawn from venipuncture, for measurement of Mg and other variables relevant for diabetes. 24 h urine collections were performed as prescribed previously [16]. Samples of blood and urine were stored at $-80\ ^\circ C$ for later analysis.

Table 1. Baseline characteristics of patients with type 2 diabetes mellitus (T2D) by a breakup of prevalent coronary heart disease (CHD).

		Total Population	No CHD	CHD	p Value
	n	$n = 450$	$n = 350$ (78%)	$n = 100$ (22%)	
Patient characteristics					
Age, years	450	63 ± 9	62 ± 9	66 ± 7	<0.001
Male, n (%)	450	261 (58)	190 (54)	71 (71)	0.003
Diabetes duration, years	450	11 (7–18)	11 (7–17)	13 (7–20)	0.15
Systolic blood pressure, mmHg	449	136 ± 16	136 ± 16	136 ± 19	0.81
Diastolic blood pressure, mmHg	449	74 ± 9	75 ± 9	72 ± 10	0.01
Heart rate, beats/min	444	74 ± 13	75 ± 13	69 ± 11	<0.001
Body surface area, m^2	448	2.10 ± 0.22	2.10 ± 0.23	2.07 ± 0.19	0.27
Urinary creatinine excretion, μmol/24 h	446	13.8 ± 4.8	13.8 ± 5.0	13.8 ± 4.2	0.97
Complications					
Cerebrovascular disease, n (%)	450	47 (11)	87 (22)	13 (27)	0.44
Peripheral artery disease, n (%)	450	44 (10)	80 (20)	20 (44)	<0.001
Retinopathy, n (%)	447	106 (24)	78 (23)	32 (32)	0.05
Neuropathy, n (%)	450	157 (36)	116 (33)	46 (46)	0.02
Diabetic nephropathy, n (%)	446	183 (42)	131 (38)	58 (58)	<0.001
eGFR < 60 mL/min·1.73 m^2	450	101 (23)	74 (21)	30 (30)	0.06
Microalbuminuria, n (%)	445	131 (30)	92 (27)	44 (44)	0.001
Lifestyle					
Body mass index, kg/m^2	448	32.8 ± 6.2	33.1 ± 6.4	32.1 ± 5.6	0.15
Body mass index $\geq$ 30 kg/m^2, n (%)	448	290 (65)	233 (67)	57 (58)	0.12
Smoking, former or current, n (%)	450	306 (70)	235 (67)	78 (78)	0.04
Alcohol	424				
No alcohol, n (%)		148 (36)	123 (37)	32 (34)	0.80
0–13 units per week, n (%)		206 (50)	159 (48)	49 (52)	
$\geq$14 units per week, n (%)		61 (15)	47 (14)	14 (15)	
Adherence guideline physical activity, n (%)	433	249 (59)	201 (60)	52 (54)	0.34
Pharmacological treatment					
Insulin use, n (%)	450	275 (63)	218 (62)	68 (68)	0.30
Statin use, n (%)	450	331 (76)	254 (73)	86 (86)	0.006
Beta blocker treatment, n (%)	450	202 (46)	131 (37)	77 (77)	<0.001
RAAS inhibition, n (%)	450	289 (66)	225 (64)	73 (73)	0.10
Calcium antagonists, n (%)	450	98 (22)	66 (19)	36 (36)	<0.001
Thiazide diuretics, n (%)	450	136 (31)	108 (31)	29 (29)	0.72
Loop diuretics, n (%)	450	75 (17)	48 (14)	33 (33)	<0.001
Number of antihypertensives	450	2 (1–3)	2 (1–3)	3 (2–4)	<0.001
Magnesium parameters					
Dietary magnesium intake *, mg/day	438	305 ± 46	309 ± 47	292 ± 40	0.001
Urinary magnesium excretion, mmol/24 h	402	3.94 ± 2.05	4.03 ± 2.05	3.66 ± 2.02	0.13
Plasma magnesium concentration, mmol/L	432	0.77 ± 0.09	0.78 ± 0.08	0.76 ± 0.09	0.06
Hypomagnesemia, n (%)	432	73 (17)	53 (16)	20 (20)	0.35
Serum values					
Total cholesterol, mmol/L	447	4.0 ± 0.9	4.1 ± 0.9	3.8 ± 1.1	0.04
HDL cholesterol, mmol/L	445	1.1 ± 0.3	1.2 ± 0.4	1.0 ± 0.3	<0.001
LDL cholesterol, mmol/L	428	2.0 ± 0.7	2.0 ± 0.7	1.9 ± 0.8	0.25
HbA1c, mmol/mol	448	57 ± 12	57 ± 12	58 ± 12	0.43
Dietary intake					
Total energy intake, kcal/day	438	1922 ± 629	1904 ± 649	1932 ± 630	0.71
Urinary sodium excretion, mmol/24 h	444	185 ± 79	183 ± 67	197 ± 84	0.14
Urinary potassium excretion, mmol/24 h	439	77 ± 25	78 ± 26	77 ± 21	0.87
Calcium intake, mg/day	438	969 ± 441	979 ± 467	905 ± 358	0.16
Fiber intake, g/day	438	20.9 ± 6.6	20.8 ± 7.0	20.4 ± 6.1	0.60
Cholesterol, g/day	438	194 ± 96	195 ± 101	188 ± 79	0.51
Total fat intake, g/day	438	79 ± 39	78 ± 34	81 ± 34	0.52
Total protein intake, g/day	438	79 ± 23	79 ± 24	76 ± 22	0.18
Total carbohydrate intake, g/day	438	207 ± 69	205 ± 72	209 ± 67	0.61

CHD: coronary heart disease, eGFR: estimated glomerular filtration rate (CKD-EPI), HDL: high density lipoprotein, LDL: low density lipoprotein, HbA1c: glycated hemoglobin. * Dietary magnesium intake was adjusted for total energy intake using the residual method.

2.4. Magnesium Measurements

We calculated dietary Mg intake using a semi-quantitative food frequency questionnaire (FFQ), inquiring about the intake of 177 items during the last month, taking seasonal variations into account [18]. The FFQ was developed and validated at the Wageningen University, and has been updated several times. For each food item, the frequency was recorded in times per day, week, or month. The number of servings was expressed in natural units (e.g., a slice of bread or a whole apple) or household measures (e.g., cup or spoon). Both questionnaires were self-administered and filled in at home. The filled-in questionnaires were checked for completeness by a trained researcher, and inconsistent answers were verified with the patients. If the patient could not remember an exact number, the trained researcher approximated the intake as closely as possible during the interview. Dietary data was converted into daily nutrient intake using the Dutch Food Composition Table of 2013 [19]. We calculated the average intake of Mg by multiplying the frequency of consumption of each food item by its Mg content in the Dutch Food Composition Table of 2013 [19], and summing the amount of Mg across all food items. We calculated Mg intake from different food categories by multiplying the frequency of consumption of each food item in that specific category by its Mg content, and summing across all food items in that category. Food items of the FFQ included in each category are listed in supplementary Table S1.

Plasma and urinary Mg were measured in stored plasma samples in routine laboratory measurements using the xylidyl blue method. Buffer/Ethylenediaminetetraacetic acid was added to mask calcium. After incubation, xylidyl blue was added to form a purple complex with Mg. Mg concentration was determined by the photometric measurement of xylidyl blue extinction. The detection range for plasma Mg was 0.1–5 mmol/L, and for 24 h urinary Mg the range was 0.5–25 mmol/L. There were no patients with values outside of the detection ranges. Hypomagnesemia was defined as serum Mg concentration <0.70 mmol/L.

2.5. Main Study Outcome

Coronary heart disease (CHD) is defined as physician-diagnosed unstable angina pectoris or myocardial infarction, percutaneous coronary intervention, or a coronary artery bypass graft in the medical history. Medical history was checked for CHD during the interview at the baseline visit, and was later reviewed in the hospital electronic patient files on three different occasions, by three different physician researchers, who were unaware of the magnesium data.

2.6. Statistics

All statistical analyses were performed using the Statistical Package for the Social Sciences (SPSS), version 23.0. Normally-distributed data are presented as mean ± standard deviation. Skewed variables are expressed as median (interquartile range). Dichotomous variables are presented in number and percentage. Dietary intake of Mg was adjusted for energy intake by the residual method [20].

Differences between T2D patients with and without CHD were determined using the Student t (normal distribution), Mann–Whitney U (skewed distribution), or Chi-Square (categorical variables) test. In order to examine parameters associated with magnesium intake, we divided the population into sex-specific quartiles of adjusted magnesium intake. Differences between the quartiles were assessed using one-way ANOVA (normal distribution), Kruskal–Wallis (skewed distribution), or Chi-Square (categorical variables) analysis.

Correlations between Mg parameters were assessed using Pearson's correlation coefficient.

We calculated the prevalence ratio (95% CI) of CHD by sex-specific quartiles of (1) dietary Mg intake; (2) 24 h urinary Mg excretion; and (3) plasma Mg concentration, using multivariable Cox proportional hazard models, with the time to event set at 1 for all patients. The models were adjusted for the potential confounding of lifestyle parameters (BMI, smoking, alcohol, and physical activity) and nutritional intake (24 h urinary sodium excretion and 24 h urinary potassium excretion) [3,21].

There was a strong correlation between dietary calcium and Mg intake (R = 0.70), therefore we did not adjust for calcium intake in the final model. Effect modification was checked for gender, BMI, smoking, and alcohol, and no significant effect modification was found ($p > 0.20$ for all interaction terms). Sensitivity analyses were performed by excluding patients with diabetic kidney disease, and prevalence ratios were similar as in the primary analyses.

Additionally, we performed multivariable Cox proportional hazard models, and calculated the prevalence ratios of CHD for each 10 mg increment of dietary Mg intake from different sources (cereals, dairy, coffee, potatoes, meat, legumes and nuts, fruit, vegetables, and other). The models were adjusted for potential confounding of lifestyle parameters (age, BMI, smoking, alcohol, and physical activity) and Mg intake from the miscellaneous sources.

3. Results

In total, 450 patients with T2D were included in DIALECT-1. Baseline characteristics are shown in Table 1. In short, patients were 63 ± 9 years old, and the majority of the population was male (57%). The population represents T2D in secondary health care, with a median diabetes duration of 11 (7–18) years, and a high prevalence of diabetic nephropathy (42%).

There were 100 (22%) CHD cases diagnosed in our population (Table 1). T2D patients with CHD were older (66 ± 7 vs. 62 ± 9 years, $p < 0.001$), were more often men (71% vs. 54%, $p = 0.003$), and more often had peripheral artery disease (44% vs. 20%, $p < 0.001$), and nephropathy (58% vs. 38%, $p < 0.001$) than patients without CHD. There were no differences in lifestyle parameters between those with and without CHD. Regarding pharmacological treatment, those with CHD more often used beta-blockers (77% vs. 37%, $p < 0.001$), and loop diuretics (33% vs. 14%, $p < 0.001$) than those without CHD. This was paralleled by a lower diastolic blood pressure (72 ± 10 mmHg vs. 75 ± 9 mmHg, $p = 0.01$) and heart rate (69 ± 11 beats/min vs. 75 ± 13 beats/min, $p < 0.001$) in patients with CHD. Systolic blood pressure was 136 ± 16 mmHg, and did not differ between the groups. Although patients with CHD more often used statins (86% vs. 73%, $p = 0.006$), serum LDL was similar in the groups (2.0 ± 0.7 mmol/L), and serum HDL cholesterol was lower in those with CHD (1.0 ± 0.3 mmol/L vs. 1.2 ± 0.4 mmol/L, $p < 0.001$) compared to those without CHD.

Mean energy-adjusted dietary Mg intake was 305 ± 46 mg/day, and was lower in those with CHD (adjusted standardized beta = -0.14, $p = 0.003$). Mean 24 h urinary Mg excretion was 3.94 ± 2.05 mmol/24 h, and mean plasma Mg concentration was 0.77 ± 0.09 mmol/L; neither differed statistically significantly between those with and without CHD (Table 1). Hypomagnesemia (plasma Mg < 0.7 mmol/L) was present in 73 patients (17%), of which 11 patients (3%) had a plasma Mg of <0.6 mmol/L.

Dietary Mg intake was significantly correlated with 24 h urinary Mg excretion (Pearson R = 0.24, $p < 0.001$), but not with plasma Mg (R = 0.02, $p = 0.64$). 24 h urinary Mg excretion was significantly correlated with plasma Mg (R = 0.13, $p < 0.008$).

Systolic blood pressure was lowest in the highest gender-specific quartile of energy-adjusted magnesium intake (4th quartile 133 ± 13 vs. 1st quartile 137 ± 17 mmHg; Supplementary Table S2), and the number of antihypertensive drugs used was lowest in this quartile as well (4th quartile 2 (0–3) vs. 2 (1–3) in other quartiles, $p = 0.008$). Serum HbA1c and cholesterol levels were similar in all Mg intake quartiles. There was a trend towards higher urinary potassium excretion, dietary calcium, fiber, protein, and carbohydrate intake, as well as a lower dietary intake of fat in each of the higher quartiles of magnesium intake.

3.1. Association between Dietary Magnesium Intake, 24 h Urinary Magnesium Excretion, Plasma Magnesium Concentration, and the Prevalence of Coronary Heart Disease

The highest quartile of Mg intake was significantly associated with a lower prevalence ratio (PR) of CHD than the lowest quartile of Mg intake (0.40 (0.20, 0.77); Table 2). When adjusting for age and lifestyle parameters (BMI, smoking, alcohol, and physical activity), the PR remained largely unchanged (0.42 (0.22, 0.82)). After adjustment for dietary intake of other micronutrients (total energy intake, sodium, and potassium), the PR became (0.40 (0.20, 0.79)), and the *p*-trend was 0.01.

There was a similar trend towards a lower prevalence of CHD in the highest quartile of 24 h urinary Mg excretion, which was not statistically significant (PR 0.63 (0.33, 1.19)). After adjustment for lifestyle and nutritional factors, the PR remained similar (0.63 (0.32, 1.26)). Also, the highest quartile of plasma Mg concentration had a non-significant trend towards a lower prevalence of CHD (unadjusted PR 0.60 (0.31, 1.14), adjusted PR 0.62 (0.32, 1.20)). The PR ratios for dietary Mg intake, urinary Mg excretion and plasma Mg concentration did not change after further adjustment for other classic CHD risk factors, namely systolic blood pressure and LDL cholesterol (data not shown).

Table 2. Prevalence ratios (95% CI) for associations between dietary, urinary and plasma Magnesium and coronary heart disease in type 2 diabetes from the DIAbetes and LifEstyle Cohort Twente (DIALECT) (*n* = 450).

	Quartile 1	Quartile 2	Quartile 3	Quartile 4	*p*-Trend
Dietary Mg intake *, mg/day	254 ± 25	291 ± 7	315 ± 8	361 ± 39	
n cases/*n* total	33/109	25/110	23/110	13/109	
Model 1 [a]	1.00	0.71 (0.42, 1.22)	0.64 (0.37, 1.10)	0.40 (0.20, 0.77)	0.005
Model 2 [b]	1.00	0.72 (0.42, 1.23)	0.69 (0.40, 1.21)	0.42 (0.22, 0.82)	0.01
Model 3 [c]	1.00	0.71 (0.41, 1.23)	0.72 (0.41, 1.27)	0.40 (0.20, 0.79)	0.01
Urinary Mg excretion, mmol/24 h	1.81 ± 0.63	3.05 ± 0.32	4.32 ± 0.57	6.64 ± 1.75	
n cases/*n* total	24/101	24/100	19/101	15/100	
Model 1 [a]	1.00	0.95 (0.54, 1.67)	0.73 (0.39, 1.35)	0.63 (0.33, 1.19)	0.24
Model 2 [b]	1.00	1.28 (0.71, 2.30)	0.96 (0.51, 1.82)	0.74 (0.39, 1.42)	0.33
Model 3 [c]	1.00	1.27 (0.70, 2.30)	0.85 (0.44, 1.65)	0.63 (0.32, 1.26)	0.13
Plasma Mg concentration, mmol/L	0.67 ± 0.06	0.75 ± 0.02	0.80 ± 0.02	0.88 ± 0.04	
n cases/*n* total	29/113	22/106	27/111	16/102	
Model 1 [a]	1.00	0.91 (0.52, 1.60)	1.03 (0.60, 1.77)	0.60 (0.31, 1.14)	0.15
Model 2 [b]	1.00	0.91 (0.51, 1.62)	1.09 (0.63, 1.89)	0.58 (0.30, 1.12)	0.17
Model 3 [c]	1.00	0.91 (0.51, 1.63)	1.12 (0.65, 1.94)	0.62 (0.32, 1.20)	0.26

[a] Model 1: Crude model [b] Model 2: Adjusted for age (years), BMI (kg/m^2), smoking (never, former or current), alcohol consumption (none, 1–13 units per week, ≥14 units per week), physical activity (not adherent to guideline, adherent to guideline). [c] Model 3: Model 2 + Total energy intake (kcal), 24 h urinary sodium excretion (mmol/24 h) and 24 h urinary potassium excretion (mmol/24 h). * Dietary magnesium intake was adjusted for total energy intake using the residual method.

3.2. Analysis on Source of Magnesium Intake and Prevalence of CHD

We performed an explorative analysis whether there was an association between Mg intake from specific dietary sources and CHD. The largest dietary contributors to total dietary Mg intake for patients with T2D (Figure 1) were cereals at 22% (16–26%), dairy at 14% (10–20%), coffee at 9% (6–13%), potatoes at 7% (4–10%), meat at 6% (5–8%), legumes and nuts at 6% (4–11%), fruit at 5% (3–8%), and vegetables with 3% (2–5%). We found no statistically significant association between Mg intake from specific food groups and CHD (Table 3). However, there was a non-significant trend towards a lower prevalence of CHD for every 10 mg increase of dietary Mg intake derived from vegetables (PR 0.75 (0.52, 1.08)).

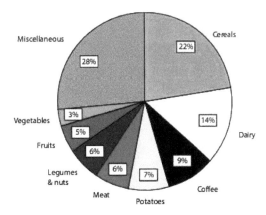

Figure 1. Sources of magnesium intake from different food product categories in patients with T2D.

Table 3. Prevalence ratios (95% CI) for associations between magnesium intake from different food sources in type 2 diabetes patients from the DIALECT cohort (n = 450).

	Model 1 [a]	Model 2 [b]	Model 3 [c]
Source of magnesium intake	PR (95% CI)	PR (95% CI)	PR (95% CI)
Magnesium intake from cereals *, 10 mg/day	1.02 (0.94, 1.10)	1.02 (0.94, 1.10)	0.95 (0.86, 1.05)
Magnesium intake from dairy *, 10 mg/day	0.95 (0.87, 1.03)	0.95 (0.87, 1.03)	0.92 (0.84, 1.01)
Magnesium intake from coffee *, 10 mg/day	0.95 (0.83, 1.06)	0.95 (0.83, 1.08)	0.96 (0.84, 1.10)
Magnesium intake from potatoes *, 10 mg/day	1.03 (0.87, 1.22)	1.02 (0.86, 1.21)	0.97 (0.80, 1.16)
Magnesium intake from meat *, 10 mg/day	0.91 (0.70, 1.20)	0.91 (0.69, 1.19)	0.80 (0.59, 1.09)
Magnesium intake from legumes & nuts *, 10 mg/day	0.96 (0.89, 1.05)	0.96 (0.88, 1.06)	0.95 (0.86, 1.05)
Magnesium intake from fruit *, 10 mg/day	1.00 (0.81, 1.23)	0.98 (0.79, 1.20)	0.96 (0.78, 1.19)
Magnesium intake from vegetables *, 10 mg/day	0.71 (0.51, 1.01)	0.71 (0.50, 1.01)	0.75 (0.52, 1.08)
Magnesium intake from miscellaneous sources *, 10 mg/day	0.95 (0.89, 1.02)	0.95 (0.89, 1.03)	0.90 (0.82, 0.99)

[a] Model 1: Crude model [b] Model 2: Adjusted for age (years), BMI (kg/m^2), smoking (never, former/current), alcohol consumption (none, 1–13 units per week, $\geq$14 units per week), physical activity (not adherent to guideline, adherent to guideline).[c] Model 3: Model 2 + Total energy intake (kcal), magnesium intake from the other sources (cereals (mg/day), dairy (mg/day), coffee (mg/day), potatoes (mg/day), meat (mg/day), legumes and nuts (mg/day), fruit (mg/day), vegetables (mg/day), and other (mg/day)). * Magnesium intake from food sources was adjusted for total energy intake using the residual method. An increment of 10 mg magnesium intake per day was used to calculate PR.PR, prevalence ratio; CI, confidence interval.

4. Discussion

We found inverse associations for dietary Mg intake, 24 h urinary Mg excretion, and plasma Mg concentration with the prevalence of CHD in patients with T2D. As far as we know, this is the first study in T2D patients which simultaneously reports on these three Mg parameters in relation to CHD. The inverse association between dietary Mg intake and the prevalence of CHD we found was strongest for Mg intake derived from vegetables, albeit not statistically significant.

The mean dietary Mg intake we report (305 $\pm$ 46 mg/day) was somewhat lower than the median Mg intake in the general Dutch population, which is around 350 mg/day [22], but was comparable to median Mg intake of population studies in the U.S. (308 mg/day) [4]. We found that in the Dutch population, cereals, dairy, and coffee intake were the largest contributors to total Mg intake, at 22%, 14%, and 9% respectively. This was somewhat different from the U.K. population, where cereals (34%), meat (19%), and dairy (18%) intake were the most important contributors [23]. In contrast, in the U.S. population the most important food groups were vegetables (13%), milk (8%), and meat (7%) [24]. It should be noted that different groupings of food products renders a head-to-head comparison between these percentages difficult. The 24 h urinary Mg excretion we report (4.0 $\pm$ 2.1 mmol/24 h) was in line with the general population the Netherlands (4.2 $\pm$ 1.7 mmol/24 h for men and 3.5 $\pm$ 1.4 mmol/24 h for women) [5]. Plasma Mg concentration (0.77 $\pm$ 0.09 mmol/L) was similar to an earlier report about Dutch diabetes patients (0.74 $\pm$ 0.10 mmol/L) [25]. The prevalence of hypomagnesemia we found (17%) was in the range of the reported prevalence of hypomagnesemia in patients with T2D, between 14% and 48% [10,11], and emphasizes that clinical vigilance for hypomagnesemia is warranted in T2D, because it is associated with increased insulin resistance and faster renal function decline [26].

We are the first to report an inverse association between dietary Mg intake and the prevalence of CHD in T2D. In contrast, a large meta-analysis in non-T2D patients demonstrated no association between dietary Mg intake and incident CHD [9]. However, low dietary Mg intake was associated with a higher risk of stroke, heart failure, new-onset diabetes, and all-cause mortality [9]. It is known that in T2D renal wasting of Mg occurs [27]. Additionally, Mg supplementation in T2D can improve insulin sensitivity and metabolic control [28]. Possibly, an adequate Mg intake in patients with T2D is even more important than in those without T2D, in order to maintain an adequate Mg status and prevent diabetes-related complications. These data fuel the hypothesis that magnesium intake is beneficial in T2D patients.

In addition, when investigating Mg intake from specific food sources, we found the strongest inverse association between Mg derived from vegetables and CHD, albeit not quite reaching statistical significance. To our knowledge, the association with vegetable-derived Mg intake and CHD has not been described before. When studying Mg intake and Mg status, it is important to consider bioavailability of ingested Mg for intestinal uptake, as this might vary considerably depending on the source of Mg intake [29]. Possibly, bioavailability from Mg in vegetables is greater than from other food sources; however, this issue would have to be addressed an in-depth mechanistic study. Nevertheless, our data illustrate that when studying the association between micronutrients and outcomes, intake of different food groups is also important. As vegetable intake in our population was low [30], and vegetable intake only accounted for 3% of total Mg intake in this population, increasing vegetable intake is a good opportunity to not only increase Mg intake, but also to improve overall diet quality. It should be noted that in our study, it is difficult to distinguish between the protective effects of overall vegetable intake and those from vegetable-derived Mg intake. Other vegetable-derived components like antioxidants, but also potassium and vitamin K, might contribute to or interact with Mg in the eventual association with CHD [31–34]. Maybe the possible cohort effect from these micronutrients and Mg could amplify such protection. Since such an analysis is beyond the scope and available data of the current study, future studies are necessary to further investigate mechanisms behind vegetable intake and risk of coronary heart disease.

Additionally, we found that lower 24 h urinary Mg excretion was associated with more prevalent CHD. In line with this finding, in the general population an inverse association between Mg excretion and CHD was reported [5]. Potential renal Mg wasting in T2D renders the interpretation of urinary Mg excretion difficult. High urinary Mg excretion could, on the one hand, reflect a high dietary Mg intake; on the other hand, though, it could reflect the hypermagnesuria found in T2D [10,11]. This could explain why, in our cohort, dietary Mg intake is more strongly associated with CHD than 24 h urinary excretion.

In parallel, lower plasma Mg concentration was also associated with prevalent CHD. In T2D, the association between plasma Mg concentration and CHD was investigated previously, and conflicting results were reported [14,15]. In non-T2D subjects, conflicting results on the association between plasma Mg have been reported as well; however, a meta-analysis demonstrated an inverse association between plasma Mg and incident CHD [8]. As Mg is mainly an intracellular cation, and therefore plasma Mg only reflects 1% of bodily Mg stores, the validity of using plasma Mg as a marker for Mg status has been questioned; Mg deficiency has been reported in patients without overt hypomagnesemia [11,35].

Our paper was not designed to unravel mechanisms behind the inverse associations between Mg intake, Mg status, and CHD. However, several mechanisms have been proposed that could underlie this association. First, animal studies have consistently shown that higher Mg status inhibits vascular calcification [36,37]. In human subjects, serum Mg and dietary Mg intake were inversely associated with the degree of coronary calcification [4,6]. Second, low Mg status might be associated with cardiac arrhythmias [38]. Lastly, increased CHD risk might be mediated through the association between low

Mg status or intake and increased traditional CHD risk factors, such as blood pressure [39] and insulin resistance [12].

Our paper is the first to simultaneously report the association between dietary Mg intake, factors of Mg status (24 h urinary Mg excretion and plasma Mg), and CHD in patients with established T2D. The robustness of our findings is established through the fact that all three Mg parameters were inversely associated with CHD. The main limitation of our paper is the cross-sectional design, which only allowed us to study associations and not causality, and therefore there is a risk of reverse causality bias. Another limitation is that the FFQ we used in our study was not validated to estimate magnesium intake. However, because there was a moderate correlation between dietary Mg intake and urinary Mg excretion, we deemed the results sufficiently valid.

Our study has several clinical implications. First, we show that Mg intake is of the utmost importance with relation to T2D. Patients with T2D are at risk of developing hypomagnesemia, as Mg intake in our population was somewhat lower in comparison to the general population. Additionally, patients with T2D have increased renal Mg excretion [27]. We show that Mg intake and Mg status is reduced in those with CHD, possibly indicating that higher Mg intake is associated with a lower risk of CHD. The best opportunity to increase Mg intake is to increase intake of Mg-rich vegetables. As Mg intake in the highest quartile is approximately 100 mg/day higher than in the lowest quartile, in clinical practice this could correspond with increasing vegetable intake by, for example, 200 g spinach, or 100 g rucola lettuce and two avocados per day. Alternatively, previous research has shown that several dietary patterns might reduce CHD risk or improve cardiac function, such as the Mediterranean diet; the Dietary Approaches to Stop Hypertension diet; or a high-protein, intermittent fasting, low-calorie diet [40–42]. We add to these findings by illustrating that Mg is an important component in such diets. For future studies, it would be of interest to investigate how Mg and other beneficial nutritional approaches could reinforce each other in the pursuit of the reduction of CHD in diabetes patients. Additionally, future mechanistic studies should be done to investigate how vegetable-derived nutrients, particularly Mg, might reduce CHD risk.

5. Conclusions

In a cohort of patients with established T2D, dietary magnesium intake, 24 h urinary magnesium excretion, and plasma magnesium concentration were inversely associated with the prevalence of coronary heart disease. Increasing dietary magnesium intake, especially through increasing vegetable intake, may reduce the risk of CHD in patients with established T2D.

Table S1: Overview of food items included in each food category, Table S2: Baseline characteristics of patients with T2D by a breakup of dietary magnesium intake.

Acknowledgments: We thank Else van den Berg, Willeke van Kampen, Sanne van Huizen, Anne Davina, Manon Harmelink and Jolien Jaspers for their contribution to patient inclusion. We thank Jelle Sanderman for supervising laboratory measurements. This work was performed without external financial support.

Author Contributions: S.H.B., G.N., S.S.S.-M. and G.D.L. conceived and designed the study; C.M.G. and S.H.B. included patients; C.M.G. and S.S.S.-M. analyzed the data; S.J.L.B., G.N. and G.D.L. contributed reagents/materials/analysis tools; C.G. wrote the paper.

References

1. Rana, J.S.; Liu, J.Y.; Moffet, H.H.; Jaffe, M.; Karter, A.J. Diabetes and Prior Coronary Heart Disease are Not Necessarily Risk Equivalent for Future Coronary Heart Disease Events. *J. Gen. Intern. Med.* **2016**, *31*, 387–393. [CrossRef] [PubMed]

2. Emerging Risk Factors Collaboration; Sarwar, N.; Gao, P.; Seshasai, S.R.; Gobin, R.; Kaptoge, S.; Di Angelantonio, E.; Ingelsson, E.; Lawlor, D.A.; Selvin, E.; et al. Diabetes Mellitus, Fasting Blood Glucose Concentration, and Risk of Vascular Disease: A Collaborative Meta-Analysis of 102 Prospective Studies. *Lancet* **2010**, *375*, 2215–2222. [PubMed]

3. Chiuve, S.E.; Sun, Q.; Curhan, G.C.; Taylor, E.N.; Spiegelman, D.; Willett, W.C.; Manson, J.E.; Rexrode, K.M.; Albert, C.M. Dietary and Plasma Magnesium and Risk of Coronary Heart Disease among Women. *J. Am. Heart Assoc.* **2013**, *2*, e000114. [CrossRef] [PubMed]

4. Hruby, A.; O'Donnell, C.J.; Jacques, P.F.; Meigs, J.B.; Hoffmann, U.; McKeown, N.M. Magnesium Intake is Inversely Associated with Coronary Artery Calcification: The Framingham Heart Study. *JACC Cardiovasc. Imaging* **2014**, *7*, 59–69. [CrossRef] [PubMed]

5. Joosten, M.M.; Gansevoort, R.T.; Mukamal, K.J.; van der Harst, P.; Geleijnse, J.M.; Feskens, E.J.; Navis, G.; Bakker, S.J.; PREVEND Study Group. Urinary and Plasma Magnesium and Risk of Ischemic Heart Disease. *Am. J. Clin. Nutr.* **2013**, *97*, 1299–1306. [CrossRef] [PubMed]

6. Posadas-Sanchez, R.; Posadas-Romero, C.; Cardoso-Saldana, G.; Vargas-Alarcon, G.; Villarreal-Molina, M.T.; Perez-Hernandez, N.; Rodriguez-Perez, J.M.; Medina-Urrutia, A.; Jorge-Galarza, E.; Juarez-Rojas, J.G.; et al. Serum Magnesium is Inversely Associated with Coronary Artery Calcification in the Genetics of Atherosclerotic Disease (GEA) Study. *Nutr. J.* **2016**, *15*, 22. [CrossRef] [PubMed]

7. Sakaguchi, Y.; Hamano, T.; Nakano, C.; Obi, Y.; Matsui, I.; Kusunoki, Y.; Mori, D.; Oka, T.; Hashimoto, N.; Takabatake, Y.; et al. Association between Density of Coronary Artery Calcification and Serum Magnesium Levels among Patients with Chronic Kidney Disease. *PLoS ONE* **2016**, *11*, e0163673. [CrossRef] [PubMed]

8. Wu, J.; Xun, P.; Tang, Q.; Cai, W.; He, K. Circulating Magnesium Levels and Incidence of Coronary Heart Diseases, Hypertension, and Type 2 Diabetes Mellitus: A Meta-Analysis of Prospective Cohort Studies. *Nutr. J.* **2017**, *16*, 60. [CrossRef] [PubMed]

9. Fang, X.; Wang, K.; Han, D.; He, X.; Wei, J.; Zhao, L.; Imam, M.U.; Ping, Z.; Li, Y.; Xu, Y.; et al. Dietary Magnesium Intake and the Risk of Cardiovascular Disease, Type 2 Diabetes, and all-Cause Mortality: A Dose-Response Meta-Analysis of Prospective Cohort Studies. *BMC Med.* **2016**, *14*, 210. [CrossRef] [PubMed]

10. Gommers, L.M.; Hoenderop, J.G.; Bindels, R.J.; de Baaij, J.H. Hypomagnesemia in Type 2 Diabetes: A Vicious Circle? *Diabetes* **2016**, *65*, 3–13. [CrossRef] [PubMed]

11. Pham, P.C.; Pham, P.M.; Pham, S.V.; Miller, J.M.; Pham, P.T. Hypomagnesemia in Patients with Type 2 Diabetes. *Clin. J. Am. Soc. Nephrol.* **2007**, *2*, 366–373. [CrossRef] [PubMed]

12. Fang, X.; Han, H.; Li, M.; Liang, C.; Fan, Z.; Aaseth, J.; He, J.; Montgomery, S.; Cao, Y. Dose-Response Relationship between Dietary Magnesium Intake and Risk of Type 2 Diabetes Mellitus: A Systematic Review and Meta-Regression Analysis of Prospective Cohort Studies. *Nutrients* **2016**, *8*, 739. [CrossRef] [PubMed]

13. Hruby, A.; Meigs, J.B.; O'Donnell, C.J.; Jacques, P.F.; McKeown, N.M. Higher Magnesium Intake Reduces Risk of Impaired Glucose and Insulin Metabolism and Progression from Prediabetes to Diabetes in Middle-Aged Americans. *Diabetes Care* **2014**, *37*, 419–427. [CrossRef] [PubMed]

14. Liao, F.; Folsom, A.R.; Brancati, F.L. Is Low Magnesium Concentration a Risk Factor for Coronary Heart Disease? The Atherosclerosis Risk in Communities (ARIC) Study. *Am. Heart J.* **1998**, *136*, 480–490. [CrossRef]

15. Peters, K.E.; Chubb, S.A.; Davis, W.A.; Davis, T.M. The Relationship between Hypomagnesemia, Metformin Therapy and Cardiovascular Disease Complicating Type 2 Diabetes: The Fremantle Diabetes Study. *PLoS ONE* **2013**, *8*, e74355. [CrossRef] [PubMed]

16. Gant, C.M.; Binnenmars, S.H.; Berg, E.V.D.; Bakker, S.J.L.; Navis, G.; Laverman, G.D. Integrated Assessment of Pharmacological and Nutritional Cardiovascular Risk Management: Blood Pressure Control in the DIAbetes and LifEstyle Cohort Twente (DIALECT). *Nutrients* **2017**, *9*, 709. [CrossRef] [PubMed]

17. Wendel-Vos, G.C.; Schuit, A.J.; Saris, W.H.; Kromhout, D. Reproducibility and Relative Validity of the Short Questionnaire to Assess Health-Enhancing Physical Activity. *J. Clin. Epidemiol.* **2003**, *56*, 1163–1169. [CrossRef]

18. Feunekes, G.I.; Van Staveren, W.A.; De Vries, J.H.; Burema, J.; Hautvast, J.G. Relative and Biomarker-Based Validity of a Food-Frequency Questionnaire Estimating Intake of Fats and Cholesterol. *Am. J. Clin. Nutr.* **1993**, *58*, 489–496. [CrossRef] [PubMed]

19. Rijksinstituut voor Volksgezondheid en Milieu. *NEVO-Tabel (Dutch Food Composition Table): Nederlands Voedingsstoffenbestand, version 4.0*; Rijksinstituut voor Volksgezondheid en Milieu: Bilthoven, The Netherlands, 2013.

20. Willett, W.C.; Stampfer, M. Implications of total energy intake for epidemiologic analyses. In *Nutritional Epidemiology*; Willett, W.C., Ed.; Oxford University Press: New York, NY, USA, 1998; pp. 273–301.

21. Zhang, W.; Iso, H.; Ohira, T.; Date, C.; Tamakoshi, A.; JACC Study Group. Associations of Dietary Magnesium Intake with Mortality from Cardiovascular Disease: The JACC Study. *Atherosclerosis* **2012**, *221*, 587–595. [CrossRef] [PubMed]

22. Van Rossum, C.; Fransen, H.; Verkaik-Kloosterman, J.; Buurma-Rethans, E.; Ocke, M. *Dutch National Food Consumption Survey 2007–2010: Diet of Children and Adults Aged 7 to 69 Years*; National Institute for Public Health and the Environment: Bilthoven, The Netherlands, 2011.

23. Davies, B.E. The UK Geochemical Environment and Cardiovascular Diseases: Magnesium in Food and Water. *Environ. Geochem. Health* **2015**, *37*, 411–427. [CrossRef] [PubMed]

24. Ford, E.S.; Mokdad, A.H. Dietary Magnesium Intake in a National Sample of US Adults. *J. Nutr.* **2003**, *133*, 2879–2882. [CrossRef] [PubMed]

25. Kurstjens, S.; de Baaij, J.H.; Bouras, H.; Bindels, R.J.; Tack, C.J.; Hoenderop, J.G. Determinants of Hypomagnesemia in Patients with Type 2 Diabetes Mellitus. *Eur. J. Endocrinol.* **2017**, *176*, 11–19. [CrossRef] [PubMed]

26. Grober, U.; Schmidt, J.; Kisters, K. Magnesium in Prevention and Therapy. *Nutrients* **2015**, *7*, 8199–8226. [CrossRef] [PubMed]

27. McNair, P.; Christensen, M.S.; Christiansen, C.; Madsbad, S.; Transbol, I. Renal Hypomagnesaemia in Human Diabetes Mellitus: Its Relation to Glucose Homeostasis. *Eur. J. Clin. Investig.* **1982**, *12*, 81–85. [CrossRef]

28. Rodriguez-Moran, M.; Guerrero-Romero, F. Oral Magnesium Supplementation Improves Insulin Sensitivity and Metabolic Control in Type 2 Diabetic Subjects: A Randomized Double-Blind Controlled Trial. *Diabetes Care* **2003**, *26*, 1147–1152. [CrossRef] [PubMed]

29. Schuchardt, J.P.; Hahn, A. Intestinal Absorption and Factors Influencing Bioavailability of Magnesium-an Update. *Curr. Nutr. Food Sci.* **2017**, *13*, 260–278. [CrossRef] [PubMed]

30. Gant, C.M.; Binnenmars, S.H.; Harmelink, M.; Soedamah-Muthu, S.S.; Bakker, S.J.L.; Navis, G.J.; Laverman, G.D. Real-Life Achievement of Lipid-Lowering Treatment Targets in the DIAbetes and LifEstyle Cohort Twente: Systemic Assessment of Pharmacological and Nutritional Factors. *Nutr. Diabetes* **2018**, in press.

31. Zhu, X.; Zuo, L. Characterization of Oxygen Radical Formation Mechanism at Early Cardiac Ischemia. *Cell Death Dis.* **2013**, *4*, e787. [CrossRef] [PubMed]

32. Keyzer, C.A.; Vermeer, C.; Joosten, M.M.; Knapen, M.H.; Drummen, N.E.; Navis, G.; Bakker, S.J.; de Borst, M.H. Vitamin K Status and Mortality After Kidney Transplantation: A Cohort Study. *Am. J. Kidney Dis.* **2015**, *65*, 474–483. [CrossRef] [PubMed]

33. Riphagen, I.J.; Keyzer, C.A.; Drummen, N.E.A.; de Borst, M.H.; Beulens, J.W.J.; Gansevoort, R.T.; Geleijnse, J.M.; Muskiet, F.A.J.; Navis, G.; Visser, S.T.; et al. Prevalence and Effects of Functional Vitamin K Insufficiency: The PREVEND Study. *Nutrients* **2017**, *9*, 1334. [CrossRef] [PubMed]

34. Kieneker, L.M.; Gansevoort, R.T.; Mukamal, K.J.; de Boer, R.A.; Navis, G.; Bakker, S.J.; Joosten, M.M. Urinary Potassium Excretion and Risk of Developing Hypertension: The Prevention of Renal and Vascular End-Stage Disease Study. *Hypertension* **2014**, *64*, 769–776. [CrossRef] [PubMed]

35. Barbagallo, M.; Di Bella, G.; Brucato, V.; D'Angelo, D.; Damiani, P.; Monteverde, A.; Belvedere, M.; Dominguez, L.J. Serum Ionized Magnesium in Diabetic Older Persons. *Metabolism* **2014**, *63*, 502–509. [CrossRef] [PubMed]

36. Alesutan, I.; Tuffaha, R.; Auer, T.; Feger, M.; Pieske, B.; Lang, F.; Voelkl, J. Inhibition of Osteo/Chondrogenic Transformation of Vascular Smooth Muscle Cells by $MgCl_2$ Via Calcium-Sensing Receptor. *J. Hypertens.* **2017**, *35*, 523–532. [CrossRef] [PubMed]

37. Kircelli, F.; Peter, M.E.; Sevinc Ok, E.; Celenk, F.G.; Yilmaz, M.; Steppan, S.; Asci, G.; Ok, E.; Passlick-Deetjen, J. Magnesium Reduces Calcification in Bovine Vascular Smooth Muscle Cells in a Dose-Dependent Manner. *Nephrol. Dial. Transplant.* **2012**, *27*, 514–521. [CrossRef] [PubMed]

38. Verduyn, S.C.; Vos, M.A.; van der Zande, J.; van der Hulst, F.F.; Wellens, H.J. Role of Interventricular Dispersion of Repolarization in Acquired Torsade-De-Pointes Arrhythmias: Reversal by Magnesium. *Cardiovasc. Res.* **1997**, *34*, 453–463. [CrossRef]

39. Dibaba, D.T.; Xun, P.; Song, Y.; Rosanoff, A.; Shechter, M.; He, K. The Effect of Magnesium Supplementation on Blood Pressure in Individuals with Insulin Resistance, Prediabetes, or Noncommunicable Chronic Diseases: A Meta-Analysis of Randomized Controlled Trials. *Am. J. Clin. Nutr.* **2017**, *106*, 921–929. [CrossRef] [PubMed]

40. Rosato, V.; Temple, N.J.; La Vecchia, C.; Castellan, G.; Tavani, A.; Guercio, V. Mediterranean Diet and Cardiovascular Disease: A Systematic Review and Meta-Analysis of Observational Studies. *Eur. J. Nutr.* **2017**. [CrossRef] [PubMed]

41. Fung, T.T.; Chiuve, S.E.; McCullough, M.L.; Rexrode, K.M.; Logroscino, G.; Hu, F.B. Adherence to a DASH-Style Diet and Risk of Coronary Heart Disease and Stroke in Women. *Arch. Intern. Med.* **2008**, *168*, 713–720. [CrossRef] [PubMed]

42. Zuo, L.; He, F.; Tinsley, G.M.; Pannell, B.K.; Ward, E.; Arciero, P.J. Comparison of High-Protein, Intermittent Fasting Low-Calorie Diet and Heart Healthy Diet for Vascular Health of the Obese. *Front. Physiol.* **2016**, *7*, 350. [CrossRef] [PubMed]

3

TRPM6 is Essential for Magnesium Uptake and Epithelial Cell Function in the Colon

Francesca Luongo[1], Giuseppe Pietropaolo[1], Mathieu Gautier[2], Isabelle Dhennin-Duthille[2], Halima Ouadid-Ahidouch[2], Federica I. Wolf[1],* and Valentina Trapani[1],*

[1] Istituto di Patologia Generale, Università Cattolica del Sacro Cuore, Fondazione Policlinico Universitario "Agostino Gemelli" IRCCS, I-00168 Rome, Italy; francesca.luongo@unicatt.it (F.L.); giuseppepietrop1993@libero.it (G.P.)

[2] Laboratoire de Physiologie Cellulaire et Moléculaire-EA4667, UFR Sciences, Université de Picardie Jules Verne, F-80039 Amiens, France; mathieu.gautier@u-picardie.fr (M.G.); isabelle.dhennin-Duthille@u-picardie.fr (I.D.-D.); ha-sciences@u-picardie.fr (H.O.-A.)

* Correspondence: federica.wolf@unicatt.it (F.I.W.); valentina.trapani@unicatt.it (V.T.)

Abstract: Intestinal magnesium (Mg) uptake is essential for systemic Mg homeostasis. Colon cells express the two highly homologous transient receptor potential melastatin type (TRPM) 6 and 7 Mg^{2+} channels, but their precise function and the consequences of their mutual interaction are not clear. To explore the functional role of TRPM6 and TRPM7 in the colon, we used human colon cell lines that innately express both channels and analyzed the functional consequences of genetic knocking-down, by RNA interference, or pharmacological inhibition, by NS8593, of either channel. TRPM7 silencing caused an increase in Mg^{2+} influx, and correspondingly enhanced cell proliferation and migration, while downregulation of TRPM6 did not affect significantly either Mg^{2+} influx or cell proliferation. Exposure to the specific TRPM6/7 inhibitor NS8593 reduced Mg^{2+} influx, and consequently cell proliferation and migration, but Mg supplementation rescued the inhibition. We propose a model whereby in colon cells the functional Mg^{2+} channel at the plasma membrane may consist of both TRPM7 homomers and TRPM6/7 heteromers. A different expression ratio between the two proteins may result in different functional properties. Altogether, our findings confirm that TRPM6 cannot be replaced by TRPM7, and that TRPM6/7 complexes and TRPM6/7-mediated Mg^{2+} influx are indispensable in human epithelial colon cells.

Keywords: cell migration; cell proliferation; intestine; ion imaging; magnesium channel; magnesium homeostasis; MagT1; NS8593; TRPM7; wound healing

1. Introduction

Magnesium (Mg) is involved in virtually all major metabolic and signaling pathways in the cell, and disturbances of Mg homeostasis accompany a variety of diseases [1]. Despite recent advancements in understanding the critical role of Mg in health and disease, the molecular mechanisms governing cellular and systemic Mg balance remain debated. Systemic Mg homeostasis primarily depends on the concerted actions of the intestine responsible for Mg uptake from food, and the kidneys, that regulate urinary Mg excretion [1]. Classical physiological experiments with different animal species have identified two Mg transport systems in the intestinal epithelium: An active transcellular and a passive paracellular pathway [2,3]. The paracellular pathway, which is driven by the electrochemical gradient, is responsible for bulk Mg absorption and takes place mostly in the small intestine, whereas fine-tuning occurs in the cecum and colon via transcellular transport. The transcellular route consists of apical Mg entry, mediated by Mg permeable channels, and a basolateral extrusion step involving putative Na^+/Mg^{2+} exchangers.

In the last two decades, several proteins have been proposed to facilitate Mg transport [4], but the biological roles of most of them continue to arouse dispute. The best-characterized transporters are the transient receptor potential melastatin (TRPM) 6 and 7 cation channels. Both TRPM6 and TRPM7 contain a transmembrane TRP channel segment fused to a cytosolic α-type serine/threonine protein kinase domain, but the functional relationship and the potential interplay between the channel and kinase moieties are still debated [5]. TRPM7 is ubiquitously expressed in human tissues and has been proposed as an indispensable cellular Mg entry pathway since TRPM7-deficient cell lines have intracellular Mg deficiency and severe cell growth defects [6,7]. The highly homologous TRPM6 channel has a more restricted expression: The highest levels are found in the distal convoluted tubule of the kidney and in the distal small intestine and colon, in murine as well as human tissues [8,9]. Interestingly, TRPM6 expression in the kidney and intestine is regulated by dietary Mg availability [8–11]. The critical role of TRPM6 for systemic Mg homeostasis became evident when loss-of-function mutations in the TRPM6 gene were discovered in patients with a rare form of hereditary hypomagnesemia (hypomagnesemia with secondary hypocalcemia, HSH) [12,13]. Although the etiology of low Mg levels in HSH was initially ascribed to renal Mg wasting, recent findings challenged this view suggesting that a defect in the intestinal Mg uptake might be of primary relevance [14]. Consequently, it is crucial to identify the key molecular players of intestinal Mg absorption and their regulation.

It is intriguing that transporting epithelia such as colon mucosa express both TRPM6 and TRPM7. Pioneering work showed that the two proteins are not redundant, and the functional ion channel at the plasma membrane is a multimeric complex consisting of either TRPM7 homotetramers or TRPM6/7 heterotetramers, each possessing different biophysical properties [15–17]. However, most findings were derived from heterologous expression models and resulted in considerable controversy on the relationship between the two channels and their exact functional role (for an up-to-date review, see Reference [5]). Recent data from our group seem to corroborate the view that TRPM6, rather than TRPM7, might have a central role in the colon; indeed, we showed that dietary Mg exerts a protective effect on colonic mucosa by upregulating TRPM6 expression in an in vivo model [18]. In the present work, we sought to scrutinize the exact role of each of the two sister channels in the colon. We decided to use human colon cell lines that innately express both channels, and, therefore, may well epitomize the physiological context. In our model cell lines, we dissected the contribution of each channel, by specifically RNA interference (RNAi) silencing either of them, and analyzing the functional consequences in terms of magnesium influx, proliferation, and migration. We present data suggesting that an alteration in the ratio between differently assorted tetramers might constitute a flexible way to modulate cation influx and affect related signaling pathways.

2. Materials and Methods

2.1. Cell Culture

Human colon carcinoma HT29, HCT116, and RKO cells were routinely grown in Dulbecco's modified Eagle's medium (DMEM) supplemented with 10% fetal bovine serum (FBS), 2 mM glutamine, 100 U/mL penicillin, and 100 µg/mL streptomycin in a 5% CO_2 humidified atmosphere at 37 °C. Human colon carcinoma Caco-2 cells were grown in the same medium supplemented with 20% FBS. To assess cell proliferation in conditions of different Mg availability, Mg-free DMEM (Invitrogen) was supplemented as for routine culture plus the desired amounts of $MgSO_4$. To obtain a transient downregulation of TRPM7, we used a short interfering RNA (siRNA) targeting the nucleotide sequence 5'-GTCTTGCCATGAAATACTC-3' (Dharmacon Research Inc., Chicago, IL, USA). For silencing TRPM6, predesigned siRNAs against human TRPM6 were purchased from Qiagen. Specific siRNAs were transfected into cells (50 ng per 400,000 cells) using HiPerFect Transfection Reagent (Qiagen Srl., Milan, Italy) following the manufacturer's protocol. Non-silencing, scrambled sequences were used as controls (CTRL). NS8593 hydrochloride salt was purchased from Sigma Aldrich; a stock solution was made in dimethyl sulfoxide (DMSO) and stored in aliquots at $-20\ °C$. To assess proliferation, cells were counted on a Thoma chamber in duplicate samples at given time points.

2.2. Western Blot

Cells were lysed in radioimmunoprecipitation assay (RIPA) buffer (50 mM Tris, pH = 8, 150 mM NaCl, 1 mM ethylenediaminetetraacetic acid (EDTA), 1% NP-40, 0.05% sodium deoxycholate, and 0.1% SDS) supplemented with protease inhibitors (10 µg/mL leupeptin, 20 µg/mL aprotinin, 1 mM phenylmethanesulfonyl fluoride, 1 mM $NaVO_4$, and 100 mM NaF). Protein concentrations were determined using the Bradford protein assay (Bio-Rad Laboratories Srl., Segrate (MI), Italy). Cell extracts (50 µg) were resolved by SDS-PAGE (8%), transferred to polyvinylidene fluoride (PVDF) membranes, and probed with rabbit monoclonal anti-TRPM7 (1:1000, Abcam Ltd., Cambridge, UK), rabbit polyclonal anti-TRPM6 (1:500, Biorbyt Ltd., Cambridge, UK), rabbit polyclonal anti-tubulin or actin (1:1000, Sigma-Aldrich Srl., Milan, Italy) primary antibodies. Horseradish peroxidase-conjugated secondary antibodies (GE Healthcare Srl., Milan, Italy) were detected by use of the ECL Prime Western Blotting Detection Reagent (GE Healthcare Srl, Milan, Italy) and the ChemiDoc XRS system (Bio-Rad Laboratories Srl., Segrate (MI) Italy).Densitometric analysis was performed by using the National Institutes of Health (NIH) ImageJ software.

2.3. Mg^{2+} Influx Measurements

Subconfluent cells grown on 35-mm microscopy dishes (µ-dish, ibidi GmbH, Martinsried, Germany) were loaded with 3 µM Mag-Fluo-4-AM (Thermo Fisher Scientific, Monza (MI), Italy), and imaged in a Na^+, Ca^{2+} and Mg^{2+}-free buffer at a confocal laser scanning microscope, as previously described [19]. Cytosolic fluorescence signals were recorded as time series of 5 min at a sampling frequency of 30 frames/min. The baseline was monitored for 30 s, then $MgSO_4$ was added drop wise to a final concentration of 20 mM. Changes in intracellular Mg levels at single cell level were estimated by the mean fluorescent increment $\Delta F/F$ [20]. Image analysis was performed by Leica Confocal Software on 10 representative cells in each microscopic field, and experiments were repeated independently at least three times.

2.4. Cell Cycle Analysis

Cells were fixed in 70% ethanol and stored at 4 °C until analysis. Prior to analysis, cell pellets were resuspended in 0.2 mg/mL of propidium iodide (PI) in Hank's balanced salt solution containing 0.6% NP-40 and RNase (1 mg/mL). The cell suspension was then filtered and analyzed for DNA content on a Coulter EPICS 753 flow cytometer, as previously described [21]. The percentage of cells in different phases of the cell cycle was determined using ModFit analysis software (version 5.2, Verity Software House Inc., Topsham, ME, USA).

2.5. Scratch Assay

A scratch assay was performed as previously reported [18]. Cells were seeded in culture inserts (ibidi GmbH, 70,000 cells/well insert) and cultured for 24 h to allow attachment. Insert removal created a 500-µm-wide cell-free gap between two confluent cell monolayers. Wound closure was monitored with an Eclipse TE2000-S microscope (Nikon Instruments Spa, Campo Bisenzio (FI), Italy) for up to 48 h, and images were analyzed using the NIH ImageJ software. Results were expressed as the percentage of the initial gap area that was covered by cells after the indicated time.

2.6. Statistical Analysis

All experiments were repeated independently three times. Prism software (version 5.01, GraphPad Software Inc., La Jolla, CA, USA) was used for all statistical analyses. Statistical significance was evaluated using unpaired Student's t test. Differences were considered statistically significant for a p value < 0.05, and significance levels were assigned as follows: * for $p < 0.05$, ** for $p < 0.01$.

3. Results

3.1. Cell Characterization

First, we assessed a panel of human colon cell lines (HT29, HCT116, RKO and Caco-2) for TRPM6 and TRPM7 protein expression using Western blot. As expected, all tested lines expressed both channels, though to various levels (Figure 1A,B). We focused on HT29 cells, which expressed the highest TRPM6 levels, but confirmed selected experiments in HCT116 cells. In HT29 cells, we also verified that proliferation was strictly dependent on extracellular Mg availability (Figure 1C).

Figure 1. Human colon cells express both transient receptor potential melastatin type TRPM6 and TRPM7 and depend on extracellular Mg availability for growing. A representative Western blot ($n = 3$) is shown for (**A**) TRPM7 and (**B**) TRPM6 in a panel of human colon cell lines. Tubulin was used as a loading control. (**C**) HT29 cell proliferation in conditions of low (0.1 mM), normal (0.8 mM) and high (10 mM) Mg availability. Cells were grown in Mg-free Dulbecco's modified Eagle's medium (DMEM) supplemented as for routine culture plus the indicated amounts of $MgSO_4$ and counted at 24, 48 and 72 h in duplicates ($n = 3$). * $p < 0.05$ by unpaired Student's t test.

To downregulate specifically the expression of either channel, we used transient siRNA transfection and assessed mRNA and protein expression by real-time reverse transcriptase polymerase chain reaction (RT-PCR) and Western blot, respectively. Significant TRPM7 knock-down was achieved at the mRNA level and was confirmed at the protein level in both HT29 and HCT116 cells (Figure 2A,

Figures S1 and S2). TRPM7 silencing did not affect TRPM6 expression (Figure 2A). Transfection of TRPM6-specific siRNA resulted in knock-down of TRPM6 expression with no effects on TRPM7 expression in HT29 cells (Figure 2B). Similar results were obtained in HCT116 cells (not shown).

Figure 2. Specific short interfering RNA (siRNA) transfection efficiently downregulates TRPM7 and TRPM6 in human colon cells. HT29 cells were transfected with either (**A**) TRPM7 or (**B**) TRPM6-specific siRNA, and protein expression of both channels was evaluated by western blot 48 h after transfection. Non-silencing, scrambled sequences were used as controls (CTRL). Tubulin was used as a loading control. A representative blot is shown ($n = 3$). Note that TRPM7 silencing does not affect TRPM6 expression and vice versa. See Figure S1 in supplementary materials for complete blots, and Figure S2 in supplementary materials for mRNA expression by real time RT-PCR and additional data on HCT116 cells.

These data prove that RNAi can achieve specific and significant downregulation of each channel and allow the distinguishing of the contribution of TRPM6 vs. TRPM7 to given cell functions.

3.2. Contribution of TRPM7 to Colon Cell Functions

Next, we transfected cells with TRPM7-specific siRNA and evaluated the effects on cation influx and most closely related functions, such as proliferation and migration, in both HT29 and HCT116 cells. Results for HT29 cells are shown in Figure 3, while principal findings for HCT116 cells are reported in Figure S3. In preliminary experiments, TRPM7-silenced cells paradoxically exhibited a significant increase in constitutive divalent cation influx as assessed by the Mn^{2+} quenching technique (Figure S3A). Since the Mn^{2+} quenching assay does not discriminate the divalent species involved, to determine whether the transmembrane flux was due to an Mg^{2+} entry, we performed live imaging of cells loaded with the Mg-specific fluorescent probe Mag-Fluo-4. Fluorescence imaging confirmed that TRPM7-silenced cells had a higher Mg^{2+} uptake (Figure 3A). In addition, TRPM7-silenced cells showed a significantly faster proliferation rate, as assessed by cell counting (Figure 3B), and confirmed by a higher percentage of cells in the S phase of the cell cycle (Figure 3C). Finally, we performed a scratch assay to evaluate the effect of TRPM7 downregulation on wound healing capacity, which encompasses both proliferation and migration properties. We found that TRPM7-silenced cells closed the cell-free gap much more efficiently than control cells (Figure 3D,E).

Figure 3. Contribution of TRPM7 to Mg^{2+} influx and Mg-dependent colon cell functions. HT29 cells were transiently silenced for TRPM7 as detailed in Materials and Methods. For HCT116 cells, see Figure S2. (**A**) Mg^{2+} influx capacity, as assessed 72 h after siRNA transfection. Mag-Fluo-4-loaded cells were challenged with 20 mM Mg (arrow) and time course of single-cell fluorescence was followed by live confocal imaging. The mean fluorescence ($\Delta F/F$) of 10 cells $\pm$ standard error (SE) from a representative experiment is reported ($n = 3$). (**B**) Cell proliferation. Cells were counted at the indicated times after siRNA transfection; mean $\pm$ SE of three independent experiments is shown. (**C**) Cell cycle distribution, as assessed 72 h after siRNA transfection. The percentage of cells in each phase was evaluated by flow cytometry; results are from a representative experiment ($n = 3$). (**D**) Cell migration. Cells were silenced and grown to confluence in well inserts for 24 h. Insert removal created a 500-μm-wide cell-free gap, whose closure was monitored by microscopy. Representative images of the wound after 24 h in CTRL and siRNA TRPM7 cells are shown. (**E**) Cell migration. Quantification of the cell-covered area from three independent wound healing assays. Results are expressed as the percentage of the initial gap area that was covered by cells after 24 h. * $p < 0.05$, ** $p < 0.01$ by unpaired Student's t test.

Altogether, these results provide a consistent picture whereby downregulation of TRPM7 in TRPM6-expressing colon cells paradoxically results in strengthening of the characteristics usually associated to TRPM7 expression in other tissues, namely cation entry, proliferation and migration.

3.3. Contribution of TRPM6 to Colon Cell Functions

We moved on to examine TRPM6 contribution to the same cellular functions by transfecting a TRPM6-specific siRNA in HT29 cells. In marked contrast to TRPM7-silenced cells, downregulation of TRPM6 did not appear to affect significantly Mg^{2+} influx, as measured by Mag-Fluo-4 imaging (Figure 4A). Correspondingly, proliferation rate of TRPM6-silenced cells did not differ considerably from that of control cells (Figure 4B).

Figure 4. Contribution of TRPM6 to Mg^{2+} influx and cell proliferation in colon cells. HT29 cells were transiently silenced for TRPM6 and assessed at the indicate times after transfection. (**A**) Mg^{2+} influx capacity, as assessed 72 h after siRNA transfection. Mag-Fluo-4-loaded cells were challenged with 20 mM Mg (arrow) and time course of single-cell fluorescence was followed by live confocal imaging. The mean fluorescence ($\Delta F/F$) of 10 cells $\pm$ SE from a representative experiment is reported ($n = 3$). (**B**) Cell proliferation. Cells were counted in duplicates; mean $\pm$ SE of three independent experiments is shown.

We conclude that partial downregulation of TRPM6 on a background of normal TRPM7 expression is not sufficient to alter significantly Mg^{2+} entry and cell proliferation.

3.4. Contribution of TRPM6/7 Channels

In the light of the results reported in the previous sections, we hypothesized that the non-redundant role of TRPM6 and TRPM7 in colon cells might be due to the formation of heteromeric channels. It is known that, in cells expressing both TRPM6 and TRPM7, the functional ion channel at the plasma membrane may consist of both TRPM7 homomers and TRPM6/7 heteromers [5]. To support the idea that Mg^{2+} influx through TRPM6/7 channels is critical for colon cell function, we used pharmacological inhibition by NS8593, a specific TRPM6/7 inhibitor [22,23]. In the presence of 30 µM NS8593, colon cells exhibited a reduced Mg^{2+} influx capacity, as evidenced by a markedly delayed and slower uptake kinetics (Figure 5A). Correspondingly, NS8593-treated cells had a decreased proliferation rate (Figure 5B), and a lower percentage of cells in the S phase of the cell cycle (Figure 5C). Furthermore, NS8593 significantly inhibited wound healing capacity (Figure 5D,E). Importantly, inhibition by NS8593 on cell proliferation and migration was successfully rescued by Mg^{2+} supplementation (10 mM).

Figure 5. Contribution of TRPM6/7 channels to Mg^{2+} influx and cell proliferation. NS8593 was used at 30 μM. (**A**) Mg^{2+} influx capacity. Mag-Fluo-4-loaded cells were challenged with 20 mM Mg (arrow) in the presence of NS8593, and time course of single-cell fluorescence was followed by live confocal imaging. The mean fluorescence ($\Delta F/F$) of 10 cells $\pm$ SE from a representative experiment is reported ($n = 3$). (**B**) Cell proliferation. Following NS8593 treatment, cells were counted at the indicated times; mean $\pm$ SE of three independent experiments is shown. (**C**) Cell cycle distribution. Percentage of cells in each phase was evaluated by flow cytometry 48 h after NS8593 treatment. Results are from a representative experiment ($n = 3$). (**D**) Cell migration. Cells were grown to confluence in inserts that were subsequently removed leaving a 500-μm-wide cell-free gap; NS8593 was added 4 h before insert removal. Wound closure was monitored by microscopy; representative images of the wound after 48 h in CTRL and NS8593-treated cells are shown. (**E**) Quantification of the cell-covered area ($n = 3$); results are expressed as the percentage of the initial gap area that was covered by cells after 48 h. * $p < 0.05$ by unpaired Student's t test.

Therefore, we conclude that in colon cells Mg^{2+} uptake and related cellular functions strictly depend on formation of TRPM6/7 heteromers, which are the physiological active form of the channel.

4. Discussion

In the present paper, we report the molecular characterization of Mg^{2+} uptake in colon cell lines and demonstrate that the presence of the TRPM6 channel is essential to guarantee intestinal Mg absorption and Mg-dependent epithelial functions. Surprisingly, we show that TRPM7 downregulation resulted in increased Mg^{2+} influx, and consequently faster cell proliferation and migration of colon cells (Figure 3). This is opposed to a vast body of literature indicating that in several other cell types TRPM7 expression is positively associated with proliferation and migration, in particular in tumor cells [24,25]. The most straightforward explanation for an increased Mg^{2+} influx in the face of a decreased TRPM7 expression would be that TRPM7 downregulation triggered an up-regulation in other Mg-transporting proteins, as previously demonstrated in different models [26,27]. Although we cannot rule out the involvement of still undisclosed players, we have convincing evidence that TRPM7-silenced cells displayed unchanged expression of the two major candidates, i.e., TRPM6 (Figure 2A) or MagT1 (Figure S1B). In contrast to TRPM7 knocking-down, TRPM6 silencing did not appear to affect significantly Mg^{2+} uptake and proliferation in colon cells (Figure 4).

To explain the apparent paradox in our results, we must take into account the coexistence of significant levels of both TRPM6 and TRPM7 in all tested cells. This implies that the functional ion channel at the plasma membrane may consist of both TRPM7 homomers and TRPM6/7 heteromers. The prevalence of either form may depend on the expression ratio between the two proteins, and may result in different functional properties.

It was originally proposed that native TRPM6 functions primarily as a subunit of heteromeric TRPM6/7 complexes [15], and this model has been corroborated by recent data [14,23,28]. The emerging picture is that TRPM6 and TRPM7 differentially contribute to regulatory characteristics of the heteromeric TRPM6/7 channel, so that the activity of the complex will hardly be affected by physiological intracellular concentrations of Mg^{2+} and Mg-ATP [23] or by osmotic changes [28]. This mechanism appears to be an indispensable prerequisite for efficient transcellular Mg^{2+} transport in intestinal cells, where a high and constant Mg^{2+} uptake should be uncoupled from cellular metabolism of Mg^{2+} and Mg-ATP [23], and should remain unaffected by frequent osmotic changes [28]. Such a functional fingerprint is probably not required in other cell types, which indeed only express TRPM7.

Our data fit perfectly in this model: Silencing either TRPM7 or TRPM6 is in fact a way to alter the relative abundance of the two proteins, and consequently will affect the ratio between differently assorted tetramers in favor of TRPM6/7 heteromers or TRPM7 homomers, respectively (Figure 6). We propose that TRPM7 downregulation tips the balance towards increased relative abundance of TRPM6/7 complexes, which are responsible for the observed increase in Mg^{2+} influx and Mg-dependent cell functions. Accordingly, in electrophysiological measurements current amplitudes of TRPM6/7 complexes were found to be higher than those of TRPM7 homomers [15,23,29]. In contrast, TRPM6 downregulation should favor TRPM7 homomerization and result in overall reduced Mg^{2+} influx and cell proliferation. Although we did not find a remarkable effect of TRPM6 downregulation (Figure 4), it must be noted that we only achieved a partial TRPM6 downregulation, which may be compatible with retaining sufficient levels of TRPM6/7 channels to foster Mg^{2+} entry and cell proliferation. However, when we used NS8593 as a potent and specific way to block channel activity regardless of its composition, we did obtain the expected reduction in Mg^{2+} uptake and cell growth (Figure 5). Furthermore, the observed inhibition was rescued by Mg supplementation, which proves that as long as sufficient Mg^{2+} entry occurs, cellular Mg homeostatic mechanisms are able to sustain cell proliferation and migration even with reduced TRPM6/7 function(s). Altogether, our findings confirm that TRPM6/7 complexes and TRPM6/7-mediated Mg^{2+} influx are absolutely necessary in human epithelial colon cells. More specifically, TRPM6 has an indispensable role in controlling Mg^{2+} entry and cell proliferation, and other ion channels, including the highly homologous TRPM7 channel, cannot replace its function.

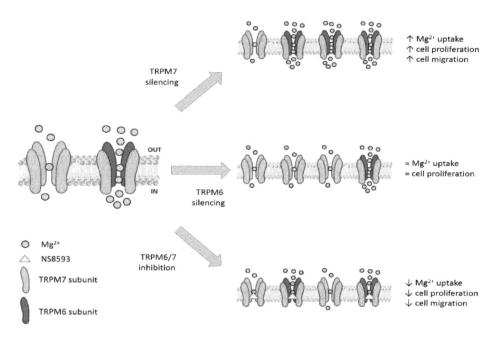

Figure 6. Suggested model for the role of TRPM6 in intestinal Mg absorption. Colon cancer cells express both TRPM7 and TRPM6, which can assemble into functional homomers or heteromers at the plasma membrane (left). The different regulation of TRPM7 and TRPM6/7 channels in physiological conditions determines higher Mg^{2+} fluxes through TRPM6/7 heteromers. Thus, the ratio between differently assorted tetramers affects cation influx and related signaling pathways (right panels). Partial TRPM7 silencing favors formation of TRPM6/7 channels, thereby increasing Mg^{2+} influx, and consequently cell proliferation and migration (upper right panel). In turn, partial TRPM6 knocking-down promotes assembly of TRPM7 homomers, which sustain basal Mg^{2+} influx and proliferation (middle right panel). Pharmacological inhibition of assembled channels decreases overall Mg^{2+} influx, and downstream functions (lower middle panel).

The main strength of our work is that we carried out our functional characterization in a completely naïve cell model, without resorting to heterologous expression systems. In the past, overexpression of recombinant proteins has greatly contributed to investigating TRPM6 and TRPM7 currents and regulation, but also generated conflicting and still unexplained results regarding TRPM6 [5]. Our results are limited to few prototypal human colon cell lines, and need further investigation before they can be generalized. In particular, the proof of concept of our hypothesis would require determination of the absolute expression levels of TRPM7 and TRPM6 as well as of the exact stoichiometric architecture of TRPM6/7 heteromers, which is technically very challenging.

Despite its limitations, our interpretation is completely in line with wider and more sophisticated studies demonstrating that TRPM6 is essential for intestinal magnesium absorption and systemic Mg balance. [14]. As for TRPM7, to the best of our knowledge, no studies investigated either mineral homeostasis in TRPM7-deficient adult mice or specific ablation of TRPM7 in the intestine. However, we would not expect to reproduce our results in a TRPM7 KO system, because the complete absence of TRPM7 would also impair TRPM6 proper localization and function [14,15]. Interestingly, heterozygous TRPM7 knock-in mice devoid of the kinase domain or activity display an altered systemic Mg homeostasis [7,30]. Although relative levels of TRPM7 homomers vs. TRPM6/7 heteromers might change in heterozygous mice, this situation cannot be exactly matched with our working model, since the current thinking is that the TRPM7 kinase moiety may function as a sensor of the organismal Mg status [30]. Overall, we cannot compare our in vitro data with any existing model. Nevertheless, the peculiarity, and paradoxically, the strength, of our model is that we only partially knock-down expression of either channel, thereby modulating the assortment of the functional complexes on a background of concurrent TRPM6 and TRPM7 expression.

5. Conclusions

In conclusion, our data confirm the existing view that maintenance of systemic Mg homeostasis requires a constant Mg supply that can be warranted only by TRPM6/7 heteromers in the intestine, and provide a simple and effective model to investigate the functional relationship between TRPM6 and TRPM7.

Author Contributions: Conceptualization: F.I.W. and V.T. Formal analysis: F.L. and V.T. Funding acquisition: H.O.-A. and F.I.W. Investigation: F.L., G.P., M.G., I.D.-D. and V.T. Resources: H.O.-A. and F.I.W. Supervision: H.O.-A., F.I.W. and V.T. Writing—original draft: V.T. Writing—review & editing: F.L., H.O.-A., F.I.W. and V.T.

Acknowledgments: Confocal imaging was performed at the LABCEMI (Laboratorio Centralizzato di Microscopia Ottica ed Elettronica), Università Cattolica del Sacro Cuore, Fondazione Policlinico Universitario "Agostino Gemelli" IRCCS, Rome, Italy.

References

1. De Baaij, J.H.; Hoenderop, J.G.; Bindels, R.J. Magnesium in man: Implications for health and disease. *Physiol. Rev.* **2015**, *95*, 1–46. [CrossRef] [PubMed]

2. Dai, L.J.; Ritchie, G.; Kerstan, D.; Kang, H.S.; Cole, D.E.; Quamme, G.A. Magnesium transport in the renal distal convoluted tubule. *Physiol. Rev.* **2001**, *81*, 51–84. [CrossRef] [PubMed]

3. Quamme, G.A. Recent developments in intestinal magnesium absorption. *Curr. Opin. Gastroenterol.* **2008**, *24*, 230–235. [CrossRef] [PubMed]

4. Quamme, G.A. Molecular identification of ancient and modern mammalian magnesium transporters. *Am. J. Physiol. Cell Physiol.* **2010**, *298*, C407–C429. [CrossRef] [PubMed]

5. Chubanov, V.; Mittermeier, L.; Gudermann, T. Role of kinase-coupled TRP channels in mineral homeostasis. *Pharmacol. Ther.* **2018**, *184*, 159–176. [CrossRef] [PubMed]

6. Schmitz, C.; Perraud, A.L.; Johnson, C.O.; Inabe, K.; Smith, M.K.; Penner, R.; Kurosaki, T.; Fleig, A.; Scharenberg, A.M. Regulation of vertebrate cellular Mg^{2+} homeostasis by TRPM7. *Cell* **2003**, *114*, 191–200. [CrossRef]

7. Ryazanova, L.V.; Rondon, L.J.; Zierler, S.; Hu, Z.; Galli, J.; Yamaguchi, T.P.; Mazur, A.; Fleig, A.; Ryazanov, A.G. TRPM7 is essential for Mg^{2+} homeostasis in mammals. *Nat. Commun.* **2010**, *1*, 109. [CrossRef] [PubMed]

8. Groenestege, W.M.; Hoenderop, J.G.; van den Heuvel, L.; Knoers, N.; Bindels, R.J. The epithelial Mg^{2+} channel transient receptor potential melastatin 6 is regulated by dietary Mg^{2+} content and estrogens. *J. Am. Soc. Nephrol.* **2006**, *17*, 1035–1043. [CrossRef] [PubMed]

9. Lameris, A.L.; Nevalainen, P.I.; Reijnen, D.; Simons, E.; Eygensteyn, J.; Monnens, L.; Bindels, R.J.; Hoenderop, J.G. Segmental transport of Ca^{2+} and Mg^{2+} along the gastrointestinal tract. *Am. J. Physiol. Gastrointest. Liver Physiol.* **2015**, *308*, G206–G216. [CrossRef] [PubMed]

10. Rondón, L.J.; Groenestege, W.M.; Rayssiguier, Y.; Mazur, A. Relationship between low magnesium status and TRPM6 expression in the kidney and large intestine. *Am. J. Physiol. Regul. Integr. Comp. Physiol.* **2008**, *294*, R2001–R2007. [CrossRef] [PubMed]

11. Van Angelen, A.A.; San-Cristobal, P.; Pulskens, W.P.; Hoenderop, J.G.; Bindels, R.J. The impact of dietary magnesium restriction on magnesiotropic and calciotropic genes. *Nephrol. Dial. Transplant.* **2013**, *28*, 2983–2993. [CrossRef] [PubMed]

12. Schlingmann, K.P.; Weber, S.; Peters, M.; Nejsum, L.N.; Vitzthum, H.; Klingel, K.; Kratz, M.; Haddad, E.; Ristoff, E.; Dinour, D.; et al. Hypomagnesemia with secondary hypocalcemia is caused by mutations in TRPM6, a new member of the TRPM gene family. *Nat. Genet.* **2002**, *31*, 166–170. [CrossRef] [PubMed]

13. Walder, R.Y.; Landau, D.; Meyer, P.; Shalev, H.; Tsolia, M.; Borochowitz, Z.; Boettger, M.B.; Beck, G.E.; Englehardt, R.K.; Carmi, R.; Sheffield, V.C. Mutation of TRPM6 causes familial hypomagnesemia with secondary hypocalcemia. *Nat. Genet.* **2002**, *31*, 171–174. [CrossRef] [PubMed]

14. Chubanov, V.; Ferioli, S.; Wisnowsky, A.; Simmons, D.G.; Leitzinger, C.; Einer, C.; Jonas, W.; Shymkiv, Y.; Bartsch, H.; Braun, A.; et al. Epithelial magnesium transport by TRPM6 is essential for prenatal development and adult survival. *Elife* **2016**, *5*, e20914. [CrossRef] [PubMed]

15. Chubanov, V.; Waldegger, S.; Mederos y Schnitzler, M.; Vitzthum, H.; Sassen, M.C.; Seyberth, H.W.; Konrad, M.; Gudermann, T. Disruption of TRPM6/TRPM7 complex formation by a mutation in the TRPM6

gene causes hypomagnesemia with secondary hypocalcemia. *Proc. Natl. Acad. Sci. USA* **2004**, *101*, 2894–2899. [CrossRef] [PubMed]

16. Schmitz, C.; Dorovkov, M.V.; Zhao, X.; Davenport, B.J.; Ryazanov, A.G.; Perraud, A.L. The channel kinases TRPM6 and TRPM7 are functionally nonredundant. *J. Biol. Chem.* **2005**, *280*, 37763–37771. [CrossRef] [PubMed]
17. Li, M.; Jiang, J.; Yue, L. Functional characterization of homo- and heteromeric channel kinases TRPM6 and TRPM7. *J. Gen. Physiol.* **2006**, *127*, 525–537. [CrossRef] [PubMed]
18. Trapani, V.; Petito, V.; Di Agostini, A.; Arduini, D.; Hamersma, W.; Pietropaolo, G.; Luongo, F.; Arena, V.; Stigliano, E.; Lopetuso, L.R.; et al. Dietary magnesium alleviates experimental murine colitis through upregulation of the transient receptor potential melastatin 6 channel. *Inflamm. Bowel Dis.* **2018**, in press. [CrossRef] [PubMed]
19. Trapani, V.; Arduini, D.; Luongo, F.; Wolf, F.I. EGF stimulates Mg^{2+} influx in mammary epithelial cells. *Biochem. Biophys. Res. Commun.* **2014**, *454*, 572–575. [CrossRef] [PubMed]
20. Trapani, V.; Schweigel-Röntgen, M.; Cittadini, A.; Wolf, F.I. Intracellular magnesium detection by fluorescent indicators. *Methods Enzymol.* **2012**, *505*, 421–444. [PubMed]
21. Wolf, F.I.; Trapani, V.; Simonacci, M.; Boninsegna, A.; Mazur, A.; Maier, J.A. Magnesium deficiency affects mammary epithelial cell proliferation: Involvement of oxidative stress. *Nutr. Cancer* **2009**, *61*, 131–136. [CrossRef] [PubMed]
22. Chubanov, V.; Mederos y Schnitzler, M.; Meißner, M.; Schäfer, S.; Abstiens, K.; Hofmann, T.; Gudermann, T. Natural and synthetic modulators of SK (K(ca)2) potassium channels inhibit magnesium-dependent activity of the kinase-coupled cation channel TRPM7. *Br. J. Pharmacol.* **2012**, *166*, 1357–1376. [CrossRef] [PubMed]
23. Ferioli, S.; Zierler, S.; Zaißerer, J.; Schredelseker, J.; Gudermann, T.; Chubanov, V. TRPM6 and TRPM7 differentially contribute to the relief of heteromeric TRPM6/7 channels from inhibition by cytosolic Mg^{2+} and Mg·ATP. *Sci. Rep.* **2017**, *7*, 8806. [CrossRef] [PubMed]
24. Trapani, V.; Arduini, D.; Cittadini, A.; Wolf, F.I. From magnesium to magnesium transporters in cancer: TRPM7, a novel signature in tumour development. *Magnes. Res.* **2013**, *26*, 149–155. [PubMed]
25. Gautier, M.; Perrière, M.; Monet, M.; Vanlaeys, A.; Korichneva, I.; Dhennin-Duthille, I.; Ouadid-Ahidouch, H. Recent advances in oncogenic roles of the TRPM7 chanzyme. *Curr. Med. Chem.* **2016**, *23*, 4092–4107. [CrossRef] [PubMed]
26. Deason-Towne, F.; Perraud, A.L.; Schmitz, C. The Mg^{2+} transporter MagT1 partially rescues cell growth and Mg^{2+} uptake in cells lacking the channel-kinase TRPM7. *FEBS Lett.* **2011**, *585*, 2275–2278. [CrossRef] [PubMed]
27. Cazzaniga, A.; Moscheni, C.; Trapani, V.; Wolf, F.I.; Farruggia, G.; Sargenti, A.; Iotti, S.; Maier, J.A.; Castiglioni, S. The different expression of TRPM7 and MagT1 impacts on the proliferation of colon carcinoma cells sensitive or resistant to doxorubicin. *Sci. Rep.* **2017**, *7*, 40538. [CrossRef] [PubMed]
28. Zhang, Z.; Yu, H.; Huang, J.; Faouzi, M.; Schmitz, C.; Penner, R.; Fleig, A. The TRPM6 kinase domain determines the Mg·ATP sensitivity of TRPM7/M6 heteromeric ion channels. *J. Biol. Chem.* **2014**, *289*, 5217–5227. [CrossRef] [PubMed]
29. Chubanov, V.; Schlingmann, K.P.; Wäring, J.; Heinzinger, J.; Kaske, S.; Waldegger, S.; Mederos y Schnitzler, M.; Gudermann, T. Hypomagnesemia with secondary hypocalcemia due to a missense mutation in the putative pore-forming region of TRPM6. *J. Biol. Chem.* **2007**, *282*, 7656–7667. [CrossRef] [PubMed]
30. Ryazanova, L.V.; Hu, Z.M.; Suzuki, S.; Chubanov, V.; Fleig, A.; Ryazanov, A.G. Elucidating the role of the TRPM7 alpha-kinase: TRPM7 kinase inactivation leads to magnesium deprivation resistance phenotype in mice. *Sci. Rep.* **2014**, *4*, 7599. [CrossRef] [PubMed]

4

Dietary Magnesium and Cardiovascular Disease: A Review with Emphasis in Epidemiological Studies

Nuria Rosique-Esteban [1,2], Marta Guasch-Ferré [1,2,3], Pablo Hernández-Alonso [1,2] and Jordi Salas-Salvadó [1,2,*]

[1] Human Nutrition Unit, Department of Biochemistry and Biotechnology,
Faculty of Medicine and Health Sciences, University Hospital of Sant Joan de Reus,
Pere Virgili Institute for Health Research, Rovira i Virgili University, St/Sant Llorenç 21, 43201 Reus, Spain;
nuria.rosique@urv.cat (N.R.-E.); mguasch@hsph.harvard.edu (M.G.-F.); pablo.hernandez@urv.cat (P.H.-A.)
[2] CIBERobn Physiopathology of Obesity and Nutrition, Institute of Health Carlos III (ISCIII), 28029 Madrid, Spain
[3] Department of Nutrition, Harvard T.H. Chan School of Public Health, Boston, MA 02115, USA
* Correspondence: jordi.salas@urv.cat

Abstract: Magnesium (Mg) is an essential dietary element for humans involved in key biological processes. A growing body of evidence from epidemiological studies, randomized controlled trials (RCTs) and meta-analyses have indicated inverse associations between Mg intake and cardiovascular diseases (CVD). The present review aims to summarize recent scientific evidence on the topic, with a focus on data from epidemiological studies assessing the associations between Mg intake and major cardiovascular (CV) risk factors and CVD. We also aimed to review current literature on circulating Mg and CVD, as well as potential biological processes underlying these observations. We concluded that high Mg intake is associated with lower risk of major CV risk factors (mainly metabolic syndrome, diabetes and hypertension), stroke and total CVD. Higher levels of circulating Mg are associated with lower risk of CVD, mainly ischemic heart disease and coronary heart disease. Further, RCTs and prospective studies would help to clarify whether Mg intake and Mg circulating levels may also protect against other CVDs and CVD death.

Keywords: magnesium; cardiovascular; type 2 diabetes; metabolic syndrome; mortality; death; epidemiological studies; inflammation; oxidation

1. Introduction

Magnesium (Mg) is an essential mineral for human health, representing the fourth most abundant mineral in the body. It is involved in important metabolic processes including ATP-dependent biochemical reactions, synthesis of DNA, RNA expression, cell signaling at muscle and nerve levels, and glucose and blood pressure (BP) control, among others (Figure 1) [1]. To guarantee the correct functioning of these processes, humans require a continuous supply of Mg from exogenous sources, i.e., dietary intake. Nuts, seeds, legumes, whole-grain cereals, leafy vegetables or water are well-recognized dietary sources of Mg (Table 1), regular consumption of which enables reaching the recommended dietary allowance currently set in 420 mg/day for adult men and 320 mg/day for adult women [2]. Mg requirements vary across age, sex and physiological situations (Figure 1). Dietary surveys in Europe and United States have shown that daily allowance of Mg are unmet in a large proportion of the population, probably as a result of following Western dietary patterns [2]. Several publications and recent meta-analyses have revealed inverse associations of dietary Mg intake with the risk of cardiovascular disease (CVD); cardiovascular (CV) risk factors including type 2 diabetes (T2D), metabolic syndrome (MetS) or hypertension; and total mortality [3]. Similarly, chronic Mg deficiency (defined as circulating $[Mg^{2+}] < 1.8$ mg/dL) has been associated with increased risk of several cardio-metabolic conditions [4,5]. A low inter-correlation between dietary Mg and circulating $[Mg^{2+}]$ has been described [6], possibly as a result of the tight homeostatic regulation of $[Mg^{2+}]$ through renal reabsorption and excretion, although the determinants of variation within the normal physiologic range are not well understood. For instance, genetic variations in single nucleotide polymorphisms may account for less than 2% of the variance in serum $[Mg^{2+}]$ [7], and the understanding of the influence of endocrine factors on Mg homeostasis need to be clarified [8]. Additionally, serum Mg only represents a minimal proportion of the Mg present in the entire body and thus intracellular $[Mg^{2+}]$ may be a more accurate method reflecting Mg status yet with additional difficulties to be measured [9]. Despite of this, and their low inter-correlation, both Mg intake and circulating $[Mg^{2+}]$ have been repeatedly associated with CV health [3–5], and therefore both are of great research interest.

	Age range	Males	Females	Pregnancy	Lactation
Recommended Daily Allowances for Magnesium	From birth to 6 mo	30 mg*	30 mg*		
	7-12 mo	75 mg*	75 mg*		
	1-3 y	80 mg	80 mg		
	4-8 y	130 mg	130 mg		
	9-13 y	240 mg	240 mg		
	14-18 y	410 mg	360 mg	400 mg	360 mg
	19- 30 y	400 mg	310 mg	350 mg	310 mg
	31-50 y	420 mg	320 mg	360 mg	320 mg
	>50 y	420 mg	320 mg		

Biological functions	• Enzyme cofactor in > 300 biochemical reactions • Energy production • DNA and RNA synthesis • Structural function of proteins, nucleic acids and mitochondria • Muscle contraction/relaxation, vasomotor tone, heart rhythm

Figure 1. Summary of current Recommended Daily Allowances (RDAs) for magnesium intake [2] and key biological functions of magnesium. Abbreviations: mo, months; y, years. * indicates Adequate Intake.

Table 1. List of foods and food groups from plant and animal origin with their corresponding magnesium content (mg/100 g edible food).

Food from Plant Origin		Food from Animal Origin	
Nuts and Seeds	Mg mg/100 g	**Dairy and Eggs**	Mg mg/100 g
Pumpkin seeds, dried	592	Parmesan cheese	44
Flaxseed	392	Feta cheese	19
Sesame seeds, roasted	356	Whole-fat milk	13
Almonds, raw	270	Plain whole-fat yogurt	12
Cashew nuts, roasted	260	Whole fresh egg	12
Walnuts	158		
Pistachio nuts, roasted	109		
Legumes		**Fish and seafood**	
Peanuts, roasted	178	Cod, cooked	133
Soybeans, cooked	86	Salmon, cooked	122
Chickpeas, cooked	48	Canned anchovies	69
Kidney beans, cooked	45	Shrimps, cooked	37
Lentils, cooked	36		
Vegetables and fruits		**Meat and meat products**	
Sun-dried tomatoes	194	Chicken breast, cooked	34
Spinach, cooked	87	Turkey, cooked	32
Kale, cooked	57	Veal, cooked	34
Dates	54	Rabbit, cooked	21
Fresh parsley	50		
Baked potatoes with skin	43		
Whole grains			
Buckwheat flour	251		
Amaranth grain	248		
Quinoa grain	197		
Oats	177		
Spelt	136		
Barley	133		

Data obtained from the US Department of Agriculture (USDA), Nutrient Database for Standard Reference, Release 28 [10].

The present review aims to summarize the most up-to-date scientific evidence on dietary Mg intake and circulating Mg, in relation to CVD. To this end, efforts have been made to describe most recent meta-analyses of prospective studies and RCTs on the topic, as well as current literature on Mg intake and CV risk factors. Recent investigations relating circulating Mg and CVD and plausible biological mechanisms underlying the potential beneficial role of dietary Mg intake on CV health have been reviewed. Because the present review is not based on a systematic search, some articles may not have been identified and publication bias should be acknowledged. However, all the authors independently conducted the literature search.

2. Dietary Magnesium and Cardiovascular Disease Risk Factors

Experimental and observational studies have shown that higher Mg intake can exert beneficial effects on CV risk factors by improving glucose and insulin metabolism, enhancing endothelium-dependent vasodilation, ameliorating lipid profile and by its actions as an antihypertensive and anti-inflammatory agent [11].

2.1. Type 2 Diabetes and Metabolic Syndrome

Mg plays an important role in glucose and insulin metabolism, likely via insulin resistance (IR) pathways and directly affecting glucose transporter protein activity 4 (GLUT 4) [12]. A large body of observational literature has suggested that higher Mg intake is associated with a lower risk of T2D and MetS. Indeed, several meta-analyses on this topic have already been conducted. The most recent one included 637,922 individuals with 26,828 T2D cases from twenty-five cohort studies. Results of this meta-analysis indicated that compared with those participants in the lowest Mg consumption category, the risk of T2D was reduced by 17% across all the studies; 19% in women and 16% in men. In addition, a linear dose–response relationship was observed between Mg intake and T2D, such that risk was 8%–13% lower per 100 mg/day increment in intake [13]. Previous meta-analyses evaluating Mg intake and T2D have also found consistent inverse associations [14,15]. More recently, a large prospective cohort study including more than 200,000 participants followed for over 28 years from the Nurses' Health Study (NHS) I, NHS II and Health Professionals' Follow-up study (HPFS) showed that, in pooled analysis across the three cohorts, those with the highest Mg intake (intake ranging from 350 to 500 mg/day) had 15% lower risk of T2D compared to those in the lowest Mg intake group (Hazard Ratio (HR) in the highest vs. the lowest quintile: 0.85 (95% CI 0.80–0.91)) [16]. This evidence has been further confirmed by clinical trials on Mg supplementation indicating beneficial effects of Mg on markers of glucose and insulin metabolism in individuals with and without T2D [17–19]. Findings from a recent meta-analysis of RCTs on the effects of supplemental Mg have demonstrated a significant effect of Mg on the Homeostatic model assessment of insulin resistance (HOMA-IR) index (weighted mean difference (WMD): -0.67, 95% CI: -1.20, -0.14); however, reductions in IR and fasting glucose were only observed when trials had a follow-up larger than four months [17].

IR is indeed one of the underlying causes of a cluster of risk factors for CVD, namely MetS. Evidence exists suggesting that there are potential benefits of dietary Mg in preventing MetS and its components [20,21]. A recent meta-analysis on this topic has summarized the evidence of nine observational studies including 31,876 participants [22]. Results indicated that higher consumption of Mg was associated with a lower risk of MetS (Odds Ratio (OR): 0.73, 95% CI, (0.62–0.86)) compared to participants in the lowest categories of Mg consumption. However, this meta-analysis combined the estimates from cross-sectional and prospective cohort studies altogether, and the association between components of the MetS and Mg intake was not assessed because it was not reported in the majority of the included studies [22]. However, for example, in a study conducted in a sample of 535 participants, Mg intake was inversely associated not only with the MetS but significant inverse relationships were observed between Mg intake, and body mass index (BMI) (OR: 0.47, 95% CI: 0.22–1.00, p for trend = 0.03), and fasting glucose (OR: 0.41, 95% CI 0.22–0.77, p for trend = 0.005) [23]. Two other review articles published in 2014 also summarized the associations between Mg intake and MetS in several studies [24,25]. Ju et al. [24] found an inverse dose–response association when pooling the data of nine observational studies, and Dibaba et al. [25] also observed consistent inverse associations between Mg intake and MetS when combining the data of six cross-sectional studies.

Overall, data from observational studies suggest a beneficial role of Mg intake in T2D prevention, whereas results from intervention studies have shown beneficial effects on HOMA-IR and fasting glucose. Given that these are surrogate biomarkers, further RCTs of Mg intake should focus on evaluating major endpoints, such as T2D incidence. Findings from studies on dietary Mg and MetS point to an inverse association with the prevalence of MetS, but further larger and long-term prospective studies and RCTs are needed to elucidate the role of Mg intake on MetS and its components.

2.2. Hypertension and Endothelial Function

High blood pressure or hypertension has been established as a strong risk factor for CVD. Among others, a diet rich in Na^+ and an inadequate dietary intake of other minerals including K^+, Ca^+ and Mg has been linked to hypertension [26]. Previous evidence has indicated that Mg deficiency might affect BP, thus leading to hypertension, and oral Mg supplementation may act as a mild antihypertensive agent [27]. In a recent meta-analysis on this topic, the authors have pooled the estimates on dietary Mg and hypertension of six prospective cohort studies including 20,119 cases and 180,566 participants [13]. The summary estimate indicated a statistically significant inverse association between dietary Mg and hypertension risk (pooled RR comparing extreme categories = 0.92; 95% CI: 0.86, 0.98) without apparent evidence of heterogeneity between studies. The range of dietary Mg intake among the included studies was 96–425 mg/day, and the follow-up ranged from 4 to 15 years. In addition, a 100 mg/day increment in Mg intake was associated with a 5% reduction in the risk of hypertension (RR = 0.95; 95% CI: 0.90, 1.00) [13]. These findings were consistent with those from RCTs examining the effect of Mg supplementation on BP. The most recent meta-analysis has identified eleven RCTs including 543 participants with preclinical or non-communicable diseases who were followed for a range of 1–6 months [28]. The weighted overall effects indicated that the group who was supplemented with oral Mg had a significantly greater reduction in both systolic BP (Standardized Mean Difference (SMD): -0.20; 95% CI: -0.37, -0.03) and diastolic BP (SMD: -0.27; 95% CI: -0.52, -0.03) than did the control group. Mg supplementation resulted in a mean reduction of 4.18 mmHg in systolic BP and 2.27 mmHg in diastolic BP [28]. Previous meta-analysis and systematic reviews on dietary Mg, BP and hypertension have also suggested potential benefits of dietary Mg [29,30], yet showing a more moderate effect, possibly as a result of combining individuals with and without chronic diseases in the pooled analysis.

Hypertension is indeed an important risk factor for endothelial dysfunction, and an essential step in the pathogenesis of atherosclerosis that ultimately may lead to coronary artery disease (CHD). Mg is involved in several essential physiological biochemical and cellular processes regulating CV function; in addition, it plays a crucial role in modulating vascular smooth muscle tone and endothelial function [31]. Several observational studies and clinical trials have evaluated the relationship between dietary Mg and biomarkers of endothelial function. As an illustration, in a cross-sectional study of 657 women of the NHS, in the age-adjusted linear regression analyses, Mg intake was inversely associated with plasma concentrations of E-selectin ($p = 0.001$), and soluble intercellular adhesion molecule 1 (sICAM-1) ($p = 0.03$). After further adjustment for physical activity, smoking status, alcohol use, postmenopausal hormone use, and BMI, dietary Mg intake remained inversely associated with E-selectin [32]. In another report of the Women's Health Initiative Observational Study including 3713 postmenopausal women, dietary Mg intake was inversely associated with plasma concentrations of soluble vascular cell adhesion molecule 1 (sVCAM-1) and E-selectin, independent of known risk factors for metabolic outcomes. Specifically, an increase of 100 mg/day Mg was inversely associated with sVCAM-1 (-0.04 ± 0.02 ng/mL; $p = 0.07$) [33]. Finally, a randomized, double-blind, placebo-controlled trial has indicated that oral Mg supplementation (30 mmol Mg/day) for six months resulted in a significant improvement in endothelium-dependent brachial artery flow-mediated vasodilation in 50 patients with coronary artery disease, indicating a beneficial effect of Mg on endothelial function [34].

In summary, several lines of evidence have suggested a potential beneficial link between high dietary Mg and low blood pressure, particularly among those individuals with either preclinical or non-communicable diseases. Furthermore, Mg intake seems to improve endothelial function but more studies are needed to confirm these associations in the long-term.

2.3. Lipid Profile

Dyslipidemia, one of the components of MetS, is a modifiable risk factor for the development of atherosclerosis and CVD [35]. Besides the potential benefits of dietary and supplemental Mg on IR, BP and endothelial function, several studies have also indicated that dietary Mg may be linked to an improvement in lipid profile including a decrease in low-density lipoprotein (LDL) cholesterol and triglycerides levels and an increase in high-density lipoprotein (HDL) cholesterol [36,37]. In a cross-sectional study, Guerrero-Romero et al. compared 192 individuals with MetS with 384 healthy age- and sex-matched controls. Of all of the MetS components, hypomagnesemia was most closely related with dyslipidemia (OR: 2.8; 95% CI: 1.3, 2.9) and hypertension (OR: 1.9; 95% CI: 1.4, 2.8) [38]. Similarly, in a cross-sectional analysis of the Tehran Lipid and Glucose Study including 2504 participants which evaluated the associations between dietary Mg and MetS and its components, Mg intake (mean intake of 349 mg/day) was inversely associated with triglycerides ($\beta = -0.058$, $P = 0.009$) [39]. In another recent cross-sectional study including 4443 individuals from the European Prospective Investigation into Cancer (EPIC)-Norfolk cohort, higher Mg intake was inversely associated with total cholesterol (p for trend = 0.02 men and 0.04 women) [40]. However, the evidence from longitudinal observational studies on dietary Mg and lipid profile biomarkers is limited. Most of the evidence regarding Mg and blood lipids comes from RCTs on oral Mg supplementation. A recent meta-analysis of RCTs did not show significant effects of Mg on plasma concentrations of total cholesterol, LDL-cholesterol, HDL-cholesterol and triglycerides [41]. The authors suggested that this may be explained by the inter-study heterogeneity due to the different formulations and salts of Mg used across the studies and the heterogeneity of the studied populations [41]. Nonetheless, the authors reported a significant reduction on LDL-cholesterol and triglyceride concentrations after Mg supplementation in a subgroup of studies in participants with hypercholesterolemia and hypertriglyceridemia, respectively. Thus, results suggested that according to the metabolic status, Mg may affect the lipid profile [41]. Moreover, in a randomized trial were 214 participants were administered a Mg-rich diet (1142 ± 225 mg/day) and 216 participants followed their usual diet (438 ± 118 mg/day) for 12 weeks, there was a significant decrease in total serum cholesterol (10.7%), LDL-cholesterol (10.5%) and triglycerides (10.1%) in participants following a Mg-rich diet compared to the baseline concentrations; no such changes were evident in participants following a usual diet. HDL-cholesterol showed a marginal mean decrease of 0.8 mg/dL in the control group and 2.0 mg/dL increase in the intervention group [36].

In conclusion, evidence from RCTs have suggested plausible beneficial effects of oral Mg supplementation for improving some lipid parameters, but improvements were only evident in individuals with dyslipidemia. Therefore, longer and larger trials and prospective cohort studies on this topic are still required.

3. Dietary Magnesium and Cardiovascular Disease

Most of the scientific literature on dietary Mg intake and CVD derive from prospective studies. Recently, an increasing number of meta-analyses have summarized previous literature on this topic, thus providing a more concise and public health-directed overview. The present section focuses on the evidence from epidemiological studies in relation with dietary Mg intake and major CVD events, as well as with CV death.

3.1. Stroke

Current scientific evidence on dietary Mg and the risk of stroke is mostly available from prospective cohort studies in North American, European and, to a lesser degree, from Asian populations. Previous and more recent meta-analyses have exemplified the available data [3,42–44], reporting similar results on the dose-dependent protective effect of Mg intake on stroke risk. While previous meta-analyses have reported between 2% and 13% protection against total stroke for an increment of 100 mg/day intake of dietary Mg [42–44], Fang et al. have confirmed this protective effect in the most updated analysis conducted in 2016, including fourteen prospective cohort studies [3]. In this updated meta-analysis, the authors have also reported 22% lower risk of stroke (RR: 0.88; 95% CI, 0.82, 0.95) in those individuals in the highest vs. the lowest categories of dietary Mg intake, which is in agreement with findings reported in previous studies [43]. It is important to highlight that these meta-analyses have shown null to low heterogeneity between studies, they have found no evidence of publication bias and they included studies adjusting for several potential confounders. Taken together, current evidence from prospective studies in large populations across the world indicated a dose-dependent inverse association between dietary Mg and stroke incidence.

3.2. Coronary Heart Disease

Coronary Heart Disease (CHD) in relation with dietary Mg intake has been extensively investigated in large population cohorts in America and Asia, including the NHS, the HPFS and the Shanghai Women's and Men's Healthy study, among other cohorts [6,45–49]. However, most of these studies did not show a significant association when comparing the highest vs. the lowest category of Mg intake in relation to the risk of CHD in either men or women. For instance, in an analysis of more than 86,000 healthy American nurses, no significant associations were found comparing the highest vs. the lowest quintile of Mg intake on total and non-fatal CHD over a median of 28 years of follow-up [6]. In this study, and similar to other analysis in the same cohort [47], Mg intake included those from food sources and supplements, whereas the rest of the investigations only included Mg intake from foods [45,46,48]. A pooled analysis by Fang and collaborators [3] including nine different prospective cohorts have revealed inverse borderline associations with the highest category of Mg intake on CHD risk (RR: 0.90; 95% CI, 0.80, 0.99), with low heterogeneity across studies. In an additional dose–response analysis, the authors reported non-significant associations for higher Mg intake on CHD, with low to medium heterogeneity among studies. On the contrary, a recently published prospective study conducted in a large cohort of community-based Japanese adults [49] with a total of 1283 cases of CHD has revealed a protection against CHD in men in the fourth (HR: 0.70 95% CI, 0.50, 0.99) and fifth quintile (HR: 0.66 95% CI, 0.44, 0.97) of Mg intake compared to the lowest quintile (*P* for linear trend = 0.036). Overall, current evidence on Mg intake and CHD suggests a non-significant inverse association in most of the populations studied. Nevertheless, additional prospective studies and clinical trials on this topic should focus on addressing plausible age, sex and country differences.

3.3. Heart Failure

Epidemiological evidence on the associations between dietary Mg and heart failure (HF) are currently limited to two independent American and Japanese cohort studies [50,51]. Although large risk reductions in HF incidence have been reported in the highest vs. lowest Mg intake among black American individuals and Japanese women, the associations were non-significant for Japanese men [51]. These differences may be due to the lower Mg intake in Japanese men compared to their American counterparts (294 and 474 mg/day, respectively), or due to biological differences between the study populations. Nevertheless, a recently published meta-analysis [3] including these two independent cohorts has shown a strong inverse association with HF for the highest vs. the lowest categories (RR: 0.69; 95% CI, 0.52, 0.91) and also per an increment of 100 mg/day of Mg intake (RR: 0.78, 95% CI, 0.69, 0.89), both with no apparent heterogeneity. Further data from prospective studies and clinical trials in other countries and ethnicity-specific populations is required to have an extensive insight on the possible role of Mg in preventing HF.

3.4. Atrial Fibrillation

The associations between dietary Mg intake and atrial fibrillation, a common cardiac arrhythmia, have barely been explored in epidemiological and experimental settings. To the best of our knowledge, only one prospective cohort study has, so far, addressed this topic [52]. The authors followed more than 14,000 middle-aged American whites and African American participants from the ARIC study for 20.6 years, reporting 1755 incident cases of atrial fibrillation. Compared to the middle quintile (median dietary Mg: 223.2–264.8 mg/day), those individuals in the highest (median dietary Mg: ≥320.1 mg/day) or the lowest quintile of Mg intake (median dietary Mg < 180.9 mg/day)—exclusively from dietary sources, as assessed by food frequency questionnaire—did not show significantly higher or lower incidence of atrial fibrillation. These results were found regardless of sex or ethnicity, as the authors reported no significant interactions with dietary Mg. Despite these results, previous experimental studies under controlled conditions in individuals with similar characteristics have demonstrated that dietary-induced Mg depletion can induce heart rhythm changes with few participants showing atrial flutter and fibrillation [53], and that subsequent Mg repletion with supplements reverse these heart rhythm changes. These limited and mixed results illustrate the need of more epidemiological and experimental evidences to elucidate the link between dietary Mg intake and atrial fibrillation across different populations.

3.5. Cardiovascular Death

Several epidemiological studies across North American [6,47,54–56], Asian [48,51], and, to a lesser degree, European populations [57] of middle-aged men and women have prospectively evaluated the associations between dietary Mg intake and risk of CV death yielding inconclusive results. With the purpose of summarizing the existing evidence on the topic, two meta-analyses have been published to date [58,59]. In a first meta-analysis, Xu et al. [58] included a total of six prospective studies comprising more than 200,000 men and women with a follow-up ranging between 10 and 26 years. In the pooled analysis, those participants in highest category of Mg intake comparted to those in the lowest category, showed no significant differences regarding total CV death risk, yet high heterogeneity across studies was detected. However, further inspection of subgroup analyses revealed a 29% protection only in women (RR: 0.71; 95% CI, 0.60, 0.84).

In a more recent updated meta-analysis [59] including more than 400,000 adults from different cohorts who were followed for 5 to 28 years, the summary estimate comparing individuals at the higher vs. the lowest categories of dietary Mg intake showed a protection of 14% (HR: 0.86; 95% CI, 0.81, 0.91) against the risk of CV death, with high heterogeneity among studies and no evidence of publication bias. Subgroup analyses revealed that this protection corresponded to 16% in women and 8% in men. Further inspection of the subtypes of CVD death showed that dietary Mg intake was inversely and significantly associated with lower risk for CHD, heart failure and sudden cardiac death. Additional dose–response analysis showed a protection of 25% (HR: 0.75; 95% CI, 0.58, 0.99) in women for the increment of 100 mg/day of Mg intake.

Overall, current evidence in relation to dietary Mg intake and death for total CVD and CV subtypes shows a protective role, particularly in women. Nevertheless, the results derived from meta-analyses should be interpreted with caution given the high heterogeneity found across the studies. Further RCTs on dietary Mg intake should focus on assessing CV hard endpoints to clarify current available evidence aroused from prospective studies.

4. Circulating Magnesium and Cardiovascular Disease

Several prospective studies have analyzed the associations between peripheral levels of Mg or urine Mg excretion (Mg status) and the risk of several CVD including cardiac arrhythmias, congestive HF, CHD, stroke, sudden death and death from all these causes.

Although a poor correlation between dietary Mg and plasma levels of this mineral has been reported in several prospective studies [6,45], evidence exists demonstrating that very low Mg diets may lead to low serum Mg levels, and a recent meta-analysis of RCTs demonstrated significant dose and time responses of circulating $[Mg^{2+}]$ and 24 h urine Mg excretion to oral Mg supplementation [60].

Therefore, in this section, we summarize the epidemiological evidence in the literature analyzing the association between low circulating (serum/plasma) $[Mg^{2+}]$ or urinary Mg excretion and CVDs.

4.1. Cardiovascular Disease, Coronary Disease and Stroke

The most recent systematic review and meta-analysis analyzing the associations between peripheral $[Mg^{2+}]$ and CVD identified significant associations of circulating Mg and risk of CVD events [4]. Circulating $[Mg^{2+}]$ (per 0.2 mmol/L increment) was associated with a 30% lower risk of CVD, with trends towards a lower risk of ischemic heart disease (IHD) and fatal IHD. This meta-analysis, including a total of 313,041 individuals and documenting 4106 CVD, 3215 IHD, and 1528 fatal IHD events, provides the most robust evidence to date of the associations between circulating $[Mg^{2+}]$ across their usual physiologic ranges with CVD risk. However, a moderate heterogeneity between the studies analyzed was reported.

Since then, two additional large prospective studies examining this relation have been conducted. Chiuve et al. [6] conducted a nested case–control analysis in the context of the NHS with 458 cases of incident CHD matched to controls. Higher plasma $[Mg^{2+}]$ was associated in an L-shaped fashion with lower risk of CHD, although this association was not independent of CVD biomarkers. In contrast, in the Prevention of Renal and Vascular End-Stage Disease (PREVEND) study—a prospective population-based cohort study—low urinary Mg excretion was independently associated with a higher risk of IHD incidence. Nevertheless, no significant associations were observed between plasma levels of this mineral and IHD incidence or death [61].

In relation to stroke, several cross-sectional and retrospective case–control studies have reported lower serum $[Mg^{2+}]$ in those individuals with acute stroke compared with healthy controls. However, in these studies Mg was not measured before stroke diagnosis and thus hypomagnesemia may have been a consequence rather than a cause of stroke in these patients. No prospective association between serum $[Mg^{2+}]$ and risk of stroke was reported in the ARIC Study cohort after adjusting by several confounders (based on 577 ischemic stroke cases in men and women with 16 years of follow-up) [62]. In the NHS, plasma Mg levels were not associated with the risk of ischemic stroke in women [63]. However, women with $[Mg^{2+}]$ levels < 0.82 mmol/L had a 57% higher risk of ischemic stroke, and this association remained unchanged after controlling for other factors associated with Mg levels and stroke risk.

4.2. Atrial Fibrillation and Sudden Death

Low serum $[Mg^{2+}]$ has been linked to an increased risk of atrial fibrillation (AF) after cardiac surgery. However, it is unknown whether hypomagnesemia predisposes to AF in the general population. Two prospective studies have analyzed the association between serum $[Mg^{2+}]$ and AF risk in healthy populations and in individuals at risk of CVD. In the context of the Framingham Health Study, low serum $[Mg^{2+}]$ was moderately associated with the development of AF in individuals without previous history of CVD [64]. In the ARIC cohort, an L-shaped association between serum $[Mg^{2+}]$ and incident AF was also identified, with the highest risk of AF in those individuals with low serum $[Mg^{2+}]$, and a lower risk at more normal and elevated $[Mg^{2+}]$ levels [52]. This association, not different among white and African populations, was evident even after adjustment for the most important recognized risk factors of AF.

4.3. Left Ventricular Hypertrophy and Heart Failure

A few lines of evidence suggest that low circulating $[Mg^{2+}]$ may predict left ventricular hypertrophy or HF among population-based individuals. For example, low serum $[Mg^{2+}]$ has been demonstrated to predict higher increase in left ventricular mass over five years of follow-up in the population-based longitudinal Study of Health in Pomerania including 1348 individuals with echocardiographic data [65]. This prognostic impact was regardless of sex, age and traditional CV risk factors including prevalent hypertension. In relation to cardiac insufficiency, in the ARIC Study, a North American population-based cohort, low serum $[Mg^{2+}]$ and high serum phosphorus and calcium concentrations were independently associated with greater risk of incident HF after controlling for several potential confounders, with the association remaining consistent across sex and ethnicity [66]. In a population-based prospective study of middle-aged Finnish men without HF at baseline, the Kuopio Ischemic Heart Disease Study, a decreased risk for incident HF with increasing serum $[Mg^{2+}]$ was also reported [67]. This association persisted after controlling for baseline characteristics, predictors of incident HF, metabolic and renal biomarkers, and other related micronutrients.

4.4. Atherosclerosis and Coronary Artery Calcification

In few epidemiological studies, low circulating $[Mg^{2+}]$ was inversely associated with atherosclerosis and coronary artery calcification. For example, in the ARIC study, decreased serum $[Mg^{2+}]$ were associated with increased mean carotid wall thickness in women [68]. Hashimoto et al. [69] analyzed 728 subjects from the general Japanese population and also found that serum $[Mg^{2+}]$ to be inversely associated with intima-media thickness of the common carotid artery, and with the presence of atherosclerotic plaque. In two recent cross-sectional studies conducted in Korean and Mexican populations free from CVD, low serum $[Mg^{2+}]$ were also associated with coronary artery calcification [70,71].

4.5. Cardiovascular Death

In a systematic review and meta-analysis, using the results of four studies including 27,293 individuals and 1528 cases the association between circulating $[Mg^{2+}]$ and fatal IHD risk has been evaluated [4], showing a trend towards a lower risk in those individuals with lower $[Mg^{2+}]$, with substantial between-study heterogeneity. In secondary analyses using fixed effects, circulating $[Mg^{2+}]$ were associated with a significantly lower risk of fatal IHD. Nevertheless, meta-regression analysis did not show statistically significant sources of heterogeneity, although statistical power to identify heterogeneity was limited because only four studies were included in the analysis.

Peripheral $[Mg^{2+}]$ were also inversely associated with fatal CHD in the NHS [6], and with fatal stroke in the NHANES I Epidemiologic Follow-up Study [72]. Low serum $[Mg^{2+}]$ were also associated with an increased risk of CHD death and sudden cardiac death in a recent European prospective population-based cohort study [73].

Finally, in a recent systematic review and meta-analysis of studies conducted in HF patients, hypermagnesemia with serum $[Mg^{2+}] \geq 1.05$ mmol/L was associated with an increased risk of CVD death and all-cause death, but this was not observed for hypomagnesemia [74]. However, these findings were limited to elderly patients with chronic HF who had reduced left ventricular systolic function.

5. Plausible Mechanisms Connecting Magnesium and Cardiovascular Disease

The inverse association between Mg intake and IR, hyperglycemia, dyslipidemia, hypertension, and markers of inflammation may justify the protective effect of dietary Mg on CVD. As reviewed in previous sections, several RCTs and epidemiological studies have widely indicated that higher dietary Mg intake and/or circulating $[Mg^{2+}]$ are associated with lower risk of CVD, such as IHD and sudden cardiac death. Given the participation of Mg^{2+} in a wide range of biological pathways and outcomes, it is not surprising that alterations in Mg homeostasis may influence different disease status, such as T2D and hypertension, together with CV events (Figure 2). Numerous studies have reported an increased oxidative stress during Mg-deficiency (Mg-D), including enhanced erythrocyte, tissue, and lipoprotein peroxidation, implicated in the early stages and progression of CVDs [75–79].

Figure 2. Mechanisms linking magnesium abnormalities (intake or circulating levels) with molecular outcomes leading to CV risk factors that may induce CV disease. Abbreviations: CV, cardiovascular; Mg, magnesium; T2D, type 2 diabetes.

In this paper, we have mainly focused in outcomes related to CVD and/or their risk factors. Studies investigating these mechanisms have mostly focused on the effects of Mg supplementation or circulating $[Mg^{2+}]$ levels on inflammation and/or oxidative processes. However, specific in vitro and/or in vivo research has also been conducted to explore the overall processes affecting CV outcomes or CV risk factors (Figure 2).

5.1. Oxidative and Inflammatory Stress

Already at the beginning of the 20th century, after the discovery of Mg as an essential nutrient, Mg-D was linked to inflammation [80]. It is well-characterized that a previous phase of Mg depletion renders cells—particularly myocardial tissue—more sensitive to oxidative stress [75–77]. However, supplementation with Mg led to an increase in antioxidant blood concentrations [75,81,82]. It has been hypothesized either that Mg-D induces oxidative stress due to its pro-inflammatory effect, or that Mg itself possess antioxidant properties, scavenging oxygen radicals [75,76]. Mg-D may also induce a pro-inflammatory response by modulation of the intracellular Ca^{2+} concentration, release of neurotransmitters, or the activation of nuclear factor-kB implicated in the regulation of immune and inflammatory responses [76].

Freedman and collaborators demonstrated during the nineties the participation of free radicals in Mg-D cardiomyopathy and the incapacity of Mg-deficient animals to withstand an in vivo oxidative stress [78,79]. They evaluated the effect on Syrian hamsters being fed for 14 days with a Mg-deficient diet or a Mg-supplemented control diet, showing that Mg-D increases the susceptibility of the CV system to oxidative stress [79]. However, researchers also found that the concentration of nitric oxide (NO) is markedly increased in plasma of Mg-deficient rats, thus providing an additional cause of oxidative lesions through formation of peroxynitrite [83].

In vitro studies were also performed and the effect of Mg-deficient culture on endothelial cell susceptibility to oxidative stress was examined. Bovine endothelial cells were cultured in either control sufficient (0.8 mM) or deficient (0.4 mM) levels of $MgCl_2$. Results derived from this investigation suggest that in vitro Mg-D enhances free radical-induced intracellular oxidation and cytotoxicity in endothelial cells [84]. To further explore these effects, Wiles et al. examined the exposure of acute Mg-D to this cell type. Decreasing $[Mg^{2+}]$ ($\leq$0.25 mM) significantly increased endothelial cell oxidant production relative to control $[Mg^{2+}]$ (1 mM). This suggested that acute Mg-D is sufficient for the induction of endothelial cells oxidant production, the extent of which may determine, at least in part, the extent of endothelial cells dysfunction/injury associated with chronic Mg-D [85].

Severe dietary Mg restriction (9% of the recommended dietary allowance (RDA) is sufficient to induce a pro-inflammatory neurogenic response in rats [86]. Thus, Kramer and collaborators evaluated in 2003 whether less severe dietary Mg restriction modulates the extent of both the neurogenic/oxidative responses in vivo and ischemia/reperfusion injury in vitro. Male Sprague-Dawley rats maintained on Mg (40% RDA) or Mg (100% RDA) diets during the first three weeks were compared with the 9% RDA Mg group. They found that erythrocyte glutathione and plasma malondialdehyde levels revealed a direct relationship between the severity of oxidative stress and hypomagnesemia. Thus, suggesting that varying dietary Mg intake directly influences the magnitude of the neurogenic/oxidative responses in vivo and the resultant myocardial tolerance to ischemia/reperfusion stress [87]. Because it has been demonstrated that Mg-D promotes inflammation in vivo, Bernardini and collaborators evaluated the effect of different $[Mg^{2+}]$ on microvascular 1G11 cells [88]. They reported that low $[Mg^{2+}]$ inhibits endothelial growth and migration, while it increases some inflammatory- and endothelial-related markers (IL-1a, IL-6, NO and VCAM), whereas high $[Mg^{2+}]$ stimulates cell proliferation and migration. This result demonstrated a direct role of Mg in the modulation of microvascular functions and provided a molecular explanation to the link among Mg, angiogenesis and inflammation observed in in vivo CV models [88].

5.2. Lipid Profile and Peroxidation

Rayssiguier and collaborators demonstrated for the first time in 1993, using Wistar rats, that dietary Mg-D affects susceptibility of lipoproteins and tissues to peroxidation [89]. The destruction of membrane lipids and the end-products of such lipid peroxidation reactions are especially dangerous for the viability of cells and tissues, hence comprising a crucial step in the pathogenesis of several CVD [90]. Several years later, Morrill et al. monitored changes in rat lipid extracts of aortic and cerebrovascular smooth muscle as extracellular $[Mg^{2+}]$ was being reduced. They found, within the pathophysiological range of Mg^{2+}, a progressive reduction in fatty acid chain length and double bond content—which results in fatty acid truncation—as $[Mg^{2+}]$ is lowered. A decrease in lipid oxidation in the presence of elevated $[Mg^{2+}]$ could contribute to the apparent protective role of increased Mg intake on vascular function in humans [91].

Postprandial accumulation of triglyceride-rich lipoproteins (TGRLP) is an important characteristic of hyperlipidemia associated with Mg-D in animal models. Control and Mg-deficient rats were fed for eight days on adequate or Mg-D diets. Researchers tested the susceptibility of TGRLP isolated from control and treated rats to cell-dependent peroxidation and the effect of these lipoproteins on in vitro cultured vascular smooth muscle cells (VSMC). Results showed a higher oxidation in the case of Mg-deficient rats. This outcome warrants the atherogenic properties of Mg-D, which is accompanied by hyperlipidemia and which affects two important linked pathways: lipoprotein peroxidation and VSMC proliferation [92]. Moreover, additional results proved that TGRLP-oxidative damage is not the result of a decrease in vitamin E antioxidant status [93].

Altura and collaborators investigated in vivo the etiology of cardiac diseases. They examined the effects of Mg depletion on myocardial bioenergetic, carbohydrate, lipid and phospholipid metabolism. Rat myocardial biopsies were studied after being fed for 3 months with a dietary Mg restriction (20% normal dietary intake). Dietary Mg-D resulted in a drop in myocardial glycogen, glucose 6-phosphate, glycerol phosphate, as well as the contents of different phospholipids, illustrating impaired phospholipid metabolism and mitochondrial oxidation of long-chain fatty acids. These observations are consistent with the principle that prolonged low $[Mg^{2+}]$ can result in marked reduction in O_2 and substrate delivery to the cardiac myocytes, with concomitant changes in membrane phospholipids (potentially resulting in a pro-oxidant state) probably as a result of coronary vasoconstriction [94].

5.3. Glucose Homeostasis/Type 2 Diabetes

The means whereby hypomagnesemia may promote or worsen existing T2D have not been fully unraveled. It has been suggested that Mg^{2+} regulates cellular glucose metabolism directly as it serves as an important cofactor for various enzymes and acts as a second messenger for insulin [95]. Importantly, it was also observed that insulin enhances intracellular Mg^{2+} uptake and this in turn mediates diverse effects ascribed to insulin [95]. Furthermore, low $[Mg^{2+}]$ may induce altered cellular glucose transport, reduced pancreatic insulin secretion, defective post-receptor insulin signaling and/or altered insulin–insulin receptor interactions [96] and thus aggravate the processes related to IR, important risk factor for CVD [95].

5.4. Endothelial Function, Blood Pressure and Hypertension

In spite of considerable research, the exact underlying causes for altered Mg metabolism in hypertensive individuals remain unclear [97]. It is assumed that inadequate dietary Mg intake or a malfunction on its metabolism can lead to vasospasm and endothelial damage [98]. Therefore, as it has already introduced before, Mg-D might affect BP and/or endothelial function, which may promote hypertension.

In an in vitro study, Maier et al. cultured human umbilical vein endothelial cells for various times in media containing different $[Mg^{2+}]$ (2–10 mM) and compared them to the corresponding controls (1 mM). High $[Mg^{2+}]$ stimulated endothelial proliferation and enhanced the mitogenic response to angiogenic factors. In addition, high $[Mg^{2+}]$ did not modulate the levels of plasminogen activator inhibitor-1, but enhanced the synthesis of NO, in part through the up-regulation of endothelial nitric oxide synthase. Thus, as it induces the synthesis of NO, Mg supplementation could be a helpful management approach in hypertension as well as in preventing thrombosis [99].

The effect of dietary Mg supplementation on BP and CV function has also been evaluated in vivo. Normotensive rats and mineralocorticoid-salt (DOCA-salt) hypertensive rats were fed for 5 weeks with a purified diet containing either a normal or Mg-supplemented diet (1.5 or 10 g/kg diet). Mg supplementation significantly lowered BP levels in hypertensive rats, but not in normotensive rats, and heart rate was not affected in either group. These findings suggested that the lowering effect of Mg supplementation on BP in hypertensive rats may be related to a vascular effect of Mg that reduces vascular tone [100]. To further test the effect of its supplementation on the development of hypertension in spontaneously hypertensive rats (SHR), Touyz et al. designed an in vivo study. Ten-week-old SHR and control Wistar-Kyoto rats (WKY) were divided into four groups which were fed for 17 weeks: WKY, WKY with Mg supplementation (650 mg/L), SHR, and SHR with Mg supplementation (650 mg/L). From 13 weeks of age, BP was significantly elevated in SHR compared with age-matched WKY. BP was significantly reduced in SHR after 10 weeks of Mg supplementation. From 18 weeks of age, serum and intracellular $[Mg^{2+}]$ levels were significantly lower in SHR than in WKY. Mg supplementation was able to normalize intracellular [Mg^{2+}] and [Ca^{2+}] in SHR. Overall, these results showed that mid-term Mg supplementation significantly attenuates, but does not prevent, the development of hypertension in SHR [101]. Importantly, Blache et al. tested the long-term effect of Mg-D. Rats were fed for 22 months with moderately deficient (150 mg/kg), standard (800 mg/kg), or supplemented (3200 mg/kg) Mg diets. Compared to the standard and supplemented diets, Mg-D enriched diet significantly increased BP, plasma IL-6, fibrinogen, and erythrocyte lysophosphatidylcholine. Thus, Mg-D induced a chronic impairment of redox status associated with inflammation, which could significantly contribute to increased oxidized lipids and promote hypertension and vascular disorders with aging. Extrapolating these results to the human situation and considering that Mg-D has been reported to be remarkably common—particularly among elderly individuals—Mg supplementation may be useful as an adjuvant therapy in preventing CVD [77].

5.5. Cardiovascular Disease Events: Arrhythmia and Acute Myocardial Infarction

Probably the most widely accepted and practiced use of Mg in CV medicine is for the prevention and/or treatment of cardiac arrhythmias [31]. Anti-arrhythmogenic properties of Mg may involve changes in the activity of some ionic channels, such as Ca^{2+} and K^+ [102]. Both extracellular and cytosolic Mg^{2+} has significant effects on cardiac ion channels, which in turn may have important consequences on the duration of action potential, cell excitability and contractility [102]. Mg^{2+} exerts its antiarrhythmic effect via modulation of myocardial excitability. However, very few studies have evaluated the effect of Mg^{2+} on cardiac voltage-dependent Na^+ channels. Using inside-out patches from guinea pig ventricular myocytes to measure currents through single cardiac Na^+ channels, Mubagwa et al. [103] showed that [Mg^{2+}] had no effect on inward currents but decreased the outward current amplitude in a concentration and voltage-dependent manner. This suggested that Mg^{2+} primarily exerts only an open channel blocking effect, with little or no direct allosteric modulatory action on the voltage-dependent Na^+ channels.

Data coming from autopsies indicated that patients who had died from IHD had reduced Mg^{2+} levels in myocardium and muscle compared with those who had died from non-cardiac causes. It was observed that during myocardial ischemia, total intracellular Mg^{2+} decreases while free intracellular Mg^{2+} increases [104]. In addition, ischemia per se leads to intracellular Ca^{2+} overload, which compromises myocardial function. It was speculated that Mg^{2+} administration reduces Ca^{2+} overload as a result of the competence between these two elements for the same binding sites. In addition, the effects of Mg^{2+} on vascular tone, its ability to improve endothelial dependent vasodilation, its anticoagulant properties, possibly through improvement of NO release [105], may all exert a beneficial effect in acute myocardial infarction. In accordance with these findings, investigators started to study Mg^{2+} replacement as an adjunctive pharmacotherapy in the context of acute myocardial infarction.

5.6. A Focus on Magnesium Receptors

Research in the mechanisms of control of vascular Mg^{2+} homeostasis revealed two cation channels of the transient receptor potential melastatin (TRPM), TRPM6 and TRPM7, as important Mg^{2+} transporters [105]. They are differentially expressed, with TRPM6 being primarily found in epithelial cells and TRPM7 occurring ubiquitously. Vascular TRPM7 is modulated by vasoactive agents, pressure, stretch, and osmotic changes and may be a novel mechanotransducer. In addition to its Mg^{2+} transporter function, TRPM7 has been implicated as a signaling kinase involved in VSMC growth, apoptosis, adhesion, contraction, important processes involved in vascular remodeling associated with hypertension and other vascular diseases [105]. Overall, TRPM7 has been shown to play an essential role in maintaining cellular Mg^{2+} homeostasis. However, more research is needed to clarify the exact mechanisms of Mg^{2+} regulation in the CV system and the implications of abnormal transmembrane Mg^{2+} transport in the pathogenesis of vascular diseases [106]. In fact, a recent randomized, double-blind clinical trial conducted in pre-hypertensive subjects compared the effect of oral Mg supplementation versus placebo treatment for four month in the expression of different Mg^{2+} transporters in leukocytes. Rodríguez-Ramírez and collaborators reported a significant increase in the TRPM6 mRNA relative expression in leukocytes from pre-hypertensive individuals following the oral Mg supplementation compared to placebo group. Conversely, non-significant differences were reported regarding TRPM7 and solute carrier family 41 member 1 (SLC41A1) mRNA relative expression [107].

Overall, Mg is an essential microelement critical in several biological processes. Its specific role on the CV system has been widely investigated. However, further in vitro and in vivo studies are needed to explore other potential molecular targets and pathways putatively modulated and influenced by dietary and circulating Mg^{2+} levels.

6. Final Conclusions

Taken together, current evidence from epidemiological studies shows that higher Mg intake, either dietary or via supplementation, is associated with a protection against major CV risk factors, including MetS, T2D and hypertension/BP, as well as against stroke and total CVDs. Nevertheless, further prospective studies and RCTs are warranted to elucidate the relation between Mg intake and MetS individual components, endothelial dysfunction, lipid profile and obesity—of which current scientific knowledge remains very scarce—and HF, CHD and CVD death in different populations. Available evidence on circulating Mg and CVDs shows that greater circulating $[Mg^{2+}]$ is also associated with lower risk of CVDs, mainly IHD and CHD, yet further insights are needed to clarify the less consistent results with other CVDs and CV death. Because Mg plays a crucial role in a wide range of biological pathways and outcomes, it is not surprising that alterations in Mg homeostasis may influence different disease status.

Importantly, the fact that Mg intake is determined using indirect methods in epidemiological studies, such as food frequency questionnaires, makes it difficult to separate the observed associations from those of other microelements that may also positively contribute to cardiometabolic health. Thus, a residual effect from the intake of other dietary microelements cannot be discarded despite the efforts for controlling this in multivariate models.

Traditionally, supplement formulations from organic Mg (aspartate, citrate, lactate and chloride) have been considered to be more bioavailable than those with inorganic Mg (oxide and sulfate), as reported by a number of studies [108]. However, this topic is currently under debate given that other studies have found no differences between these formulations, and several factors have been shown to play a role in the complex process of Mg absorption and utilization [109].

The inverse association between Mg intake and IR, hyperglycemia, dyslipidemia, hypertension, and markers of inflammation may justify the protective effect of dietary Mg on CVD. Overall, the current evidence supports the importance of adequate dietary magnesium for lowering CVD risk. In addition, these findings support the importance to increase the consumption of magnesium-rich foods, including fruits, vegetables, legumes, nuts and whole grains for the prevention of chronic diseases.

Acknowledgments: This work was supported in part by the Spanish Ministry of Health (Carlos III Health Institute) through the Fondo de Investigacion para la Salud (FIS), which is co-funded by the European Regional Development Fund. NR.-E is beneficiary of a predoctoral FI-AGAUR fellowship from the Secretaria d'Universitats i Recerca del Departament d'Economia i Coneixement de la Generalitat de Catalunya. Marta Guasch-Ferré was supported by a postdoctoral fellowship granted by the Lilly Foundation European Association of Diabetes (EASD) through the Institut d'Investigacions Sanitàries Pere i Virgili (IISPV), Tarragona, Spain.

Author Contributions: N.R.-E., M.G.-F., P.H.-A. and J.S.S. designed the review; N.R.-E., M.G.-F., P.H.-A. and J.S.S. performed the literature research; N.R.-E., M.G.-F., P.H.-A. and J.S.S. wrote the first draft of the manuscript; and all authors contributed to the editing of the manuscript. All authors approved the final version of the manuscript.

Abbreviations

ARIC	Atherosclerosis Risk in Communities
ATP	adenosine triphosphate
BMI	body mass index
BP	blood pressure
Ca^{2+}	calcium
CHD	coronary heart disease
CV	cardiovascular
CVD	cardiovascular disease
DNA	deoxyribonucleic acid
GLUT 4	glucose transporter protein activity 4
HDL	high-density lipoprotein
HF	heart failure
HR	hazard ratio
HOMA-IR	homeostatic model assessment of insulin resistance
IHD	ischemic heart disease
IL	interleukin
IR	insulin resistance
K+	potassium
LDL	low-density lipoprotein
MetS	metabolic syndrome
Mg	magnesium
Mg-D	Mg-deficiency
$[Mg^{2+}]$	magnesium concentrations
Mg^{2+}	intracellular magnesium
Na+	sodium
NO	nitric oxide
O2	oxygen
T2D	type 2 diabetes
TGRLP	triglyceride-rich lipoproteins
TRPM	transient receptor potential melastatin
RCT	randomized control trial
RDA	recommended dietary allowance
RR	Relative Risk
sICAM-1	soluble intercellular adhesion molecule 1
SLC41A1	solute carrier family 41 member 1
SHR	spontaneously hypertensive rats
UVEC	umbilical vein endothelial cells
VCAM	vascular cell adhesion protein 1
VSMC	vascular smooth muscle cells
WKY	Wistar-Kyoto rats

References

1. Gröber, U.; Schmidt, J.; Kisters, K. Magnesium in Prevention and Therapy. *Nutrients* **2015**, 8199–8226. [CrossRef] [PubMed]

2. Standing Committee on the Scientific Evaluation of Dietary Reference Intakes; Food and Nutrition Board; Institute of Medicine (IOM). *Dietary Reference Intakes for Calcium, Phosphorus, Magnesium, Vitamin D, and Fluoride*; National Academies Press: Washington, DC, USA, 1997.

3. Fang, X.; Wang, K.; Han, D.; He, X.; Wei, J.; Zhao, L.; Imam, M.U.; Ping, Z.; Li, Y.; Xu, Y.; et al. Dietary magnesium intake and the risk of cardiovascular disease, type 2 diabetes, and all-cause mortality: A dose—Response meta- analysis of prospective cohort studies. *BMC Med.* **2016**. [CrossRef] [PubMed]

4. Del Gobbo, L.C.; Imamura, F.; Wu, J.H.Y.; Otto, M.C.D.O.; Chiuve, S.E. Circulating and dietary magnesium and risk of cardiovascular disease: A systematic review and meta-analysis of prospective studies. *Am. J. Clin. Nutr.* **2013**, 160–173. [CrossRef] [PubMed]

5. Qu, X.; Jin, F.; Hao, Y.; Li, H.; Tang, T.; Wang, H.; Yan, W.; Dai, K. Magnesium and the Risk of Cardiovascular Events: A Meta-Analysis of Prospective Cohort Studies. *PLoS ONE* **2013**, *8*. [CrossRef] [PubMed]

6. Chiuve, S.E.; Sun, Q.; Curhan, G.C.; Taylor, E.N.; Spiegelman, D.; Willett, W.C.; Manson, J.E.; Rexrode, K.M.; Albert, C.M. Dietary and plasma magnesium and risk of coronary heart disease among women. *J. Am. Heart Assoc.* **2013**, 1–10. [CrossRef] [PubMed]

7. Meyer, T.E.; Verwoert, G.C.; Hwang, S.J.; Glazer, N.L.; Smith, A.V.; van Rooij, F.J.A.; Ehret, G.B.; Boerwinkle, E.; Felix, J.F.; Leak, T.S.; et al. Genome-wide association studies of serum magnesium, potassium, and sodium concentrations identify six loci influencing serum magnesium levels. *PLoS Genet.* **2010**, *6*. [CrossRef] [PubMed]

8. Saris, N.-E.L.E.A. Magnesium An update on phsyiological, clinical and analytical aspects. *Clin. Chim. Acta* **2000**, *294*, 1–26. [CrossRef]

9. Jahnen-Dechent, W.; Ketteler, M. Magnesium basics. *CKJ Clin. Kidney J.* **2012**, *5*. [CrossRef] [PubMed]

10. US Department of Agriculture, Agricultural Research Service, Nutrient Data Laboratory. USDA National Nutrient Database for Standard Reference, Release 28 (Revised). Available online: www.ars.usda.gov/ba/bhnrc/ndl (accessed on 24 January 2018).

11. Shechter, M. Magnesium and cardiovascular system. *Magnes. Res.* **2010**, *23*, 60–72. [CrossRef] [PubMed]

12. Gommers, L.M.M.; Hoenderop, J.G.J.; Bindels, R.J.M.; de Baaij, J.H.F. Hypomagnesemia in Type 2 Diabetes: A Vicious Circle? *Diabetes* **2016**, *65*, 3–13. [CrossRef] [PubMed]

13. Fang, X.; Han, H.; Li, M.; Liang, C.; Fan, Z.; Aaseth, J.; He, J.; Montgomery, S.; Cao, Y. Dose-Response Relationship between Dietary Magnesium Intake and Risk of Type 2 Diabetes Mellitus: A Systematic Review and Meta-Regression Analysis of Prospective Cohort Studies. *Nutrients* **2016**, *8*, 739. [CrossRef] [PubMed]

14. Dong, J.-Y.; Xun, P.; He, K.; Qin, L.-Q. Magnesium Intake and Risk of Type 2 Diabetes: Meta-analysis of prospective cohort studies. *Diabetes Care* **2011**, *34*, 2116–2122. [CrossRef] [PubMed]

15. Schulze, M.B.; Schulz, M.; Heidemann, C.; Schienkiewitz, A.; Hoffmann, K.; Boeing, H. Fiber and magnesium intake and incidence of type 2 diabetes: A prospective study and meta-analysis. *Arch. Intern. Med.* **2007**, *167*, 956–965. [CrossRef] [PubMed]

16. Hruby, A.; Guasch-Ferré, M.; Bhupathiraju, S.N.; Manson, J.E.; Willett, W.C.; McKeown, N.M.; Hu, F.B. Magnesium Intake, Quality of Carbohydrates, and Risk of Type 2 Diabetes: Results from Three U.S. Cohorts. *Diabetes Care* **2017**, *40*, 1695–1702. [CrossRef] [PubMed]

17. Simental-Mendía, L.E.; Sahebkar, A.; Rodríguez-Morán, M.; Guerrero-Romero, F. A systematic review and meta-analysis of randomized controlled trials on the effects of magnesium supplementation on insulin sensitivity and glucose control. *Pharmacol. Res.* **2016**, *111*, 272–282. [CrossRef] [PubMed]

18. Guerrero-Romero, F.; Rodríguez-Morán, M. Magnesium improves the beta-cell function to compensate variation of insulin sensitivity: Double-blind, randomized clinical trial. *Eur. J. Clin. Investig.* **2011**, *41*, 405–410. [CrossRef] [PubMed]

19. Song, Y.; He, K.; Levitan, E.B.; Manson, J.E.; Liu, S. Effects of oral magnesium supplementation on glycaemic control in Type 2 diabetes: A meta-analysis of randomized double-blind controlled trials. *Diabetes Med.* **2006**, *23*, 1050–1056. [CrossRef] [PubMed]

20. Guerrero-Romero, F.; Tamez-Perez, H.E.; González-González, G.; Salinas-Martínez, A.M.; Montes-Villarreal, J.; Treviño-Ortiz, J.H.; Rodríguez-Morán, M. Oral magnesium supplementation improves insulin sensitivity in non-diabetic subjects with insulin resistance. A double-blind placebo-controlled randomized trial. *Diabetes Metab.* **2004**, *30*, 253–258. [CrossRef]

21. He, K.; Liu, K.; Daviglus, M.L.; Morris, S.J.; Loria, C.M.; Van Horn, L.; Jacobs, D.R.; Savage, P.J. Magnesium intake and incidence of metabolic syndrome among young adults. *Circulation* **2006**, *113*, 1675–1682. [CrossRef] [PubMed]

22. Sarrafzadegan, N.; Khosravi-Boroujeni, H.; Lotfizadeh, M.; Pourmogaddas, A.; Salehi-Abargouei, A. Magnesium status and the metabolic syndrome: A systematic review and meta-analysis. *Nutrition* **2016**, *32*, 409–417. [CrossRef] [PubMed]

23. McKeown, N.M.; Jacques, P.F.; Zhang, X.L.; Juan, W.; Sahyoun, N.R. Dietary magnesium intake is related to metabolic syndrome in older Americans. *Eur. J. Nutr.* **2008**, *47*, 210–216. [CrossRef] [PubMed]

24. Ju, S.-Y.; Choi, W.-S.; Ock, S.-M.; Kim, C.-M.; Kim, D.-H. Dietary magnesium intake and metabolic syndrome in the adult population: Dose-response meta-analysis and meta-regression. *Nutrients* **2014**, *6*, 6005–6019. [CrossRef] [PubMed]

25. Dibaba, D.T.; Xun, P.; Fly, A.D.; Yokota, K.; He, K. Dietary magnesium intake and risk of metabolic syndrome: A meta-analysis. *Diabet. Med.* **2014**, *31*, 1301–1309. [CrossRef] [PubMed]

26. Nguyen, H.; Odelola, O.A.; Rangaswami, J.; Amanullah, A. A Review of Nutritional Factors in Hypertension Management. *Int. J. Hypertens.* **2013**, *2013*, 1–12. [CrossRef] [PubMed]

27. Touyz, R.M.; Milne, F.J.; Reinach, S.G. Intracellular Mg^{2+}, Ca^{2+}, Na^{2+} and K^+ in platelets and erythrocytes of essential hypertension patients: Relation to blood pressure. *Clin. Exp. Hypertens. A* **1992**, *14*, 1189–1209. [CrossRef] [PubMed]

28. Dibaba, D.T.; Xun, P.; Song, Y.; Rosanoff, A.; Shechter, M.; He, K. The effect of magnesium supplementation on blood pressure in individuals with insulin resistance, prediabetes, or noncommunicable chronic diseases: A meta-analysis of randomized controlled trials. *Am. J. Clin. Nutr.* **2017**, *106*, 921–929. [CrossRef] [PubMed]

29. Jee, S.H.; Miller, E.R.; Guallar, E.; Singh, V.K.; Appel, L.J.; Klag, M.J. The effect of magnesium supplementation on blood pressure: A meta-analysis of randomized clinical trials. *Am. J. Hypertens.* **2002**, *15*, 691–696. [CrossRef]

30. Kass, L.; Weekes, J.; Carpenter, L. Effect of magnesium supplementation on blood pressure: A meta-analysis. *Eur. J. Clin. Nutr.* **2012**, *66*, 411–418. [CrossRef] [PubMed]

31. Kolte, D.; Vijayaraghavan, K.; Khera, S.; Sica, D.A.; Frishman, W.H. Role of magnesium in cardiovascular diseases. *Cardiol. Rev.* **2014**, *22*, 182–192. [CrossRef] [PubMed]

32. Song, Y.; Li, T.Y.; van Dam, R.M.; Manson, J.E.; Hu, F.B. Magnesium intake and plasma concentrations of markers of systemic inflammation and endothelial dysfunction in women. *Am. J. Clin. Nutr.* **2007**, *85*, 1068–1074. [PubMed]

33. Chacko, S.A.; Song, Y.; Nathan, L.; Tinker, L.; de Boer, I.H.; Tylavsky, F.; Wallace, R.; Liu, S. Relations of dietary magnesium intake to biomarkers of inflammation and endothelial dysfunction in an ethnically diverse cohort of postmenopausal women. *Diabetes Care* **2010**, *33*, 304–310. [CrossRef] [PubMed]

34. Shechter, M.; Sharir, M.; Labrador, M.J.; Forrester, J.; Silver, B.; Bairey Merz, C.N. Oral magnesium therapy improves endothelial function in patients with coronary artery disease. *Circulation* **2000**, *102*, 2353–2358. [CrossRef] [PubMed]

35. Carr, M.C.; Brunzell, J.D. Abdominal obesity and dyslipidemia in the metabolic syndrome: Importance of type 2 diabetes and familial combined hyperlipidemia in coronary artery disease risk. *J. Clin. Endocrinol. Metab.* **2004**, *89*, 2601–2607. [CrossRef] [PubMed]

36. Singh, R.B.; Rastogi, S.S.; Sharma, V.K.; Saharia, R.B.; Kulshretha, S.K. Can dietary magnesium modulate lipoprotein metabolism? *Magnes. Trace Elem.* **1990**, *9*, 255–264. [PubMed]

37. Geiger, H.; Wanner, C. Magnesium in disease. *Clin. Kidney J.* **2012**, *5*, i25–i38. [CrossRef] [PubMed]

38. Guerrero-Romero, F.; Rodríguez-Morán, M. Low serum magnesium levels and metabolic syndrome. *Acta Diabetol.* **2002**, *39*, 209–213. [CrossRef] [PubMed]

39. Mirmiran, P.; Shab-Bidar, S.; Hosseini-Esfahani, F.; Asghari, G.; Hosseinpour-Niazi, S.; Azizi, F. Magnesium intake and prevalence of metabolic syndrome in adults: Tehran Lipid and Glucose Study. *Public Health Nutr.* **2012**, *15*, 693–701. [CrossRef] [PubMed]

40. Bain, L.K.M.; Myint, P.K.; Jennings, A.; Lentjes, M.A.H.; Luben, R.N.; Khaw, K.-T.; Wareham, N.J.; Welch, A.A. The relationship between dietary magnesium intake, stroke and its major risk factors, blood pressure and cholesterol, in the EPIC-Norfolk cohort. *Int. J. Cardiol.* **2015**, *196*, 108–114. [CrossRef] [PubMed]

41. Simental-Mendía, L.E.; Simental-Mendía, M.; Sahebkar, A.; Rodríguez-Morán, M.; Guerrero-Romero, F. Effect of magnesium supplementation on lipid profile: A systematic review and meta-analysis of randomized controlled trials. *Eur. J. Clin. Pharmacol.* **2017**, *73*, 525–536. [CrossRef] [PubMed]

42. Larsson, S.C.; Orsini, N.; Wolk, A. Dietary magnesium intake and risk of stroke: A meta-analysis of prospective studies. *Am. J. Clin. Nutr.* **2012**, *95*, 362–366. [CrossRef] [PubMed]

43. Nie, Z.-L.; Wang, Z.-M.; Zhou, B.; Tang, Z.-P.; Wang, S.-K. Magnesium intake and incidence of stroke: Meta-analysis of cohort studies. *Nutr. Metab. Cardiovasc. Dis.* **2013**, *23*, 169–176. [CrossRef] [PubMed]

44. Adebamowo, S.N.; Spiegelman, D.; Willett, W.C.; Rexrode, K.M. Association between intakes of magnesium, potassium, and calcium and risk of stroke: 2 Cohorts of US women and updated meta-analyses. *Am. J. Clin. Nutr.* **2015**, *101*, 1269–1277. [CrossRef] [PubMed]

45. Liao, F.; Folsom, A.R.; Brancati, F.L. Is low magnesium concentration a risk factor for coronary heart disease? The Atherosclerosis Risk in Communities (ARIC) Study. *Am. Heart J.* **1998**, *136*, 480–490. [CrossRef]

46. Abbott, R.D.; Ando, F.; Masaki, K.H.; Tung, K.H.; Rodriguez, B.L.; Petrovitch, H.; Yano, K.; Curb, J.D. Dietary magnesium intake and the future risk of coronary heart disease (The Honolulu heart program). *Am. J. Cardiol.* **2003**, *92*, 665–669. [CrossRef]

47. Song, Y.; Manson, J.E.; Cook, N.R.; Albert, C.M.; Buring, J.E.; Liu, S. Dietary magnesium intake and risk of cardiovascular disease among women. *Am. J. Cardiol.* **2005**, *96*, 1135–1141. [CrossRef] [PubMed]

48. Dai, Q.; Shu, X.-O.; Deng, X.; Xiang, Y.-B.; Li, H.; Yang, G.; Shrubsole, M.J.; Ji, B.; Cai, H.; Chow, W.-H.; et al. Modifying effect of calcium/magnesium intake ratio and mortality: A population-based cohort study. *Br. Med. J.* **2013**, *3*, e002111. [CrossRef] [PubMed]

49. Kokubo, Y.; Saito, I.; Iso, H.; Yamagishi, K.; Yatsuya, H.; Ishihara, J.; Maruyama, K.; Inoue, M.; Sawada, N.; Tsugane, S. Dietary magnesium intake and risk of incident coronary heart disease in men: A prospective cohort study. *Clin. Nutr.* **2017**, 1–7. [CrossRef] [PubMed]

50. Taveira, T.H.; Ouellette, D.; Gulum, A.; Choudhary, G.; Eaton, C.B.; Liu, S.; Wu, W.C. Relation of magnesium intake with cardiac function and heart failure hospitalizations in black adults. *Circ. Heart Fail.* **2016**, *9*. [CrossRef]

51. Zhang, W.; Iso, H.; Ohira, T.; Date, C.; Tamakoshi, A. Associations of dietary magnesium intake with mortality from cardiovascular disease: The JACC study. *Atherosclerosis* **2012**, *221*, 587–595. [CrossRef] [PubMed]

52. Misialek, J.R.; Lopez, F.L.; Lutsey, P.L.; Huxley, R.R.; Peacock, J.M.; Chen, L.Y.; Soliman, E.Z.; Agarwal, S.K.; Alonso, A. Serum and Dietary Magnesium and Incidence of Atrial Fibrillation in Whites and in African Americans—Atherosclerosis Risk in Communities (ARIC) Study. *Circ. J.* **2013**, *77*, 323–329. [CrossRef] [PubMed]

53. Nielsen, F.H.; Milne, D.B.; Klevay, L.M.; Gallagher, S.; Johnson, L.A. Dietary magnesium deficiency induces heart rhythm changes, impairs glucose tolerance, and decreases serum cholesterol in post menopausal women. *J. Am. Coll. Nutr.* **2007**, *26*, 121–132. [CrossRef] [PubMed]

54. Deng, X.; Song, Y.; Manson, J.E.; Signorello, L.B.; Zhang, S.M.; Shrubsole, M.J.; Ness, R.M.; Seidner, D.L.; Dai, Q. Magnesium, vitamin D status and mortality: Results from US National Health and Nutrition Examination Survey (NHANES) 2001 to 2006 and NHANES III. *BMC Med.* **2013**, *11*, 187. [CrossRef] [PubMed]

55. Levitan, E.B.; Shikany, J.M.; Ahmed, A.; Snetselaar, L.G.; Martin, L.W.; Curb, J.D.; Lewis, C.E. Calcium, magnesium and potassium intake and mortality in women with heart failure: The Women's Health Initiative. *Br. J. Nutr.* **2013**, *110*, 179–185. [CrossRef] [PubMed]

56. Chiuve, S.E.; Korngold, E.C.; Januzzi, J.L., Jr.; Gantzer, M.L.; Albert, C.M. Plasma and dietary magnesium and risk of sudden cardiac death. *Am. J. Clin. Nutr.* **2011**, 253–260. [CrossRef] [PubMed]

57. Guasch-Ferré, M.; Bulló, M.; Estruch, R.; Corella, D.; Martínez-González, M.A.; Ros, E.; Covas, M.; Arós, F.; Gómez-Gracia, E.; Fiol, M.; et al. Dietary magnesium intake is inversely associated with mortality in adults at high cardiovascular disease risk. *J. Nutr.* **2014**, *144*, 55–60. [CrossRef] [PubMed]

58. Xu, T.; Sun, Y.; Xu, T.; Zhang, Y. Magnesium intake and cardiovascular disease mortality: A meta-analysis of prospective cohort studies. *Int. J. Cardiol.* **2013**, *167*, 3044–3047. [CrossRef] [PubMed]

59. Fang, X.; Liang, C.; Li, M.; Montgomery, S.; Fall, K.; Aaseth, J.; Cao, Y. Dose-response relationship between dietary magnesium intake and cardiovascular mortality: A systematic review and dose-based meta-regression analysis of prospective studies. *J. Trace Elem. Med. Biol.* **2016**, *38*, 64–73. [CrossRef] [PubMed]

60. Zhang, X.; Del Gobbo, L.C.; Hruby, A.; Rosanoff, A.; He, K.; Dai, Q.; Costello, R.B.; Zhang, W.; Song, Y. The Circulating Concentration and 24-h Urine Excretion of Magnesium Dose- and Time-Dependently Respond to Oral Magnesium Supplementation in a Meta-Analysis of Randomized Controlled Trials. *J. Nutr.* **2016**, *146*, 595–602. [CrossRef] [PubMed]

61. Joosten, M.M.; Gansevoort, R.T.; Mukamal, K.J.; Van Der Harst, P.; Geleijnse, J.M.; Feskens, E.J.M. Urinary and plasma magnesium and risk of ischemic heart disease. *Am. J. Clin. Nutr.* **2013**, *97*, 1299–1306. [CrossRef] [PubMed]

62. Ohira, T.; Peacock, J.M.; Iso, H.; Chambless, L.E.; Rosamond, W.D.; Folsom, A.R. Serum and dietary magnesium and risk of ischemic stroke. *Am. J. Epidemiol.* **2009**, *169*, 1437–1444. [CrossRef] [PubMed]

63. Akarolo-Anthony, S.N.; Jiménez, M.C.; Chiuve, S.E.; Spiegelman, D.; Willett, W.C.; Rexrode, K.M. Plasma magnesium and risk of ischemic stroke among women. *Stroke* **2014**, *45*, 2881–2886. [CrossRef]

64. Khan, A.M.; Lubitz, S.A.; Sullivan, L.M.; Sun, J.X.; Levy, D.; Vasan, R.S.; Magnani, J.W.; Ellinor, P.T.; Benjamin, E.J.; Wang, T.J. Low serum magnesium and the development of atrial fibrillation in the community: The framingham heart study. *Circulation* **2013**, *127*, 33–38. [CrossRef] [PubMed]

65. Reffelmann, T.; Dörr, M.; Ittermann, T.; Schwahn, C.; Völzke, H.; Ruppert, J.; Robinson, D.; Felix, S.B. Low serum magnesium concentrations predict increase in left ventricular mass over 5 years independently of common cardiovascular risk factors. *Atherosclerosis* **2010**, *213*, 563–569. [CrossRef] [PubMed]

66. Lutsey, P.L.; Alonso, A.; Michos, E.D.; Loehr, L.R.; Astor, B.C.; Coresh, J.; Folsom, A.R. Serum magnesium, phosphorus, and calcium are associated with risk of incident heart failure: The Atherosclerosis Risk in Communities (ARIC). *Am. J. Clin. Nutr.* **2014**, 756–764. [CrossRef] [PubMed]

67. Kunutsor, S.K.; Khan, H.; Laukkanen, J.A. Serum magnesium and risk of new onset heart failure in men: The Kuopio Ischemic Heart Disease Study. *Eur. J. Epidemiol.* **2016**, *31*, 1035–1043. [CrossRef] [PubMed]

68. Ma, J.; Folsom, A.R.; Melnick, S.L.; Eckfeldt, J.H.; Sharrett, A.R.; Nabulsi, A.A.; Hutchinson, R.G.; Metcalf, P.A. Associations of serum and dietary magnesium with cardiovascular disease, hypertension, diabetes, insulin, and carotid arterial wall thickness: The aric study. *J. Clin. Epidemiol.* **1995**, *48*. [CrossRef]

69. Hashimoto, T.; Hara, A.; Ohkubo, T.; Kikuya, M.; Shintani, Y.; Metoki, H.; Inoue, R.; Asayama, K.; Kanno, A.; Nakashita, M.; et al. Serum magnesium, ambulatory blood pressure, and carotid artery alteration: The ohasama study. *Am. J. Hypertens.* **2010**, *23*, 1292–1298. [CrossRef] [PubMed]

70. Lee, S.Y.; Hyun, Y.Y.; Lee, K.B.; Kim, H. Low serum magnesium is associated with coronary artery calcification in a Korean population at low risk for cardiovascular disease. *Nutr. Metab. Cardiovasc. Dis.* **2015**, *25*, 1056–1061. [CrossRef] [PubMed]

71. Posadas-Sánchez, R.; Posadas-Romero, C.; Cardoso-Saldaña, G.; Vargas-Alarcón, G.; Villarreal-Molina, M.T.; Pérez-Hernández, N.; Rodríguez-Pérez, J.M.; Medina-Urrutia, A.; Jorge-Galarza, E.; Juárez-Rojas, J.G.; et al. Serum magnesium is inversely associated with coronary artery calcification in the Genetics of Atherosclerotic Disease (GEA) study. *Nutr. J.* **2015**, *15*, 22. [CrossRef] [PubMed]

72. Zhang, X.; Xia, J.; Del Gobbo, L.C.; Hruby, A.; Dai, Q.; Song, Y. Serum magnesium concentrations and all-cause, cardiovascular, and cancer mortality among U.S. adults: Results from the NHANES I Epidemiologic Follow-up Study. *Clin. Nutr.* **2017**. [CrossRef] [PubMed]

73. Kieboom, B.C.T.; Niemeijer, M.N.; Leening, M.J.G.; van den Berg, M.E.; Franco, O.H.; Deckers, J.W.; Hofman, A.; Zietse, R.; Stricker, B.H.; Hoorn, E.J. Serum Magnesium and the Risk of Death From Coronary Heart Disease and Sudden Cardiac Death. *J. Am. Heart Assoc.* **2016**, *5*, e002707. [CrossRef] [PubMed]

74. Angkananard, T.; Anothaisintawee, T.; Eursiriwan, S.; Gorelik, O.; McEvoy, M.; Attia, J.; Thakkinstian, A. The association of serum magnesium and mortality outcomes in heart failure patients. *Medicine (Baltimore)* **2016**, *95*, e5406. [CrossRef] [PubMed]

75. Barbagallo, M.; Dominguez, L.J.; Galioto, A.; Ferlisi, A.; Cani, C.; Malfa, L.; Pineo, A.; Busardo', A.; Paolisso, G. Role of magnesium in insulin action, diabetes and cardio-metabolic syndrome X. *Mol. Asp. Med.* **2003**, *24*, 39–52. [CrossRef]

76. Mazur, A.; Maier, J.A.M.; Rock, E.; Gueux, E.; Nowacki, W.; Rayssiguier, Y. Magnesium and the inflammatory response: Potential physiopathological implications. *Arch. Biochem. Biophys.* **2007**, *458*, 48–56. [CrossRef] [PubMed]

77. Blache, D.; Devaux, S.; Joubert, O.; Loreau, N.; Schneider, M.; Durand, P.; Prost, M.; Gaume, V.; Adrian, M.; Laurant, P.; et al. Long-term moderate magnesium-deficient diet shows relationships between blood pressure, inflammation and oxidant stress defense in aging rats. *Free Radic. Biol. Med.* **2006**, *41*, 277–284. [CrossRef] [PubMed]

78. Freedman, A.M.; Atrakchi, A.H.; Cassidy, M.M.; Weglicki, W.B. Magnesium deficiency-induced cardiomyopathy: Protection by vitamin E. *Biochem. Biophys. Res. Commun.* **1990**, *170*, 1102–1106. [CrossRef]

79. Freedman, A.M.; Cassidy, M.M.; Weglicki, W.B. Magnesium-deficient myocardium demonstrates an increased susceptibility to an in vivo oxidative stress. *Magnes. Res.* **1991**, *4*, 185–189. [PubMed]

80. King, D.E. Inflammation and elevation of C-reactive protein: Does magnesium play a key role? *Magnes. Res.* **2009**, *22*, 57–59. [PubMed]

81. Olatunji, L.A.; Soladoye, A.O. Increased magnesium intake prevents hyperlipidemia and insulin resistance and reduces lipid peroxidation in fructose-fed rats. *Pathophysiology* **2007**, *14*, 11–15. [CrossRef] [PubMed]

82.   Garcia, L.A.; Dejong, S.C.; Martin, S.M.; Smith, R.S.; Buettner, G.R.; Kerber, R.E. Magnesium reduces free radicals in an in vivo coronary occlusion- reperfusion model. *J. Am. Coll. Cardiol.* **1998**, *32*, 536–539. [CrossRef]

83.   Rock, E.; Astier, C.; Lab, C.; Malpuech, C.; Nowacki, W.; Gueux, E.; Mazur, A.; Rayssiguier, Y. Magnesium deficiency in rats induces a rise in plasma nitric oxide. *Magnes. Res.* **1995**, *8*, 237–242. [PubMed]

84.   Dickens, B.F.; Weglicki, W.B.; Li, Y.S.; Mak, I.T. Magnesium deficiency in vitro enhances free radical-induced intracellular oxidation and cytotoxicity in endothelial cells. *FEBS Lett.* **1992**, *311*, 187–191. [CrossRef]

85.   Wiles, M.E.; Wagner, T.L.; Weglicki, W.B. Effect of acute magnesium deficiency (MgD) on aortic endothelial cell (EC) oxidant production. *Life Sci.* **1997**, *60*, 221–236. [CrossRef]

86.   Kramer, J.H.; Mišík, V.; Weglicki, W.B. Magnesium-deficiency potentiates free radical production associated with postischemic injury to rat hearts: Vitamin E affords protection. *Free Radic. Biol. Med.* **1994**, *16*, 713–723. [CrossRef]

87.   Kramer, J.H.; Mak, I.T.; Phillips, T.M.; Weglicki, W.B. Dietary magnesium intake influences circulating pro-inflammatory neuropeptide levels and loss of myocardial tolerance to postischemic stress. *Exp. Biol. Med. (Maywood)* **2003**, *228*, 665–673. [CrossRef] [PubMed]

88.   Bernardini, D.; Nasulewic, A.; Mazur, A.; Maier, J.A.M. Magnesium and microvascular endothelial cells: A role in inflammation and angiogenesis. *Front. Biosci.* **2005**, *10*, 1177–1182. [CrossRef] [PubMed]

89.   Rayssiguier, Y.; Gueux, E.; Bussière, L.; Durlach, J.; Mazur, A. Dietary magnesium affects susceptibility of lipoproteins and tissues to peroxidation in rats. *J. Am. Coll. Nutr.* **1993**, *12*, 133–137. [CrossRef] [PubMed]

90.   Mylonas, C.; Kouretas, D. Lipid peroxidation and tissue damage. *In Vivo* **1999**, *13*, 295–309. [PubMed]

91.   Morrill, G.A.; Gupta, R.K.; Kostellow, A.B.; Ma, G.Y.; Zhang, A.; Altura, B.T.; Altura, B.M. Mg^{2+} modulates membrane lipids in vascular smooth muscle: A link to atherogenesis. *FEBS Lett.* **1997**, *408*, 191–194. [CrossRef]

92.   Bussière, L.; Mazur, A.; Gueux, E.; Nowacki, W.; Rayssiguier, Y. Triglyceride-rich lipoproteins from magnesium-deficient rats are more susceptible to oxidation by cells and promote proliferation of cultured vascular smooth muscle cells. *Magnes. Res.* **1995**, *8*, 151–157. [PubMed]

93.   Gueux, E.; Azais-Braesco, V.; Bussière, L.; Grolier, P.; Mazur, A.; Rayssiguier, Y. Effect of magnesium deficiency on triacylglycerol-rich lipoprotein and tissue susceptibility to peroxidation in relation to vitamin E content. *Br. J. Nutr.* **1995**, *74*, 849–856. [PubMed]

94.   Altura, B.M.; Gebrewold, A.; Altura, B.T.; Brautbar, N. Magnesium depletion impairs myocardial carbohydrate and lipid metabolism and cardiac bioenergetics and raises myocardial calcium content in-vivo: Relationship to etiology of cardiac diseases. *Biochem. Mol. Biol. Int.* **1996**, *40*, 1183–1190. [CrossRef] [PubMed]

95.   Takaya, J.; Higashino, H.; Kobayashi, Y. Intracellular magnesium and insulin resistance. *Magnes. Res.* **2004**, *17*, 126–136. [PubMed]

96.   Pham, P.-C.T.; Pham, P.-M.T.; Pham, S.V.; Miller, J.M.; Pham, P.-T.T. Hypomagnesemia in Patients with Type 2 Diabetes. *Clin. J. Am. Soc. Nephrol.* **2007**, *2*, 366–373. [CrossRef] [PubMed]

97.   Sontia, B.; Touyz, R.M. Magnesium transport in hypertension. *Pathophysiol. Off. J. Int. Soc. Pathophysiol.* **2007**, *14*, 205–211. [CrossRef] [PubMed]

98.   Barbagallo, M.; Dominguez, L.J.; Resnick, L.M. Magnesium metabolism in hypertension and type 2 diabetes mellitus. *Am. J. Ther.* **2007**, *14*, 375–385. [CrossRef] [PubMed]

99.   Maier, J.A.M.; Bernardini, D.; Rayssiguier, Y.; Mazur, A. High concentrations of magnesium modulate vascular endothelial cell behaviour in vitro. *Biochim. Biophys. Acta Mol. Basis Dis.* **2004**, *1689*, 6–12. [CrossRef] [PubMed]

100. Laurant, P.; Kantelip, J.P.; Berthelot, A. Dietary magnesium supplementation modifies blood pressure and cardiovascular function in mineralocorticoid-salt hypertensive rats but not in normotensive rats. *J. Nutr.* **1995**, *125*, 830–841. [PubMed]

101. Touyz, R.M.; Milne, F.J. Magnesium supplementation attenuates, but does not prevent, development of hypertension in spontaneously hypertensive rats. *Am. J. Hypertens.* **1999**, *12*, 757–765. [CrossRef]

102. Agus, M.S.D.; Agus, Z.S. Cardiovascular actions of magnesium. *Crit. Care Clin.* **2001**, *17*, 175–186. [CrossRef]

103. Mubagwa, K.; Gwanyanya, A.; Zakharov, S.; Macianskiene, R. Regulation of cation channels in cardiac and smooth muscle cells by intracellular magnesium. *Arch. Biochem. Biophys.* **2007**, *458*, 73–89. [CrossRef] [PubMed]

104. Johnson, C.J.; Peterson, D.R.; Smith, E.K. Myocardial tissue concentrations of magnesium and potassium in men dying suddenly from ischemic heart disease. *Am. J. Clin. Nutr.* **1979**, *32*, 967–970. [CrossRef] [PubMed]
105. Paravicini, T.M.; Chubanov, V.; Gudermann, T. TRPM7: A unique channel involved in magnesium homeostasis. *Int. J. Biochem. Cell Biol.* **2012**, *44*, 1381–1384. [CrossRef] [PubMed]
106. Touyz, R.M. Transient receptor potential melastatin 6 and 7 channels, magnesium transport, and vascular biology: Implications in hypertension. *Am. J. Physiol. Heart Circ. Physiol.* **2008**, *294*, H1103–H1118. [CrossRef] [PubMed]
107. Rodríguez-Ramírez, M.; Rodríguez-Morán, M.; Reyes-Romero, M.A.; Guerrero-Romero, F. Effect of oral magnesium supplementation on the transcription of TRPM6, TRPM7, and SLC41A1 in individuals newly diagnosed of pre-hypertension. A randomized, double-blind, placebo-controlled trial. *Magnes. Res.* **2017**, *30*, 80–87. [PubMed]
108. Kappeler, D.; Heimbeck, I.; Herpich, C.; Naue, N.; Höfler, J.; Timmer, W.; Michalke, B. Higher bioavailability of magnesium citrate as compared to magnesium oxide shown by evaluation of urinary excretion and serum levels after single-dose administration in a randomized cross-over study. *BMC Nutr.* **2017**, *3*, 7. [CrossRef]
109. Schuchardt, J.P.; Hahn, A. Intestinal Absorption and Factors Influencing Bioavailability of Magnesium—An Update. *Curr. Nutr. Food Sci.* **2017**, *13*, 260–278. [CrossRef] [PubMed]

5

Magnesium Levels Modify the Effect of Lipid Parameters on Carotid Intima Media Thickness

Serafi Cambray [1,*], Merce Ibarz [2], Marcelino Bermudez-Lopez [1], Manuel Marti-Antonio [1], Milica Bozic [1], Elvira Fernandez [1], Jose M. Valdivielso [1,*]
and on behalf of the NEFRONA Investigators

[1] Vascular and Renal Translational Research Group, Institute for Biomedical Research Pifarré Foundation, IRBLleida Av. Rovira Roure 80, 25198 Lleida, Spain; mbermudez@irblleida.cat (M.B.-L.); mmartia@irblleida.cat (M.M.-A.); milica.bozic@irblleida.udl.cat (M.B.); elvirafgiraldez@gmail.com (E.F.)
[2] Indicators and Specifications of the Quality in the Clinical Laboratory Group, Institute for Biomedical Research Pifarré Foundation, IRBLleida, 25198 Lleida, Spain; mibarz.lleida.ics@gencat.cat
* Correspondence: scambray@irblleida.cat (S.C.); valdivielso@irblleida.cat (J.M.V.)

Abstract: Classical risk factors of atherosclerosis in the general population show paradoxical effects in chronic kidney disease (CKD) patients. Thus, low low-density lipoprotein (LDL) cholesterol levels have been associated with worse cardiovascular outcomes. Magnesium (Mg) is a divalent cation whose homeostasis is altered in CKD. Furthermore, Mg levels have been associated with cardiovascular health. The present study aims to understand the relationships of Mg and lipid parameters with atherosclerosis in CKD. In this analysis, 1754 participants from the Observatorio Nacional de Atherosclerosis en Nefrologia (NEFRONA) cohort were included. Carotid intima media thickness (cIMT) was determined in six arterial territories, and associated factors were investigated by linear regression. cIMT correlated positively with being male, Caucasian, a smoker, diabetic, hypertensive, dyslipidemic and with increased age, BMI, and triglyceride levels, and negatively with levels of HDL cholesterol. First-order interactions in linear regression analysis showed that Mg was an effect modifier on the influence of lipidic parameters. Thus, cIMT predicted values were higher when triglycerides or LDL levels were high and Mg levels were low. On the contrary, when Mg levels were high, this effect disappeared. In conclusion, Mg acts as an effect modifier between lipidic parameters and atherosclerotic cardiovascular disease. Therefore, Mg levels, together with lipidic parameters, should be taken into account when assessing atherosclerotic risk.

Keywords: magnesium; cholesterol; atherosclerosis; first-order interaction; cardiovascular risk

1. Introduction

According to the Cardiovascular Disease Statistics from the European Society of Cardiology, in 2015 there were 11 million new cases of cardiovascular disease (CVD) reported in Europe, and the majority of countries showed an increase in cases from 1990 [1]. Its prevalence was reported to be 83.5 million people, of which 35.7 million people showed peripheral vascular disease [1]. Moreover, CVD also led to 64 million disability-adjusted life years in the European population [1].

Among risk factors associated with CVD, plasma lipids play a key role in the initiation and progression of atheromatous disease [2]. Epidemiological studies show that increased concentrations of low-density lipoprotein cholesterol (LDL-C) are associated with an increased risk of cardiovascular events [3,4], while the contrary effect has been demonstrated for high-density lipoprotein cholesterol [5] (HDL-C). Triglyceride levels are inversely associated with HDL-C levels [6] and, despite not showing atherogenic properties per se, are considered to be an important biomarker of CVD, due to their association with atherogenic remnant lipoproteins containing apo CIII [7]. Triglycerides have important implications for chronic kidney disease (CKD) patients, a population that presents a high incidence of atherosclerotic events [8]. Additionally, traditional lipid profiles are not associated with increased cardiovascular risk in this population. CKD patients present low levels of HDL-C and hypertriglyceridemia [9], but levels of LDL-C or total cholesterol are not usually modified, or are even low in advanced stages [10]. Some works point to the importance of LDL-C particle size [11] or the levels of oxidized LDL-C [12]. Nevertheless, the link between altered lipid metabolism and the higher presence of atheromasias in CKD patients is not clear.

Currently, to prevent cardiovascular events in high risk populations, most efforts have been directed towards lowering plasma LDL-C and triglycerides, by means of pharmacological treatment [13], dietary intervention [14,15], or diet supplements [16–18]. Among diet supplements, magnesium (Mg) was one of the first to be used for lowering serum lipids. During the 1980s, it was demonstrated that Mg deficiency was associated with hypertension and vascular calcifications, while increasing its dietary intake prevented atheroma in experimental animals with normal renal function [19], and in experimental uremia [20]. Later on, during the 1990s, different studies in patients showed that lower Mg plasma concentrations were associated with atherosclerosis [21], and that Mg supplementation lowered plasma cholesterol, LDL, and triglyceride concentrations [22,23]. Recent studies also found an inverse correlation between Mg levels, carotid intima–media thickness (cIMT) [24,25] and peripheral artery disease [26,27], while many epidemiological studies and clinical trials reported Mg as a key player in cardiovascular health [28–31], even in hemodialysis patients [32]. However, randomized clinical trials with Mg supplementation have yielded conflicting results [33,34]. CKD patients often present an altered Mg balance. Thus, the decrease in glomerular filtration rate (GFR) can induce Mg retention, whereas in other cases tubular dysfunction and diuretic use can induce hypomagnesemia. Therefore, the altered Mg levels, alongside the specific dyslipidemia found in those patients, make them a very interesting group to investigate the possible interactions of both variables in atherosclerosis.

Despite the fact that some data showed that Mg levels can affect cIMT and that, according to some studies, it could also affect plasma lipid concentrations, no studies have analyzed the possible interactions of both variables in atherosclerosis. In the present study, we aim to study the impact of Mg on cIMT, and how Mg interacts with plasma lipids and other known CVD risk factors in a CKD population form the Observatorio Nacional de Atherosclerosis en Nefrologia (NEFRONA) cohort.

2. Materials and Methods

2.1. Study Design

The NEFRONA study was designed to assess the utility of noninvasive vascular imaging techniques and plasma biomarkers to predict cardiovascular events and mortality in CKD patients [35,36]. Briefly, CKD and non-CKD volunteers aged 18 to 75 years were recruited throughout Spanish primary care centers and renal units from 2009 to 2012. Patients with a history of CVD, remarkable carotid stenosis, active infections (tuberculosis and human immunodeficiency virus), pregnancy, less than twelve month of life expectancy, and with any organ transplantation or carotid artery surgery were excluded from the study. Of the NEFRONA study, 1754 subjects had available serum samples to measure Mg levels. Out of those, 40 presented with missing data on CKD status or cIMT values. Thus, 1754 volunteers were used in the present study. In total, 1542 presented with CKD (629 Stage 3; 528 Stages 4–5; 385 dialysis), and 212 were non-CKD controls (glomerular filtration rate > 60 mL/min/1.73 m^2). The ethics committee of each hospital approved the protocol of the study, and all volunteers were included after signing an informed consent. The research followed the principles of the Declaration of Helsinki. Non-CKD controls were included as per the protocol of the NEFRONA study and as a reference with normal Mg and lower cIMT values.

2.2. Clinical Data and Mg Determination

A nurse and two specifically trained technicians collected the following data: gender, age, body mass index, systolic and diastolic blood pressure (SBP and DBP), pulse pressure, and smoking status. Information about presence of diabetes, hypertension, and dyslipidemia was obtained from clinical records. Fasting blood samples were also collected by the same team and were stored at −80 °C in the Biobank of the RedInRen in the University of Alcala de Henares (Madrid). Biochemical analysis was performed as described previously [37]. The determination of Mg in serum samples was performed using the Mg reagent from Beckman Coulter (Brea, CA USA; Ref. OSR6189), following the manufacturer's instructions.

2.3. Atherosclerosis Assessment

Atherosclerosis assessment was performed as previously described [38]. Briefly, carotid ultrasound measurements were performed in three territories of both carotid arteries (bifurcation, internal, and common carotid arteries). Plaques were defined according to the Mannheim Carotid Intima–Media Thickness (cIMT) Consensus and the American Society of Echocardiography as a cIMT lumen protrusion ≥ 1.5 mm [39,40]. More extended protocols and data about plaque prevalence in the entire NEFRONA cohort have been published previously [37]. In the present analysis, we used the average cIMT of the territories that did not show atheroma plaque.

2.4. Statistical Analysis

Absolute frequencies (and percentage) or mean (and standard deviation) were used to describe qualitative and quantitative variables, respectively. Pearson correlation coefficients were calculated to analyze the relationships between cIMT and Mg levels with other clinical variables. Multivariate regression linear models were used to assess the association of clinical variables with cIMT. To specifically assess the joint association of Mg with the rest of the explanatory variables on cIMT, all possible first-order interactions were considered in the model, and a backwards stepwise algorithm was used to select the significant ones. A graph showing the predicted values of cIMT when the rest of the variables of the model are set to zero, and showing the interactions of continuous values of lipid parameters and Mg levels was drawn. All analyses were performed using R, setting the threshold of significance at 0.05.

3. Results

3.1. Clinical Characteristics

The study comprised 1754 volunteers with a mean age of 58.6 ± 12.7 years. Significant differences were found between CKD stages in all the parameters of the study, except in the percentage of smokers, which was not significantly different between CKD stages. Interestingly, Mg levels increased as renal function decreased, whereas cIMT levels showed the opposite tendency. LDL levels also showed a significant tendency to decrease as renal function impairment worsened (Table 1).

Table 1. Clinical characteristics of the cohort.

Variable	All n = 1754 (100%)	Control n = 212 (12.1%)	CKD 2–3 n = 629 (35.9%)	CKD 4–5 n = 528 (30.1%)	Dialysis n = 385 (21.9%)	p-Value (CKD Groups)	p-Value (Trend CKD Groups)
Sex (Male)	1040 (59.3%)	100 (47.2%)	425 (67.6%)	299 (56.6%)	216 (56.1%)	<0.001	0.512
Race (Caucasian)	1704 (97.1%)	209 (98.6%)	620 (98.6%)	514 (97.3%)	361 (93.8%)	<0.001	<0.001
Age, years	58.6 (12.7)	51.7 (12.4)	62.15 (11.2)	58.8 (12.5)	56.4 (13.6)	<0.001	0.001
Smoker (Yes)	977 (55.7%)	123 (58%)	363 (57.7%)	279 (52.8%)	212 (55.1%)	0.347	0.211
Diabetes (Yes)	373 (21.3%)	0 (0%)	170 (27%)	127 (24.1%)	76 (19.7%)	<0.001	0.003
Hypertension (Yes)	1498 (85.4%)	67 (31.6)	569 (90.5%)	507 (96%)	355 (92.8%)	<0.001	<0.001
Dyslipidemia (Yes)	1170 (66.7%)	52 (24.5)	467 (74.2%)	399 (75.6%)	252 (65.5%)	<0.001	<0.001
BMI (kg/m^2)	28.3 (5.21)	27.7 (4.5)	29.2 (4.7)	28.5 (5.5)	26.9 (5.6)	<0.001	0.026
SBP (mmHg)	138 (20.4)	131 (17.9)	138 (18.7)	141 (18.9)	138 (24.8)	0.004	<0.001
DBP (mmHg)	79.8 (10.9)	79 (10.2)	79.6 (9.7)	81 (10.2)	79 (13.5)	<0.001	0.792
Pulse pressure (mmHg)	58.7 (16.7)	52.1 (12.6)	58.8 (15.4)	60.3 (16.8)	59.9 (19.4)	<0.001	<0.001
Total Cholesterol (mg/dL)	180 (39.9)	203 (32.3)	184 (37.5)	177 (38.5)	164 (42.2)	<0.001	<0.001
HDL Cholesterol (mg/dL)	50.1 (14.9)	52.9 (13.8)	50.8 (14.8)	50.1 (15.1)	46.9 (15.1)	<0.001	<0.001
LDL Cholesterol (mg/dL)	104 (34.0)	127 (30.2)	107 (31.6)	100 (33.0)	91.9 (34.5)	<0.001	<0.001
Triglycerides (mg/dL)	141 (84.6)	116 (71.7)	145 (83.5)	143 (88.6)	146 (85.5)	<0.001	<0.001
Glucose (mg/dL)	107 (42.1)	96 (12.4)	110 (38.4)	107 (45.1)	108 (52.5)	<0.001	0.003
Calcium (mmol/L)	2.33 (0.152)	2.34 (0.094)	2.37 (0.119)	2.34 (0.144)	2.24 (0.197)	<0.001	<0.001
Phosphorus (mmol/L)	1.259 (0.332)	1.09 (0.158)	1.06 (0.18)	1.292 (0.245)	1.55 (0.442)	<0.001	<0.001
Sodium (mmol/L)	141 (2.93)	141 (2.25)	141 (2.65)	141 (2.80)	139 (3,22)	<0.001	<0.001
Potassium (mmol/L)	4.79 (0.60)	4.4 (0.39)	4.7 (0.50)	4.9 (0.54)	4.9 (0.80)	<0.001	<0.001
Magnesium (mmol/L)	0.83 (0.15)	0.82 (0.08)	0.80 (0.12)	0.84 (0.14)	0.88 (0.22)	<0.001	<0.001
cIMT	0.73 (0.14)	0.70 (0.13)	0.75 (0.14)	0.71 (0.14)	0.72 (0.14)	<0.001	0.569

Absolute frequency (percentage) and mean (standard deviation) are shown for qualitative and quantitative variables, respectively. Abbreviations: Body Mass Index (BMI), Systolic Blood Pressure (SBP), Diastolic Blood Pressure (DBP), Carotid Intima–Media Thickness (cIMT), Chronic Kidney Disease (CKD).

3.2. Correlations of Clinical Variables with cIMT and Mg Levels

Results for the correlation matrix of cIMT and Mg levels with the clinical variables of the study are shown in Table 2. cIMT correlated positively with being male, Caucasian, smoker, diabetic, hypertensive, dyslipidemic and with increased age, BMI, and triglyceride levels. Furthermore, it correlated negatively with levels of HDL cholesterol. Interestingly, no significant correlation was found with total or LDL cholesterol levels. Mg levels positively correlated with the presence of hypertension, and negatively with being Caucasian, diabetic, and with level of BMI. The correlation matrix of the variables with cIMT was calculated for the controls (Supplementary Table S1) as a sensitivity analysis. Some of the significant correlations were lost (due to the lower sample size), but most of the coefficients were similar.

Table 2. Bivariate correlation coefficients between cIMT and Magnesium levels with other variables.

	cIMT		Magnesium	
Variable	r	p-Value	r	p-Value
Sex (Male)	0.223	<0.001	−0.003	0.906
Race (Caucasian)	0.083	0.001	−0.079	0.001
Age, years	0.528	<0.001	−0.035	0.141
Smoker	0.105	<0.001	−0.018	0.445
Diabetes	0.157	<0.001	−0.070	0.003
Hypertension	0.137	<0.001	0.053	0.028
Dyslipidemia	0.094	<0.001	0.015	0.536
BMI	0.158	<0.001	−0.053	0.027

Table 2. *Cont.*

Variable	cIMT		Magnesium	
	r	*p*-Value	r	*p*-Value
Total Cholesterol	0.021	0.392	−0.043	0.075
HDL Cholesterol	−0.071	0.007	0.001	0.967
LDL Cholesterol	0.007	0.781	−0.009	0.724
Triglycerides	0.082	0.001	0.009	0.709
Magnesium	−0.003	0.914	-	-
cIMT	-	-	−0.003	0.914

Pearson's correlation coefficients (r) and *p*-value are shown for each variable. Abbreviations: Body Mass Index (BMI), Carotid Intima–Media Thickness (cIMT).

3.3. Association of Clinical Variables with cIMT

The results from the multivariate main effects model, which included all the variables studied, showed that age, being male or a smoker, pulse pressure, potassium, and CKD stage were factors that were significantly associated with cIMT. Mg levels did not reach statistical significance in this model, underlying the fact that Mg had no association with cIMT when considering its effect in the multivariate model independently of the rest of variables (Table 3). However, interestingly, the results from the model including the interactions revealed that Mg levels were significantly associated with cIMT, when interactions with cholesterol levels (total, LDL-C, and HDL-C) and triglycerides are taken into account. Sex, age, tobacco, pulse pressure, CKD stage, and potassium levels were significantly associated with cIMT in this multivariate model (Table 4).

Table 3. Multivariate linear main effects model for cIMT.

	All Cohort		
	Beta	SE	*p*-Value
Intercept	0.14	0.18	0.43
Magnesium	0.002	0.02	0.92
Sex, male	0.034	0.007	<0.00001
Race, Caucasian	0.006	0.02	0.74
Age	0.005	0.0003	<0.00001
Current smoker	0.02	0.007	0.01
Diabetes	−0.0002	0.01	0.98
Hypertension	0.01	0.01	0.35
Dyslipidemia	−0.005	0.007	0.49
BMI	0.0003	0.0007	0.65
Pulse pressure	0.0007	0.0002	0.0004
CKD Stage, 2–3	−0.03	0.013	0.015
CKD Stage, 4–5	−0.06	0.014	0.00006
CKD Stage, dialysis	−0.016	0.015	0.31
Total Cholesterol	0.0005	0.0004	0.25
HDL Cholesterol	−0.0006	0.0005	0.24
LDL Cholesterol	−0.0002	0.0004	0.57
Triglycerides	−0.00002	0.00009	0.82
Glucose	0.0001	0.0001	0.25
Calcium	−0.001	0.006	0.82
Phosphorus	−0.002	0.004	0.59
Sodium	0.0007	0.001	0.53
Potassium	0.014	0.006	0.016

Estimated parameters (beta), standard error (SE) and *p*-value shown for each variable. Abbreviations: Body Mass Index (BMI), Chronic Kidney Disease (CKD).

Table 4. Multivariate linear effects model for cIMT with first-order interactions.

	All Cohort		
	Beta	**SE**	**p-Value**
Intercept	0.35	0.089	0.00007
Sex, male	0.04	0.007	<0.00001
Age (years)	0.006	0.0003	<0.00001
Current smoker	0.018	0.007	0.006
Pulse pressure	0.0007	0.0002	0.0002
CKD stage, 2–3	−0.027	0.01	0.01
CKD stage, 4–5	−0.05	0.01	0.00001
CKD stage, dialysis	−0.014	0.01	0.26
Magnesium	−0.12	0.099	0.23
Total Cholesterol	−0.006	0.003	0.02
HDL Cholesterol	0.006	0.003	0.03
LDL Cholesterol	0.006	0.003	0.04
Triglycerides	0.001	0.0005	0.014
Potassium	0.013	0.006	0.016
Interactions			
Magnesium→Total Cholesterol	0.008	0.003	0.011
Magnesium→HDL Cholesterol	−0.007	0.003	0.016
Magnesium→LDL Cholesterol	−0.007	0.003	0.03
Magnesium→Triglycerides	−0.0014	0.0005	0.01

Estimated parameters (beta), standard error (SE) and p-value shown for each significant variable considering interactions.

3.4. Visualization of the Association of the Interaction of Mg and Plasma Lipids with cIMT

To better visualize the interactions between plasma lipids and Mg, we performed an interaction graph for continuous data. As seen in Figure 1a, cIMT predicted values were higher when triglycerides levels were high and Mg levels were low. On the contrary, when Mg levels were higher than 1 mmol/L, the relationship between high triglyceride levels and increased cIMT disappeared. A similar tendency was seen when LDL-C levels, Mg, and cIMT were plotted (Figure 1b). The interaction between HDL-C and Mg showed that the protective effect of high HDL-C levels disappears when Mg levels are low (Figure 1c). Finally, a paradoxical effect of total cholesterol levels is depicted, predicting higher cIMT when both total cholesterol and Mg are high (Figure 1d).

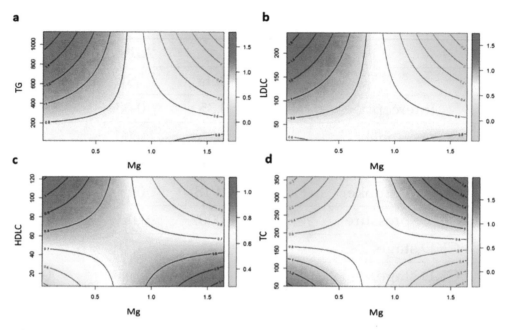

Figure 1. Interaction Graphs for Continuous Data. (**a**) Predicted cIMT with different levels of triglycerides (TG) and magnesium (Mg). (**b**) Predicted cIMT with different levels of LDL cholesterol (LDLC) and magnesium. (**c**) Predicted cIMT with different levels of HDL cholesterol (HDLC) and magnesium. (**d**) Predicted cIMT with different levels of total cholesterol (TC) and magnesium.

4. Discussion

The present study identifies, for the first time, the role of Mg as an effect modifier on the association of lipid parameters with cIMT in CKD patients. Thus, high LDL and triglyceride levels affect cIMT only when Mg levels are low. In the same model, high HDL levels associate with lower cIMT only when Mg levels are high. This result could be behind some of the paradoxical effects of lipid parameters on atherosclerosis in renal patients, in which Mg levels are often modified by the disease.

Hypertriglyceridemia and high cholesterol levels are related to atherosclerosis [2,41], and current mathematical models estimate that lipid-lowering therapies could avoid a substantial number of cardiovascular events [42]. Among the different dietary supplements proposed for lipid-lowering treatment, Mg has been used not only to prevent cardiovascular events in patients suffering from chronic kidney disease [43], but also for metabolic syndrome treatment [44] as well as to improve cardiovascular health in overweight and obese people [45]. In renal patients, however, the relationship between lipid parameters and atherosclerosis is not so clear. Thus, high LDL cholesterol levels have sometimes been found to be unrelated to cardiovascular disease in CKD patients. In other cases, the phenomenon called reverse causality has also been shown in this population, finding an association of lower LDL levels with higher cardiovascular risk [46]. Although malnutrition has been shown to partially explain this paradoxical effect, hypomagnesemia, which is associated with malnutrition, could be part of the exact mechanism [47]. The same different effect on cardiovascular risk has also been observed with HDL, which seems to lose its association with cardiovascular risk as renal function declines [48]. This report also shows that the interaction between Mg and triglycerides has an impact on cIMT. Pioneering work from the ARIC study found a relationship between serum Mg levels and cIMT that was maintained after adjusting for age, but that disappeared after adjusting for other risk factors [49]. Indeed, and in agreement with previous literature reports, Mg has been recently identified as a possible independent risk factor for carotid atherosclerosis [50], and a meta-analysis showed an inverse relationship between circulating and dietary Mg and cardiovascular risk [30]. As far as we know, none of the works that identified a relationship between serum Mg levels and cIMT have considered the impact of Mg–lipid interaction on cIMT.

One of the possible explanations for our results is that Mg is an important antioxidant, and its deficiency has been related to an increase in oxidative stress biomarkers [51], and to an increase in lipid peroxidation [52,53]. High levels of these molecules have been associated with cardiovascular events [54]. A proposed mechanism of its atherogenic potential includes the recruitment and retention of macrophages, the secretion of cytokines by macrophages and endothelial cells, the proliferation of smooth muscle cells, and lymphocyte chemotaxis [55]. Therefore, according to our findings, high Mg levels could mitigate lipid peroxidation even with high plasma lipid profiles, thereby reducing its impact on cIMT. Another possible mechanism to explain our results could be the prevention of the oxidation of LDL by Mg. There is a clear relationship between the levels of oxidized LDL and atheromatous disease [56], and CKD patients showed increased levels of oxidized LDL [57]. In addition, it has been reported that oxidized LDL concentrations are higher in subjects with low Mg levels [58,59]. Thus, future studies should aim to correlate Mg levels with oxidized LDL levels and atheromatous disease in CKD patients. Finally, it is worth mentioning that many studies have proposed an active role of Mg in retarding vascular calcification of the medial arterial layer. However, this process is not related to lipid peroxidation, but to the binding of phosphate, decreasing calcium phosphate deposition [60], and regulating smooth muscle cells transdifferentiation [61].

This study has some limitations. First, its cross-sectional nature impeded us from making predictions—only associations. Furthermore, and in order to obtain a relatively wide degree of variation in Mg levels, a population with controls, different stages of CKD, and hemodialysis were included. This last group is especially sensible for the current analysis due to its susceptibility to present atherosclerotic disease and a plethora of additional pro-atherogenic factors (such as dialysis vintage, type of dialysis, etc.) that cannot be included in the whole analysis as possible confounders. However, CKD stage was included in the logistic model and did not reach statistical significance, allowing for the extrapolation of our results to our whole population. The second limitation is that we only measured plasma Mg, whose levels could differ from intracellular Mg [62,63] (which is responsible for the majority of reactions involving it as coenzyme [31]), and from levels obtained by the twenty-four hour excretion of magnesium in urine, which could more accurately reflect Mg balance. However, on the one hand, plasma lipid peroxidation is the possible mechanism by which Mg could be involved in the modification of cardiovascular events [54], and therefore serum Mg levels could better correlate with cIMT than tissue levels. On the other hand, Mg excretion in urine should be carefully taken in CKD patients [64]; consequently, for the current study, plasma Mg is a valid quantification method. As for the strengths of the current work, we would like to hallmark the relatively large cohort, which allowed us to adjust the regression models by ten different variables.

In summary, the current study shows an interaction of Mg with lipid parameters that modifies its effect on cITM. This result could shed some light on the effect of lipid levels on atherosclerosis in conditions in which Mg levels are modified and highlight that the important effect of this mineral on cardiovascular physiology could be more complex than initially thought. Although this analysis suggests around 1 nmol/L as the cutoff point of serum Mg that could influence the deleterious effect of lipids on atherosclerosis, further specifically designed studies are needed. In conclusion, Mg levels should be measured together with lipid parameters in order to assess the risk of atherosclerosis, especially in situations in which alterations in serum Mg are expected.

Table S1: Bivariate correlation coefficients between cIMT and Magnesium levels with other variables in control volunteers.

Author Contributions: Conceptualization, S.C., E.F., and J.M.V.; methodology, M.I. and M.M.-A.; formal analysis, S.C., M.B.-L., and M.M.-A.; data curation, M.B.; writing—original draft preparation, S.C.; writing—review and editing, S.C. and J.M.V.; funding acquisition, E.F. and J.M.V. All authors have read and agreed to the published version of the manuscript.

References

1. Timmis, A.; Townsend, N.; Gale, C.; Grobbee, R.; Maniadakis, N.; Flather, M.; Wilkins, E.; Wright, L.; Vos, R.; Bax, J.; et al. European Society of Cardiology: Cardiovascular Disease Statistics 2017. *Eur. Heart J.* **2018**, *39*, 508–579. [CrossRef]

2. Ference, B.A.; Graham, I.; Tokgozoglu, L.; Catapano, A.L. Impact of Lipids on Cardiovascular Health: JACC Health Promotion Series. *J. Am. Coll. Cardiol.* **2018**, *72*, 1141–1156. [CrossRef] [PubMed]

3. Lewington, S.; Whitlock, G.; Clarke, R.; Sherliker, P.; Emberson, J.; Halsey, J.; Qizilbash, N.; Peto, R.; Collins, R. Blood cholesterol and vascular mortality by age, sex, and blood pressure: A meta-analysis of individual data from 61 prospective studies with 55,000 vascular deaths. *Lancet* **2007**, *370*, 1829–1839.

4. Ference, B.A.; Ginsberg, H.N.; Graham, I.; Ray, K.K.; Packard, C.J.; Bruckert, E.; Hegele, R.A.; Krauss, R.M.; Raal, F.J.; Schunkert, H.; et al. Low-density lipoproteins cause atherosclerotic cardiovascular disease. 1. Evidence from genetic, epidemiologic, and clinical studies. A consensus statement from the European Atherosclerosis Society Consensus Panel. *Eur. Heart J.* **2017**, *38*, 2459–2472. [CrossRef]

5. Toth, P.P.; Barter, P.J.; Rosenson, R.S.; Boden, W.E.; Chapman, M.J.; Cuchel, M.; D'Agostino, R.B., Sr.; Davidson, M.H.; Davidson, W.S.; Heinecke, J.W.; et al. High-density lipoproteins: A consensus statement from the National Lipid Association. *J. Clin. Lipidol.* **2013**, *7*, 484–525. [CrossRef]

6. Varbo, A.; Benn, M.; Tybjærg-Hansen, A.; Jørgensen, A.B.; Frikke-Schmidt, R.; Nordestgaard, B.G. Remnant cholesterol as a causal risk factor for ischemic heart disease. *J. Am. Coll. Cardiol.* **2013**, *61*, 427–436. [CrossRef]

7. Miller, M.; Stone, N.J.; Ballantyne, C.; Bittner, V.; Criqui, M.H.; Ginsberg, H.N.; Goldberg, A.C.; Howard, W.J.; Jacobson, M.S.; Kris-Etherton, P.M.; et al. Triglycerides and cardiovascular disease: A scientific statement from the American Heart Association. *Circulation* **2011**, *123*, 2292–2333. [CrossRef]

8. Sarnak, M.J.; Levey, A.S.; Schoolwerth, A.C.; Coresh, J.; Culleton, B.; Hamm, L.L.; McCullough, P.A.; Kasiske, B.L.; Kelepouris, E.; Klag, M.J.; et al. Kidney disease as a risk factor for development of cardiovascular disease: A statement from the American Heart Association Councils on Kidney in Cardiovascular Disease, High Blood Pressure Research, Clinical Cardiology, and Epidemiology and Prevention. *Circulation* **2003**, *108*, 2154–2169. [CrossRef]

9. Ferro, C.J.; Mark, P.B.; Kanbay, M.; Sarafidis, P.; Heine, G.H.; Rossignol, P.; Massy, Z.A.; Mallamaci, F.; Valdivielso, J.M.; Malyszko, J.; et al. Lipid management in patients with chronic kidney disease. *Nat. Rev. Nephrol.* **2018**, *14*, 727–749. [CrossRef]

10. Arroyo, D.; Betriu, A.; Martinez-Alonso, M.; Vidal, T.; Valdivielso, J.M.; Fernández, E. Observational multicenter study to evaluate the prevalence and prognosis of subclinical atheromatosis in a Spanish chronic kidney disease cohort: Baseline data from the NEFRONA study. *BMC Nephrol.* **2014**, *15*, 168. [CrossRef]

11. Bermudez-Lopez, M.; Forne, C.; Amigo, N.; Bozic, M.; Arroyo, D.; Bretones, T.; Alonso, N.; Cambray, S.; Del Pino, M.D.; Mauricio, D.; et al. An in-depth analysis shows a hidden atherogenic lipoprotein profile in non-diabetic chronic kidney disease patients. *Expert Opin. Ther. Targets* **2019**, *23*, 619–630. [CrossRef] [PubMed]

12. Florens, N.; Calzada, C.; Lyasko, E.; Juillard, L.; Soulage, C.O. Modified Lipids and Lipoproteins in Chronic Kidney Disease: A New Class of Uremic Toxins. *Toxins* **2016**, *8*, 376. [CrossRef] [PubMed]

13. Hegele, R.A.; Tsimikas, S. Lipid-Lowering Agents. *Circ. Res.* **2019**, *124*, 386–404. [CrossRef]

14. Yokoyama, Y.; Levin, S.M.; Barnard, N.D. Association between plant-based diets and plasma lipids: A systematic review and meta-analysis. *Nutr. Rev.* **2017**, *75*, 683–698. [CrossRef]

15. Schwingshackl, L.; Hoffmann, G. Comparison of effects of long-term low-fat vs high-fat diets on blood lipid levels in overweight or obese patients: A systematic review and meta-analysis. *J. Acad. Nutr. Diet.* **2013**, *113*, 1640–1661. [CrossRef]

16. Jorat, M.V.; Tabrizi, R.; Mirhosseini, N.; Lankarani, K.B.; Akbari, M.; Heydari, S.T.; Mottaghi, R.; Asemi, Z. The effects of coenzyme Q10 supplementation on lipid profiles among patients with coronary artery disease: A systematic review and meta-analysis of randomized controlled trials. *Lipids Health Dis.* **2018**, *17*, 230. [CrossRef]

17. Bianconi, V.; Mannarino, M.R.; Sahebkar, A.; Cosentino, T.; Pirro, M. Cholesterol-Lowering Nutraceuticals Affecting Vascular Function and Cardiovascular Disease Risk. *Curr. Cardiol. Rep.* **2018**, *20*, 53. [CrossRef]

18. Martini, D.; Chiavaroli, L.; González-Sarrías, A.; Bresciani, L.; Palma-Duran, S.A.; Dall'Asta, M.; Deligiannidou, G.E.; Massaro, M.; Scoditti, E.; Combet, E.; et al. Impact of Foods and Dietary Supplements

Containing Hydroxycinnamic Acids on Cardiometabolic Biomarkers: A Systematic Review to Explore Inter-Individual Variability. *Nutrients* **2019**, *11*, 1805. [CrossRef]

19. Rayssiguier, Y. Magnesium, lipids and vascular diseases. Experimental evidence in animal models. *Magnesium* **1986**, *5*, 182–190.

20. Kaesler, N.; Goettsch, C.; Weis, D.; Schurgers, L.; Hellmann, B.; Floege, J.; Kramann, R. Magnesium but not nicotinamide prevents vascular calcification in experimental uraemia. *Nephrol. Dial. Transplant.* **2020**, *35*, 65–73. [CrossRef]

21. Iskra, M.; Patelski, J.; Majewski, W. Concentrations of calcium, magnesium, zinc and copper in relation to free fatty acids and cholesterol in serum of atherosclerotic men. *J. Trace Elem. Electrolytes Health Dis.* **1993**, *7*, 185–188.

22. Kirsten, R.; Heintz, B.; Nelson, K.; Sieberth, H.G.; Oremek, G.; Hasford, J.; Speck, U. Magnesium pyridoxal 5-phosphate glutamate reduces hyperlipidaemia in patients with chronic renal insufficiency. *Eur. J. Clin. Pharmacol.* **1988**, *34*, 133–137. [CrossRef]

23. Singh, R.B.; Rastogi, S.S.; Mani, U.V.; Seth, J.; Devi, L. Does dietary magnesium modulate blood lipids? *Biol. Trace Elem. Res.* **1991**, *30*, 59–64. [CrossRef]

24. De Oliveira Otto, M.C.; Alonso, A.; Lee, D.H.; Delclos, G.L.; Jenny, N.S.; Jiang, R.; Lima, J.A.; Symanski, E.; Jacobs, D.R., Jr.; Nettleton, J.A. Dietary micronutrient intakes are associated with markers of inflammation but not with markers of subclinical atherosclerosis. *J. Nutr.* **2011**, *141*, 1508–1515. [CrossRef]

25. Hashimoto, T.; Hara, A.; Ohkubo, T.; Kikuya, M.; Shintani, Y.; Metoki, H.; Inoue, R.; Asayama, K.; Kanno, A.; Nakashita, M.; et al. Serum magnesium, ambulatory blood pressure, and carotid artery alteration: The Ohasama study. *Am. J. Hypertens.* **2010**, *23*, 1292–1298. [CrossRef]

26. Sun, X.; Zhuang, X.; Huo, M.; Feng, P.; Zhang, S.; Zhong, X.; Zhou, H.; Guo, Y.; Hu, X.; Du, Z.; et al. Serum magnesium and the prevalence of peripheral artery disease: The Atherosclerosis Risk in Communities (ARIC) study. *Atherosclerosis* **2019**, *282*, 196–201. [CrossRef]

27. Menez, S.; Ding, N.; Grams, M.E.; Lutsey, P.L.; Heiss, G.; Folsom, A.R.; Selvin, E.; Coresh, J.; Jaar, B.G.; Matsushita, K. Serum magnesium, bone-mineral metabolism markers and their interactions with kidney function on subsequent risk of peripheral artery disease: The Atherosclerosis Risk in Communities Study. *Nephrol. Dial. Transplant.* **2020**. [CrossRef]

28. Rosique-Esteban, N.; Guasch-Ferré, M.; Hernández-Alonso, P.; Salas-Salvadó, J. Dietary Magnesium and Cardiovascular Disease: A Review with Emphasis in Epidemiological Studies. *Nutrients* **2018**, *10*, 168. [CrossRef]

29. DiNicolantonio, J.J.; Liu, J.; O'Keefe, J.H. Magnesium for the prevention and treatment of cardiovascular disease. *Open Heart* **2018**, *5*, e000775. [CrossRef]

30. Del Gobbo, L.C.; Imamura, F.; Wu, J.H.; de Oliveira Otto, M.C.; Chiuve, S.E.; Mozaffarian, D. Circulating and dietary magnesium and risk of cardiovascular disease: A systematic review and meta-analysis of prospective studies. *Am. J. Clin. Nutr.* **2013**, *98*, 160–173. [CrossRef]

31. Severino, P.; Netti, L.; Mariani, M.V.; Maraone, A.; D'Amato, A.; Scarpati, R.; Infusino, F.; Pucci, M.; Lavalle, C.; Maestrini, V.; et al. Prevention of Cardiovascular Disease: Screening for Magnesium Deficiency. *Cardiol. Res. Pract.* **2019**, *2019*, 4874921. [CrossRef]

32. Tzanakis, I.P.; Stamataki, E.E.; Papadaki, A.N.; Giannakis, N.; Damianakis, N.E.; Oreopoulos, D.G. Magnesium retards the progress of the arterial calcifications in hemodialysis patients: A pilot study. *Int. Urol. Nephrol.* **2014**, *46*, 2199–2205. [CrossRef]

33. Woods, K.L.; Fletcher, S.; Roffe, C.; Haider, Y. Intravenous magnesium sulphate in suspected acute myocardial infarction: Results of the second Leicester Intravenous Magnesium Intervention Trial (LIMIT-2). *Lancet* **1992**, *339*, 1553–1558. [CrossRef]

34. ISIS-4. A randomised factorial trial assessing early oral captopril, oral mononitrate, and intravenous magnesium sulphate in 58,050 patients with suspected acute myocardial infarction. ISIS-4 (Fourth International Study of Infarct Survival) Collaborative Group. *Lancet* **1995**, *345*, 669–685. [CrossRef]

35. Junyent, M.; Martínez Alonso, M.; Borràs, M.; Betriu i Bars, M.; Coll, B.; Marco Mayayo, M.P.; Sarró, F.; Valdivielso Revilla, J.M.; Fernández i Giráldez, E. Usefulness of imaging techniques and novel biomarkers in the prediction of cardiovascular risk in patients with chronic kidney disease in Spain: The NEFRONA project. *Nefrologia* **2010**, *30*, 119–126.

36. Junyent, M.; Martínez, M.; Borràs, M.; Coll, B.; Valdivielso, J.M.; Vidal, T.; Sarró, F.; Roig, J.; Craver, L.; Fernández, E. Predicting cardiovascular disease morbidity and mortality in chronic kidney disease in Spain. The rationale and design of NEFRONA: A prospective, multicenter, observational cohort study. *BMC Nephrol.* **2010**, *11*, 14. [CrossRef]

37. Betriu, A.; Martinez-Alonso, M.; Arcidiacono, M.V.; Cannata-Andia, J.; Pascual, J.; Valdivielso, J.M.; Fernández, E. Prevalence of subclinical atheromatosis and associated risk factors in chronic kidney disease: The NEFRONA study. *Nephrol. Dial. Transplant.* **2014**, *29*, 1415–1422. [CrossRef]

38. Gracia, M.; Betriu, À.; Martínez-Alonso, M.; Arroyo, D.; Abajo, M.; Fernández, E.; Valdivielso, J.M. Predictors of Subclinical Atheromatosis Progression over 2 Years in Patients with Different Stages of CKD. *Clin. J. Am. Soc. Nephrol.* **2016**, *11*, 287–296. [CrossRef]

39. Stein, J.H.; Korcarz, C.E.; Hurst, R.T.; Lonn, E.; Kendall, C.B.; Mohler, E.R.; Najjar, S.S.; Rembold, C.M.; Post, W.S. Use of carotid ultrasound to identify subclinical vascular disease and evaluate cardiovascular disease risk: A consensus statement from the American Society of Echocardiography Carotid Intima-Media Thickness Task Force. Endorsed by the Society for Vascular Medicine. *J. Am. Soc. Echocardiogr.* **2008**, *21*, 93–111.

40. Touboul, P.J.; Hennerici, M.G.; Meairs, S.; Adams, H.; Amarenco, P.; Desvarieux, M.; Ebrahim, S.; Fatar, M.; Hernandez, R.H.; Kownator, S.; et al. Mannheim intima-media thickness consensus. *Cerebrovasc. Dis.* **2004**, *18*, 346–349. [CrossRef]

41. Peng, J.; Luo, F.; Ruan, G.; Peng, R.; Li, X. Hypertriglyceridemia and atherosclerosis. *Lipids Health Dis.* **2017**, *16*, 233. [CrossRef] [PubMed]

42. Cannon, C.P.; Khan, I.; Klimchak, A.C.; Sanchez, R.J.; Sasiela, W.J.; Massaro, J.M.; D'Agostino, R.B.; Reynolds, M.R. Simulation of impact on cardiovascular events due to lipid-lowering therapy intensification in a population with atherosclerotic cardiovascular disease. *Am. Heart J.* **2019**, *216*, 30–41. [CrossRef]

43. Leenders, N.H.J.; Vervloet, M.G. Magnesium: A Magic Bullet for Cardiovascular Disease in Chronic Kidney Disease? *Nutrients* **2019**, *11*, 455. [CrossRef]

44. Guerrero-Romero, F.; Jaquez-Chairez, F.O.; Rodríguez-Morán, M. Magnesium in metabolic syndrome: A review based on randomized, double-blind clinical trials. *Magnes. Res.* **2016**, *29*, 146–153. [CrossRef] [PubMed]

45. Joris, P.J.; Plat, J.; Bakker, S.J.; Mensink, R.P. Long-term magnesium supplementation improves arterial stiffness in overweight and obese adults: Results of a randomized, double-blind, placebo-controlled intervention trial. *Am. J. Clin. Nutr.* **2016**, *103*, 1260–1266. [CrossRef]

46. Massy, Z.A.; de Zeeuw, D. LDL cholesterol in CKD–to treat or not to treat? *Kidney Int.* **2013**, *84*, 451–456. [CrossRef]

47. Jahnen-Dechent, W.; Ketteler, M. Magnesium basics. *Clin. Kidney J.* **2012**, *5* (Suppl. 1), i3–i14. [CrossRef]

48. Zewinger, S.; Speer, T.; Kleber, M.E.; Scharnagl, H.; Woitas, R.; Lepper, P.M.; Pfahler, K.; Seiler, S.; Heine, G.H.; März, W.; et al. HDL cholesterol is not associated with lower mortality in patients with kidney dysfunction. *J. Am. Soc. Nephrol.* **2014**, *25*, 1073–1082. [CrossRef]

49. Ma, J.; Folsom, A.R.; Melnick, S.L.; Eckfeldt, J.H.; Sharrett, A.R.; Nabulsi, A.A.; Hutchinson, R.G.; Metcalf, P.A. Associations of serum and dietary magnesium with cardiovascular disease, hypertension, diabetes, insulin, and carotid arterial wall thickness: The ARIC study. Atherosclerosis Risk in Communities Study. *J. Clin. Epidemiol.* **1995**, *48*, 927–940. [CrossRef]

50. Rodríguez-Ortiz, M.E.; Gómez-Delgado, F.; de Larriva, A.P.A.; Canalejo, A.; Gómez-Luna, P.; Herencia, C.; López-Moreno, J.; Rodríguez, M.; López-Miranda, J.; Almadén, Y. Serum Magnesium is associated with Carotid Atherosclerosis in patients with high cardiovascular risk (CORDIOPREV Study). *Sci. Rep.* **2019**, *9*, 8013. [CrossRef]

51. Zheltova, A.A.; Kharitonova, M.V.; Iezhitsa, I.N.; Spasov, A.A. Magnesium deficiency and oxidative stress: An update. *Biomedicine* **2016**, *6*, 20. [CrossRef] [PubMed]

52. Rayssiguier, Y.; Gueux, E.; Bussière, L.; Durlach, J.; Mazur, A. Dietary magnesium affects susceptibility of lipoproteins and tissues to peroxidation in rats. *J. Am. Coll. Nutr.* **1993**, *12*, 133–137. [CrossRef] [PubMed]

53. Scibior, A.; Gołębiowska, D.; Niedźwiecka, I. Magnesium can protect against vanadium-induced lipid peroxidation in the hepatic tissue. *Oxid. Med. Cell. Longev.* **2013**, *2013*, 802734. [CrossRef] [PubMed]

54. Walter, M.F.; Jacob, R.F.; Bjork, R.E.; Jeffers, B.; Buch, J.; Mizuno, Y.; Mason, R.P. Circulating lipid hydroperoxides predict cardiovascular events in patients with stable coronary artery disease: The PREVENT

study. *J. Am. Coll. Cardiol.* **2008**, *51*, 1196–1202. [CrossRef]

55. Feingold, K.R.; Grunfeld, C. Introduction to Lipids and Lipoproteins. In *Endotext*; Feingold, K.R., Anawalt, B., Boyce, A., Eds.; MDText.com, Inc.: South Dartmouth, MA, USA, 2 February 2018.

56. Gao, S.; Liu, J. Association between circulating oxidized low-density lipoprotein and atherosclerotic cardiovascular disease. *Chronic Dis. Transl. Med.* **2017**, *3*, 89–94. [CrossRef]

57. Vaziri, N.D. Role of dyslipidemia in impairment of energy metabolism, oxidative stress, inflammation and cardiovascular disease in chronic kidney disease. *Clin. Exp. Nephrol.* **2014**, *18*, 265–268. [CrossRef]

58. Cocate, P.G.; Natali, A.J.; de Oliveira, A.; Longo, G.Z.; Rita de Cássia, G.A.; Maria do Carmo, G.P.; dos Santos, E.C.; Buthers, J.M.; de Oliveira, L.L.; Hermsdorff, H.H.M. Fruit and vegetable intake and related nutrients are associated with oxidative stress markers in middle-aged men. *Nutrition* **2014**, *30*, 660–665. [CrossRef]

59. Wegner, M.; Araszkiewicz, A.; Zozulińska-Ziółkiewicz, D.; Wierusz-Wysocka, B.; Pioruńska-Mikołajczak, A.; Pioruńska-Stolzmann, M. The relationship between concentrations of magnesium and oxidized low density lipoprotein and the activity of platelet activating factor acetylhydrolase in the serum of patients with type 1 diabetes. *Magnes. Res.* **2010**, *23*, 97–104.

60. Louvet, L.; Büchel, J.; Steppan, S.; Passlick-Deetjen, J.; Massy, Z.A. Magnesium prevents phosphate-induced calcification in human aortic vascular smooth muscle cells. *Nephrol. Dial. Transplant.* **2013**, *28*, 869–878. [CrossRef]

61. Braake, A.D.; Shanahan, C.M.; Baaij, J.F.H. Magnesium Counteracts Vascular Calcification Passive Interference or Active Modulation? *Arterioscler. Thromb. Vasc. Biol.* **2017**, *37*, 1431–1445. [CrossRef]

62. De Lourdes Lima, M.; Cruz, T.; Rodrigues, L.E.; Bomfim, O.; Melo, J.; Correia, R.; Porto, M.; Cedro, A.; Vicente, E. Serum and intracellular magnesium deficiency in patients with metabolic syndrome—Evidences for its relation to insulin resistance. *Diabetes Res. Clin. Pract.* **2009**, *83*, 257–262. [CrossRef] [PubMed]

63. Shah, S.A.; Clyne, C.A.; Henyan, N.; Migeed, M.; Yarlagadda, R.; Silver, B.B.; Kluger, J.; White, C.M. Impact of magnesium sulfate on serum magnesium concentrations and intracellular electrolyte concentrations among patients undergoing radio frequency catheter ablation. *Conn. Med.* **2008**, *72*, 261–265. [PubMed]

64. Elin, J.R. Assessment of magnessium status for diagnosis and therapy. *Magnes. Res.* **2010**, *23*, 194–198.

6

Dietary Intake of Magnesium or Calcium and Chemotherapy-Induced Peripheral Neuropathy in Colorectal Cancer Patients

Evertine Wesselink [1], Renate M. Winkels [1], Harm van Baar [1], Anne J. M. R. Geijsen [1], Moniek van Zutphen [1], Henk K. van Halteren [2], Bibi M. E. Hansson [3], Sandra A. Radema [4], Johannes H. W. de Wilt [5], Ellen Kampman [1] and Dieuwertje E. G. Kok [1,*]

[1]   Division of Human Nutrition, Wageningen University & Research, Stippeneng 4, 6708 WE Wageningen, The Netherlands; vera.wesselink@wur.nl (E.W.); renate.winkels@wur.nl (R.M.W.); harm.vanbaar@wur.nl (H.v.B.); anne.geijsen@wur.nl (A.J.M.R.G.); moniek.vanzutphen@wur.nl (M.v.Z.); ellen.kampman@wur.nl (E.K.)
[2]   Department of Internal Medicine, Admiraal de Ruyter Ziekenhuis, 's-Gravenpolderseweg 114, 4462 RA Goes, The Netherlands; h.vanhalteren@adrz.nl
[3]   Department of Surgery, Canisius Wilhelmina Ziekenhuis, Weg door het Jonkerbos 100, 6532 SZ Nijmegen, The Netherlands; b.hansson@cwz.nl
[4]   Department of Medical Oncology, Radboud University Medical Centre, Geert Grooteplein-Zuid 22, 6525 GA Nijmegen, The Netherlands; sandra.radema@radboudumc.nl
[5]   Department of Surgery, Radboud University Medical Centre, Geert Grooteplein-Zuid 22, 6525 GA Nijmegen, The Netherlands; Hans.deWilt@radboudumc.nl
*   Correspondence: dieuwertje.kok@wur.nl

Abstract: Chemotherapy-induced peripheral neuropathy (CIPN) is a common and severe side-effect in colorectal cancer (CRC) patients. This study assessed the association between habitual dietary intake of magnesium or calcium and prevalence and severity of chronic CIPN in CRC patients receiving adjuvant chemotherapy. For this prospective cohort study, 196 CRC patients were considered. Magnesium and calcium intake was determined using a food frequency questionnaire at diagnosis, during and after chemotherapy. Chronic CIPN was assessed 12 months after diagnosis using the quality of life questionnaire CIPN20. Prevalence ratios were calculated to assess the association between magnesium or calcium intake and the prevalence of CIPN. Multivariable linear regression analysis was used to assess the association between magnesium or calcium intake and severity of CIPN. CIPN was reported by 160 (82%) patients. Magnesium intake during chemotherapy was statistically significantly associated with lower prevalence of CIPN (prevalence ratio (PR) 0.53, 95% confidence interval (CI) 0.32, 0.92). Furthermore, higher dietary intake of magnesium during (β −1.08, 95% CI −1.95, −0.22) and after chemotherapy (β −0.93, 95% CI −1.81, −0.06) was associated with less severe CIPN. No associations were found for calcium intake and the prevalence and severity of CIPN. To conclude, we observed an association between higher dietary magnesium intake and lower prevalence and severity of CIPN in CRC patients.

Keywords: calcium; chemotherapy; colorectal cancer; magnesium; neuropathy; oxaliplatin

1. Introduction

Chemotherapy-induced peripheral neuropathy (CIPN) is a common side-effect in colorectal cancer (CRC) patients treated with oxaliplatin [1]. Oxaliplatin can cause both acute and chronic CIPN. Symptoms of chronic CIPN include distal paresthesia, tingling sensations and numbness. Chronic CIPN predominantly affects sensory nerves and can lead to long-term disability [1]. Occurrence and severity of chronic CIPN are related to the cumulative dose and dose-intensity of the treatment [1–3].

Six to eight months after the end of oxaliplatin treatment, 40–60% of the patients still suffer from CIPN [4–7]. In order to minimize the detrimental effects in CRC patients, it is important to understand which factors can influence the development and severity of CIPN.

Magnesium and calcium are proposed to be important in the etiology of CIPN, because they are both involved in electric excitability of neurons and muscle contraction [8]. Low circulating levels of magnesium, but not calcium, before treatment have been associated with more severe CIPN in CRC patients [3]. Besides circulating levels of magnesium and calcium, several studies focused on intravenous administration of magnesium and calcium and the severity of CIPN [9–16]. The clinical observational study of Gamelin et al. found a lower occurrence and severity of CIPN in CRC patients who received magnesium and calcium in comparison to patients who did not receive magnesium and calcium for several reasons [9]. Other observational studies in CRC patients did not find an association between intravenous magnesium and calcium infusions and CIPN [10,11].

Several randomized-controlled trials (RCTs) [11–15] studied the effect of intravenous magnesium and calcium infusions on CIPN, but results are inconclusive. Grothey et al. reported a protective effect of magnesium and calcium on the prevalence of CIPN in 102 colon cancer patients [12]. The prevalence of CIPN was 22% in the magnesium and calcium group compared to 41% in the placebo group ($p = 0.04$) [12]. On the contrary, four other RCTs conducted among 27–353 CRC patients, did not find a protective effect of magnesium and calcium infusions on CIPN [13–16]. So far, no consensus about the use of magnesium and calcium infusions to reduce or prevent CIPN has been reached [17].

Most studies conducted so far focused on acute CIPN during and directly after treatment. It has been shown that further progression of CIPN can occur months after the end of treatment [1]. Moreover, the associations between dietary magnesium or calcium intake and the prevalence and severity of chronic CIPN have not been described so far. Dietary intake in relation to CIPN is important as dietary magnesium intake is the main contributor to the magnesium status. Further insights into the relation between diet and CIPN may provide feasible opportunities for dietary strategies directed against CIPN in cancer patients. In this prospective cohort study, we assessed the association between habitual dietary intake of magnesium or calcium and the prevalence and severity of CIPN approximately six months after chemotherapy, i.e., 12 months after diagnosis, in CRC patients receiving adjuvant chemotherapy.

2. Materials and Methods

2.1. Patients

This study is embedded in the longitudinal observational study on nutritional and lifestyle factors (COLON study), which is a prospective cohort study focusing on nutritional and lifestyle factors in relation to clinical outcomes and quality of life of CRC patients in the Netherlands [18]. The design and recruitment of the COLON study has been described in detail previously [18]. In short, newly diagnosed CRC patients were recruited directly after diagnosis in 12 hospitals in the Netherlands and were followed up during and after treatment. Men and women of all ages, who were in any stage of the disease were eligible for the study. Non-Dutch speaking patients, or patients with a history of CRC or (partial) bowel resection, chronic inflammatory bowel disease, hereditary CRC syndromes (e.g., Lynch syndrome, Familial Adenomatous Polyposis, Peutz-Jegher), dementia or another mental condition that made it impossible to fill out a questionnaire correctly, were excluded from the study. Participants of the COLON study who were included between April 2012 and December 2015 and who received adjuvant chemotherapy were eligible for the current study ($n = 293$). Patients who also received neoadjuvant chemotherapy ($n = 8$), who did not start with chemotherapy ($n = 22$), or did not fill out the questionnaire on CIPN ($n = 67$) were excluded, resulting in a total of 196 newly diagnosed CRC patients eligible for the current study (Figure 1). Hospital records and linkage with the Dutch ColoRectal Audit (DCRA) [19] were used to obtain data regarding cancer type, cancer stage and type of chemotherapy. All patients provided written informed consent. All procedures followed were in accordance with the ethical standards of the institution and the COLON study was approved by the Committee on Research involving Human Subjects, region Arnhem-Nijmegen, the Netherlands (file 2009-349).

Figure 1. Flowchart representing patient selection for the current study. Colorectal cancer patients participating in the longitudinal observational study on nutritional and lifestyle factors (the COLON study) and who received adjuvant chemotherapy and filled out the quality of life questionnaire to assess chemotherapy-induced peripheral neuropathy (QLQ-CIPN16) were included in the present study. * Patients who were recruited before April 2012 were not included in this study, because the QLQ-CIPN16 questionnaire was implemented from April 2012 onwards.

2.2. Magnesium and Calcium Intake

A 204-item semi-quantitative food frequency questionnaire (FFQ) developed by the Division of Human Nutrition of Wageningen University and Research, the Netherlands, was used to assess habitual intake of magnesium and calcium from the diet during the previous month. The magnesium or calcium content of a product was determined based on data from the Dutch food composition table of 2011 [20]. Dietary intake of magnesium and calcium was calculated for each food item based on frequency of intake, number of portions and portion size, as well as the type of product (e.g., whole grain bread or brown bread). The total amount of the nutrients consumed per day was calculated by adding all items containing the respective nutrient. The dietary intake of magnesium and calcium was adjusted for total energy intake using the residual method [21]. Dietary supplement use was assessed by a dietary supplement questionnaire developed by the Division of Human Nutrition of Wageningen University and Research [18]. Intake of magnesium and calcium from dietary supplements was not considered for the current study, due to the relatively low number of supplement users and the lack of details on exact dosages, frequency and compliance. However, we performed sensitivity analyses excluding patients who reported use of dietary supplements containing magnesium or calcium. The FFQs and dietary supplement questionnaires were filled out at diagnosis and six and 12 months after diagnosis. These three time points represent the usual dietary intake before surgery, during chemotherapy and six months after chemotherapy, respectively.

2.3. Chemotherapy-Induced Peripheral Neuropathy

Prevalence and severity of chronic CIPN were assessed using the 'European Organization for Research and Treatment of Cancer Quality of Life Questionnaire to assess Chemotherapy Induced Peripheral Neuropathy' (EORTC QLQ-CIPN16). This is an abbreviated version of the QLQ-CIPN20 [22], which is used in the COLON study. This questionnaire was filled out 12 months after diagnosis, representing approximately six months after the end of chemotherapy. The QLQ-CIPN16 consists of 16 questions of which eight assessing sensory symptoms and eight assessing motor symptoms. These questions were shown to be valid and reliable to assess patient-reported CIPN [22]. Patients reported the degree to which they have experienced sensory and motor symptoms during the past week using a 4-point Likert scale. Sensory and motor scale scores from the QLQ-CIPN16 ranged from 1–32. The scores of the QLQ-CIPN16 were linear transformed to a 0–100 scale. Based on mean scores of CIPN in the general Dutch population, the presence of CIPN was defined as >3.6 for the total CIPN16 score, >3.2 for the sensory sub-score and >3.8 for the motor sub-score [23]. Furthermore, we have evaluated severity of CIPN-related symptoms by specifically focusing on the CIPN scores, with higher scores indicating more severe CIPN. Missing values were handled by the mean-person imputation method [24], however, participants were excluded from analyses when more than two items in the QLQ-CIPN16 were missing.

2.4. Data Analysis

To study the association between magnesium and calcium and the prevalence of CIPN, prevalence ratios (PR) were calculated using a Cox proportional hazards regression model, with a fixed time variable. PRs were used, since odds ratios tend to overestimate the size of the association when the outcome is common [25]. Subsequently, among patients suffering from CIPN, the association between magnesium or calcium intake and the severity of CIPN was assessed by using multivariable linear regression analysis.

The Shapiro-Wilk test was used to determine whether data were normally distributed. Dietary intake of magnesium, calcium, vitamin D, total energy, as well as CIPN scores were natural-log transformed. To adjust for potential confounding, the models were adjusted for age, gender as well as energy adjusted dietary calcium or magnesium and vitamin D intake. When a variable changed the regression coefficient of the independent variable with 10% or more, the variable was considered to be a confounder and was added as a covariate to the model. Self-reported magnesium or calcium supplement use, diabetes mellitus, physical activity, smoking, as well as B vitamins and alcohol intake did not influence the observed associations. There was a strong correlation between protein and magnesium intake ($r = 0.81$), as well as between protein and calcium intake ($r = 0.80$), therefore we did not adjust for protein intake in the final model. Sensitivity analyses were performed for oxaliplatin-containing chemotherapy (OX), patients with colon cancer and non-supplement users. Stratified analysis was done for age (<65 and ≥65 years of age) to assess possible age differences.

Statistical analyses were performed in SAS 9.4 (SAS Institute, Cary, NC, USA). Ninety-five percent confidence intervals (95% CIs), not containing 1 for the Cox regression analyses and not containing 0 for the multivariable regression analyses, represent statistically significant associations [26].

3. Results

3.1. Patients Characteristics

In total, 196 CRC patients from 12 hospitals in the Netherlands were included in this study. The majority of the patients started with OX ($n = 166$, 85%), while 23 (11%) patients received capecitabine monotherapy (Table 1). In our study population, 160 patients (82%) reported CIPN 12 months after diagnosis. Among these patients, both sensory as well as motor CIPN symptoms were commonly reported (81% and 76%, respectively). Common sensory symptoms included tingling and numbness in fingers and toes, whereas difficulty with manipulating small objects and opening jars or bottles were commonly reported motor symptoms. The severity of sensory symptoms was higher than the severity of motor symptoms (mean score 20.8 and 12.5, respectively).

The median intake of magnesium was 317 mg/day and for calcium this was 851 g/day. The most important food sources of magnesium in our population were whole grain bread and nuts. Also, coffee, dairy products, dark chocolate, banana and legumes were common sources of magnesium.

For calcium the most important food source was dairy products, especially cheese, yoghurt and milk. The intake of magnesium was below the estimated average requirement of 350 mg/day for men and 265 mg/day for women [27] in 48% of our study population at the time of diagnosis. During and after chemotherapy, 65% and 57% of the patients had an intake below the estimated average requirement, respectively. The intake of calcium was below the estimated average requirement of 800 mg/day for man <70 years and 1000 mg/day for man >70 years and 1000 mg for women [28] in 58% of our population at the time of diagnosis, 59% during treatment and 65% after treatment.

Table 1. Characteristics of colorectal cancer patients who received adjuvant chemotherapy by prevalence of chemotherapy-induced peripheral chemotherapy (CIPN).

		CIPN	
	Total Population n = 196	CIPN No n = 36 (18%)	Yes [1] n = 160 (82%)
Gender, women	71 (36%)	12 (33%)	59 (37%)
Age (years)	64.0 (59.8–68.1)	65.4 (59.0–68.2)	63.7 (59.9–68.0)
Diabetes mellitus (yes) [2]	15 (8%)	3 (8%)	12 (8%)
Physical activity (meeting norm) [3]	143 (73%)	25 (69%)	118 (74%)
Tumor stage			
Stage II	15 (8%)	2 (6%)	13 (8%)
Stage III	145 (74%)	28 (76%)	117 (73%)
Stage IV	21 (10%)	3 (9%)	18 (11%)
Missing	15 (8%)	3 (9%)	12 (8%)
Cancer site			
Colon	181 (93%)	33 (92%)	148 (93%)
Rectum	14 (7%)	3 (8%)	11 (7%)
Missing	1 (0%)	0 (0%)	1 (0%)
Type of chemotherapy			
Oxaliplatin-containing (OX)	166 (85%)	27 (75%)	139 (87%)
Capecitabine monotherapy	23 (12%)	9 (25%)	14 (9%)
Other	2 (1%)	0 (0%)	2 (1%)
Missing	5 (2%)	0 (0%)	5 (3%)
Dietary factors			
Magnesium intake from diet (mg/day) [2,4]	317 (261–383)	325 (261–396)	313 (261–380)
Use of magnesium supplements (yes)	36 (18%)	6 (17%)	30 (18%)
Calcium intake from diet (mg/day) [2,4]	851 (621–1143)	789 (597–1155)	861 (631–1123)
Use of calcium supplements (yes)	35 (18%)	6 (17%)	29 (18%)
Vitamin D intake from diet (mg/day) [2,4]	3.1 (2.4–4.1)	2.8 (2.2–3.7)	3.2 (2.4–4.2)
Total energy intake (kcal/day) [2,4]	1893 (1534–2265)	1898 (1547–2230)	1893 (1534–2285)
CIPN [5]			
Total score [6]	14.6 (6.3–26.4)	0.0 (0–2.1)	16.7 (10.4–29.2)
Sensory score [7]	16.7 (4.2–37.5)	0.0 (0–0)	20.8 (12.5–37.5)
Motor score [8]	8.3 (4.2–20.8)	0.0 (0–0)	12.5 (8.3–20.8)

Values presented are median (quartile 1–quartile 3) or number (percentage). [1] Cut-off point for CIPN total score: 3.6, [2] Assessed at diagnosis. [3] Meeting the Dutch physical activity guideline of 150 min per week of moderate intensive exercise at baseline, [4] Intake is missing for two patients, [5] Assessed 12 months after diagnosis. [6] Data for one patient missing. [7] Data for two patients missing. [8] Data for five patients missing.

3.2. Dietary Magnesium or Calcium Intake and CIPN

Dietary intake of magnesium during chemotherapy was associated with the prevalence of chronic CIPN (PR 0.53, 95% CI 0.32, 0.90) (Table 2). Among patients suffering from CIPN, a higher dietary intake of magnesium was associated with less severe symptoms of CIPN (β −1.08, 95% CI −1.95, −0.22 for the intake during chemotherapy and β −0.93, 95% CI −1.81, −0.06 for the intake after chemotherapy) (Table 3). Dietary intake of calcium was not associated with the prevalence (Table 2) and severity (Table 3) of CIPN.

Sensitivity analyses including only patients receiving OX (n = 166) or only patients with colon cancer (n = 181) or only non-supplement users (n = 160–171) showed similar results (Table 4).

Table 2. Association between dietary magnesium or calcium intake and the prevalence of chronic chemotherapy-induced neuropathy in colorectal cancer patients receiving adjuvant chemotherapy.

	n/Events	Prevalence Ratio (95% CI) Total Score CIPN16[1]	n/Events	Sensory Symptoms[1]	n/Events	Motor Symptoms[1]
Magnesium intake						
Crude model						
At diagnosis	194/158	0.81 (0.51, 1.29)	194/157	0.98 (0.64, 1.52)	194/147	0.95 (0.54, 1.67)
During chemotherapy	192/156	**0.57 (0.35, 0.92)**	192/156	0.70 (0.44, 1.12)	192/145	0.59 (0.33, 1.05)
After chemotherapy	181/147	0.67 (0.43, 1.05)	181/146	0.86 (0.57, 1.31)	181/136	0.61 (0.36, 1.03)
Full model						
At diagnosis	194/158	0.69 (0.42, 1.13)	194/157	0.84 (0.51, 1.39)	194/147	0.81 (0.43, 1.52)
During chemotherapy	192/156	**0.53 (0.32, 0.90)**	192/156	0.67 (0.40, 1.10)	192/145	0.57 (0.30, 1.09)
After chemotherapy	181/147	0.61 (0.37, 1.03)	181/146	0.84 (0.51, 1.37)	181/136	**0.51 (0.28, 0.93)**
Calcium intake						
Crude model						
At diagnosis	194/158	1.15 (0.93, 1.41)	194/157	1.20 (0.98, 1.46)	194/147	1.12 (0.89, 1.41)
During chemotherapy	192/156	0.97 (0.83, 1.13)	192/156	1.02 (0.87, 1.19)	192/145	0.89 (0.73, 1.09)
After Chemotherapy	181/147	1.03 (0.86, 1.23)	181/146	1.08 (0.90, 1.30)	181/136	0.96 (0.78, 1.17)
Full model						
At diagnosis	194/158	1.21 (0.95, 1.56)	194/157	1.24 (0.97, 1.58)	194/147	1.15 (0.88, 1.50)
During chemotherapy	192/156	1.03 (0.86, 1.23)	192/156	1.06 (0.89, 1.28)	192/145	0.92 (0.73, 1.16)
After Chemotherapy	181/147	1.08 (0.89, 1.32)	181/146	1.10 (0.89, 1.35)	181/136	0.99 (0.79, 1.24)

Analyses were performed using a Cox proportional hazard regression model, with a fixed time variable. Crude models: energy-adjusted intake of magnesium or calcium. Full model for magnesium was adjusted for, energy-adjusted dietary calcium and vitamin D intake as well as age and gender. Full model for calcium was adjusted for, energy-adjusted dietary magnesium and vitamin D intake as well as age and gender. [1] CIPN was defined as a score >3.6 for the total CIPN16 score, >3.2 for the sensory sub-score and >3.8 for the motor sub-score.

Table 3. Associations between dietary magnesium or calcium intake and severity of chronic chemotherapy-induced neuropathy in colorectal cancer patients receiving adjuvant chemotherapy.

| | | Beta (95% CI) | | | | |
	n	Total Score CIPN16	n	Sensory Symptoms	n	Motor Symptoms
Magnesium intake						
Crude model						
At diagnosis	158	−0.68 (−1.45, 0.08)	157	−1.09 (−1.90 −0.27)	147	−0.45 (−1.33, 0.43)
During chemotherapy	156	**−1.21 (−2.01, −0.41)**	156	**−1.43 (−2.30, −0.57)**	145	**−1.25 (−2.16, −0.35)**
After chemotherapy	147	**−0.81 (−1.59, −0.04)**	146	**−1.05 (−1.87, −0.22)**	136	−0.64 (−1.48, 0.21)
Full model						
At diagnosis	158	−0.65 (−1.52, 0.20)	157	**−1.10 (−2.01, −0.18)**	147	−0.36 (−1.36, 0.63)
During chemotherapy	156	**−1.08 (−1.95, −0.22)**	156	**−1.24 (−2.17, −0.32)**	145	**−1.25 (−2.24, −0.27)**
After chemotherapy	147	**−0.93 (−1.81, −0.06)**	146	**−1.11 (−2.04, −0.19)**	136	−0.76 (−1.73, 0.21)
Calcium intake						
Crude model						
At diagnosis	158	−0.20 (−0.55, 0.14)	157	−0.31 (−0.68, 0.06)	147	−0.19 (−0.56, 0.18)
During chemotherapy	156	−0.31 (−0.62, 0.00)	156	**−0.39 (−0.74, −0.04)**	145	−0.31 (−0.66, 0.04)
After chemotherapy	147	−0.19 (−0.55, 0.17)	146	−0.36 (−0.75, 0.03)	136	−0.04 (−0.42, 0.35)
Full model						
At diagnosis	158	−0.05 (−0.45, 0.35)	157	0.03 (−0.40, 0.45)	147	−0.19 (−0.61, 0.23)
During chemotherapy	156	−0.16 (−0.51, 0.19)	156	−0.14 (−0.52, 0.23)	145	−0.19 (−0.57, 0.19)
After chemotherapy	147	−0.03 (−0.42, 0.35)	146	−0.10 (−0.52, 0.32)	136	0.01 (−0.40, 0.43)

Analyses were performed using multivariable linear regression analyses. Crude models: energy-adjusted intake of magnesium or calcium. Full model for magnesium was adjusted for energy-adjusted dietary calcium and vitamin D intake as well as age and gender. Full model for calcium was adjusted for energy-adjusted dietary magnesium and vitamin D intake as well as age and gender.

Table 4. Sensitivity analyses for the associations between dietary magnesium or calcium intake and severity of chronic chemotherapy-induced neuropathy.

		Beta (95% CI)				
	n	Total Score CIPN16	n	Sensory Symptoms	n	Motor Symptoms
Patients receiving oxaliplatin-containing chemotherapy						
Magnesium						
At diagnosis	137	−0.68 (−1.58, 0.22)	138	−1.01 (−1.97, −0.05)	126	−0.48 (−0.53, 0.57)
During chemotherapy	136	−0.90 (−1.80, −0.00)	137	−1.10 (−2.06, −0.14)	125	−1.28 (−2.33, −0.24)
After chemotherapy	132	−0.94 (−1.85, −0.02)	133	−1.10 (−2.07, −0.12)	121	−0.94 (−1.98, 0.10)
Calcium						
At diagnosis	137	0.00 (−0.42, 0.42)	138	0.08 (−0.36, 0.53)	132	−0.19 (−0.63, 0.26)
During chemotherapy	136	−0.18 (−0.54; 0.18)	137	−0.11 (−0.51; 0.28)	125	−0.28 (−0.69; 0.13)
After chemotherapy	132	0.00 (−0.39, 0.41)	133	−0.06 (−0.49, 0.38)	121	0.01 (−0.43, 0.45)
Not supplement users						
Magnesium						
At diagnosis	128	−0.80 (−1.80, 0.20)	126	−0.99 (−2.08, 0.10)	119	−0.68 (−1.83, 0.48)
During chemotherapy	136	−1.24 (−2.21, −0.27)	134	−1.20 (−2.27, −0.13)	128	−1.81 (−2.90, −0.71)
After chemotherapy	129	−1.34 (−2.30, −0.37)	126	−1.29 (−2.37, −0.21)	119	−1.38 (−2.44, −0.32)
Calcium						
At diagnosis	127	−0.06 (−0.50, 0.37)	127	0.06 (−0.41, 0.53)	119	−0.08 (−0.56, 0.38)
During chemotherapy	140	−0.12 (−0.48, 0.23)	138	−0.07 (−0.45, 0.32)	132	−0.20 (−0.60, 0.20)
After chemotherapy	127	−0.00 (−0.41, 0.42)	130	−0.09 (−0.54, 0.36)	119	0.09 (−0.35, 0.53)
Colon cancer patients						
Magnesium						
At diagnosis	146	−0.66 (−1.54, 0.22)	145	−1.11 (−2.04, −0.18)	135	−0.34 (−1.37, 0.68)
During chemotherapy	145	−1.13 (−2.03, −0.23)	145	−1.34 (−2.30, −0.38)	134	−1.30 (−2.33, −0.26)
After chemotherapy	139	−0.80 (−1.71, 0.11)	137	−0.98 (−1.95, −0.02)	128	−0.66 (−1.67, 0.36)
Calcium						
At diagnosis	146	−0.00 (−0.42, 0.41)	145	0.07 (−0.37, 0.51)	135	−0.15 (−0.58, 0.28)
During chemotherapy	145	−0.11 (−0.48, 0.25)	145	−0.07 (−0.47, 0.35)	134	−0.16 (−0.57, 0.26)
After chemotherapy	139	−0.03 (−0.45, 0.39)	137	−0.11 (−0.56, 0.34)	128	0.04 (−0.41, 0.50)

Analyses were performed using multivariable linear regression analyses. Models for magnesium was adjusted for energy-adjusted dietary calcium and vitamin D intake as well as age and gender. Models for calcium was adjusted for energy-adjusted dietary magnesium and vitamin D intake as well as age and gender.

Stratified analyses for age showed statistically significant associations between magnesium intake at all three time points and the severity of CIPN for patients aged 65 and older ($n = 88$), but not for patients younger than 65 years ($n = 108$) (data not shown).

4. Discussion

The aim of this study was to assess the association between magnesium and calcium intake and CIPN in a prospective cohort of CRC patients. Dietary intake of magnesium during chemotherapy was associated with a lower prevalence of CIPN. A higher dietary intake of magnesium, but not calcium, during and after chemotherapy was associated with a lower severity of total CIPN symptoms.

The prevalence of CIPN approximately six months after chemotherapy, i.e., 12 months after diagnosis, was higher than expected (81%) in our study population consisting of 196 CRC patients treated with adjuvant chemotherapy. Argyriou et al. reported a prevalence of 40% for CIPN in CRC patients six to eight months after finalizing their treatment containing OX [1]. CIPN is related to various risk factors, including treatment schedule, dose per course, cumulative dose, time of infusion and pre-existing peripheral neuropathy [1]. These factors likely vary between studies and countries. Furthermore, difference in the prevalence of CIPN may be explained by different methods to assess CIPN. Most previous studies used criteria of the National Cancer Institute (NCI-CTCAE) or the total neuropathy score (TNSc) to assess CIPN [4–7]. These methods are based on clinical examination, while the QLQ-CIPN16 is a patient-reported assessment of CIPN. The use of the QLQ-CIPN16 is inherent to the large-scale setting of the COLON cohort study. Recent studies compared several commonly used methods to assess CIPN [29,30]. A high correlation was found for the NCI-CTCAE and the EORTC QLQ-CIPN [29,30]. Furthermore, we did expect a high prevalence of sensory symptoms, and not motor symptoms, since OX is mainly associated with chronic sensory CIPN [1,31]. Although motor symptoms were also commonly reported in our study, it should be noted that the severity of motor symptoms was relatively low in the present study (mean score 12.5 versus 20.8 for sensory symptoms).

In the present study, we found that a higher magnesium intake was associated with a lower severity of chronic CIPN, whereas no association for calcium was found. Both magnesium and calcium are involved in electric excitability of neurons and muscle contraction [8]. A potential explanation for the association between magnesium and the severity of CIPN is the role of magnesium in the neuromuscular system and nervous tissue conduction [32]. It has been supposed that CIPN is caused by the stimulating effect of OX on neural excitability due to re-configuration of sodium channels in the cell membrane [33]. Magnesium (and calcium) are hypothesized to decrease OX-induced hyper-excitability [34,35], thereby limiting damage of neurons. In addition, magnesium specifically plays a role in membrane integrity and stability [32].

In the present study, we focused for the first time on dietary intake of magnesium and calcium in relation to CIPN. It should be noted that magnesium levels in blood are tightly regulated [36]. When circulating levels of magnesium are low, other tissues such as bone and muscle provide magnesium to restore circulating magnesium levels. With a low magnesium intake, body stores of magnesium could be depleted, while circulating levels are still in the healthy range [3,37]. Among our study population, 65% of the patients had an intake below the estimated average requirement of 350 mg/day for men and 265 mg/day for women [28] during chemotherapy. Hypothetically, especially patients with a low intake of magnesium could benefit from additional intake of magnesium, as a higher intake could restore depleted body stores of magnesium and thereby increases availability of magnesium in muscles and nerves. Stratified analyses for age showed a stronger association in patients aged 65 years and older. In this group the percentages of patients with a magnesium intake below the estimated average requirement was higher compared to participants younger than 65. In addition, during chemotherapy more participants had a magnesium intake below the estimated average requirement compared to before and after chemotherapy. These results indicate that an optimal magnesium status throughout treatment is important. Further studies are needed to confirm these findings and to determine the clinical relevance of the reported association between magnesium and CIPN.

The present study has some limitations. First, intake from dietary supplements was not considered because of the relative limited number of supplement users. In addition detailed data on dosage, frequency and compliance was lacking and supplement use was not consistent over the study duration. Also, the mineral content of the drinking water was not considered. Magnesium and calcium from drinking water contribute to the total magnesium and calcium intake. In the Netherlands, magnesium and calcium content in the tap water ranges from 1.7–26.2 mg/L (1–8% of the total intake) and 15–157 mg/L (1–17% of the total intake), respectively [38]. Second, although we explored the possible interaction between magnesium or calcium and many nutrients like B vitamins, calcium, vitamin D, vitamin E and alcohol, we could not exclude the possibility that other nutrients or bioactive compounds contributed to the observed effects. Third, the prevalence of pre-existing CIPN was not taken into account. Pre-existing CIPN is a risk factor for developing chronic CIPN [1]. Diabetes mellitus is an important cause of peripheral neuropathy [39]. However, in the present study, adjustment for self-reported diabetes mellitus did not influence the observed associations. In addition, we have not been able to take specific information on treatment-related factors, such as cumulative dose of chemotherapy and use of specific medications that may have influenced magnesium status into account. However, in the specific setting of studies focusing on long-term (chronic) toxicities, dose is a complicated factor. Patients who received a low (cumulative) dose may have experienced severe (acute) toxicities which have resulted in a dose reduction or premature discontinuation of therapy. Because of severe toxicities, among which potentially CIPN, an increased risk of chronic CIPN on the long-term may be expected. On the other hand, patients who completed their scheduled treatment, and hence received a high (cumulative) dose, may also have an increased risk of CIPN because of extensive exposure to the cytotoxic regimens. Furthermore, although information on clinical and socio-demographic characteristics of patients who did not fill out the QLQ-CIPN16 ($n = 67$, 23%) was available, it remains unknown why they did not fill out the questionnaires. It could be that these patients suffered from CIPN symptoms in their hands, resulting in selection which theoretically could decrease the validity of the present study. However, we do not expect that these non-responses had a major impact on the results of our study as the overall response rate was high (77%). The sample size of this study was relatively small ($n = 196$) and restricted to CRC patients and therefore we cannot state yet if generalization of our results to other cancer patients or chemotherapeutic agents is justified. Finally, we did not measure blood levels of magnesium and calcium. It should be noted, however, that the specific objective of this study was to investigate the association between dietary intake of magnesium and CIPN. Next to that, circulating levels are tightly regulated and not representative for magnesium levels in muscles and bone [37].

The present study also has important strengths. First of all, this is the first prospective cohort study which assessed the association between habitual dietary intake of magnesium or calcium and CIPN. Our data extend and complement existing evidence regarding the association between magnesium, calcium and neuropathy. Previous studies focusing on infusions with magnesium and calcium showed inconsistent findings and relied on acute exposure, while we assessed habitual, long-term intake of magnesium and calcium. In addition, previous studies focused on acute CIPN (during and directly after chemotherapy), while we focused on chronic and persistent CIPN. Therefore, this study provides an important contribution to the limited knowledge on chronic CIPN and its association with diet before, during and after chemotherapy. Furthermore, in the present study we used the 16 items of the QLQ-CIPN20 that are considered to be valid and reliable [22]. This approach resulted in a clinically relevant estimation of the prevalence and severity of CIPN compared to the QLQ-CIPN20 [22]. Due the availability of detailed data on diet and other clinical and lifestyle factors, we could adjust for the most plausible confounders, although residual confounding can never be fully excluded.

5. Conclusions

The results of this study showed that a higher dietary magnesium intake was associated with a lower prevalence and less severe CIPN symptoms among CRC patients who received adjuvant chemotherapy. Further studies are needed to confirm our findings and to provide a solid basis for future recommendations directed towards the intake of magnesium before and during chemotherapy.

Acknowledgments: The authors would like to thank the co-workers from the following hospitals for their involvement in recruitment for the COLON study: Hospital Gelderse Vallei, Ede; RadboudUMC, Nijmegen; Slingeland Hospital, Doetinchem,; Canisius Wilhelmina Hospital, Nijmegen; Rijnstate Hospital, Arnhem; Gelre Hospitals, Apeldoorn/Zutphen; Hospital Bernhoven, Uden; Isala, Zwolle; ZGT, Almelo; Martini Hospital, Groningen; Admiraal de Ruyter Hospital, Goes/Vlissingen, all in The Netherlands. Sources of support: This project is sponsored by Wereld Kanker Onderzoek Fonds (WCRF-NL) & World Cancer Research Fund International (WCRF International 2014/1179); Alped'Huzes / Dutch Cancer Society (UM 2012–5653, UW 2013–5927; UW 2015-7946).

Author Contributions: E.W., R.M.W., E.K. and D.E.G.K. contributed to the conception and design of this study. B.M.E.H., H.K.v.H. and H.d.W. contributed to the recruitment of participants. M.v.Z., H.v.B., A.J.M.R.G. and E.W. contributed to recruitment of participants and the data collection. Statistical data analyses were done and interpreted by E.W. The manuscript was drafted by E.W. and D.E.G.K., who also had primary responsibility, and all authors critically read and revised the manuscript. All authors approved the final version of the manuscript. The datasets used and analyzed during the current study are available from the corresponding author on reasonable request.

References

1. Argyriou, A.A.; Polychronopoulos, P.; Iconomou, G.; Chroni, E.; Kalofonos, H.P. A review on oxaliplatin-induced peripheral nerve damage. *Cancer Treat. Rev.* **2008**, *34*, 368–377. [CrossRef] [PubMed]

2. Staff, N.P.; Grisold, A.; Grisold, W.; Windebank, A.J. Chemotherapy-Induced Peripheral Neuropathy: A Current Review. *Ann. Neurol.* **2017**, *81*, 772–781. [CrossRef] [PubMed]

3. Vincenzi, B.; Frezza, A.M.; Schiavon, G.; Spoto, C.; Silvestris, N.; Addeo, R.; Catalano, V.; Graziano, F.; Santini, D.; Tonini, G. Identification of clinical predictive factors of oxaliplatin-induced chronic peripheral neuropathy in colorectal cancer patients treated with adjuvant Folfox IV. *Support. Care Cancer* **2013**, *21*, 1313–1319. [CrossRef] [PubMed]

4. Attal, N.; Bouhassira, D.; Gautron, M.; Vaillant, J.N.; Mitry, E.; Lepère, C.; Rougier, P.; Guirimand, F. Thermal hyperalgesia as a marker of oxaliplatin neurotoxicity: A prospective quantified sensory assessment study. *Pain* **2009**, *144*, 245–252. [CrossRef] [PubMed]

5. André, T.; de Gramont, A.; Vernerey, D.; Chibaudel, B.; Bonnetain, F.; Tijeras-Raballand, A.; Scriva, A.; Hickish, T.; Tabernero, J.; Van Laethem, J.L.; et al. Adjuvant Fluorouracil, Leucovorin, and Oxaliplatin in Stage II to III Colon Cancer: Updated 10-Year Survival and Outcomes According to BRAF Mutation and Mismatch Repair Status of the MOSAIC Study. *J. Clin. Oncol.* **2015**, *33*, 4176–4187. [CrossRef] [PubMed]

6. De Gramont, A.; Figer, A.; Seymour, M.; Homerin, M.; Hmissi, A.; Cassidy, J.; Boni, C.; Cortes-Funes, H.; Cervantes, A.; Freyer, G.; et al. Leucovorin and fluorouracil with or without oxaliplatin as first-line treatment in advanced colorectal cancer. *J. Clin. Oncol.* **2000**, *18*, 2938–2947. [CrossRef] [PubMed]

7. Extra, J.M.; Marty, M.; Brienza, S.; Misset, J.L. Pharmacokinetics and safety profile of oxaliplatin. *Semin. Oncol.* **1998**, *25*, 13–22. [PubMed]

8. Laires, M.J.; Monteiro, C.P.; Bicho, M. Role of cellular magnesium in health and human disease. *Front. Biosci.* **2004**, *9*, 262–276. [CrossRef] [PubMed]

9. Gamelin, L.; Boisdron-Celle, M.; Delva, R.; Guérin-Meyer, V.; Ifrah, N.; Morel, A.; Gamelin, E. Prevention of oxaliplatin-related neurotoxicity by calcium and magnesium infusions: A retrospective study of 161 patients receiving oxaliplatin combined with 5-Fluorouracil and leucovorin for advanced colorectal cancer. *Clin. Cancer Res.* **2004**, *10*, 4055–4061. [CrossRef] [PubMed]

10. Knijn, N.; Tol, J.; Koopman, M.; Werter, M.J.B.P.; Imholz, A.L.T.; Valster, F.A.A.; Mol, L.; Vincent, A.D.; Teerenstra, S.; Punt, C.J.A. The effect of prophylactic calcium and magnesium infusions on the incidence of neurotoxicity and clinical outcome of oxaliplatin-based systemic treatment in advanced colorectal cancer patients. *Eur. J. Cancer* **2011**, *47*, 369–374. [CrossRef] [PubMed]

11. Kono, T.; Mamiya, N.; Chisato, N.; Ebisawa, Y.; Yamazaki, H.; Watari, J.; Yamamoto, Y.; Suzuki, S.; Asama, T.; Kamiya, K. Efficacy of Goshajinkigan for Peripheral Neurotoxicity of Oxaliplatin in Patients with Advanced or Recurrent Colorectal Cancer. *Evid.-Based Complement. Altern. Med.* **2011**, *2011*, 418481. [CrossRef] [PubMed]

12. Grothey, A.; Nikcevich, D.A.; Sloan, J.A.; Kugler, J.W.; Silberstein, P.T.; Dentchev, T.; Wender, D.B.; Novotny, P.J.; Chitaley, U.; Alberts, S.R.; et al. Intravenous calcium and magnesium for oxaliplatin-induced

sensory neurotoxicity in adjuvant colon cancer: NCCTG N04C7. *J. Clin. Oncol.* **2011**, *29*, 421–427. [CrossRef] [PubMed]

13. Hochster, H.S.; Grothey, A.; Hart, L.; Rowland, K.; Ansari, R.; Alberts, S.; Chowhan, N.; Ramanathan, R.K.; Keaton, M.; Hainsworth, J.D.; et al. Improved time to treatment failure with an intermittent oxaliplatin strategy: Results of CONcePT. *Ann. Oncol.* **2014**, *25*, 1172–1178. [CrossRef] [PubMed]

14. Loprinzi, C.L.; Qin, R.; Dakhil, S.R.; Fehrenbacher, L.; Flynn, K.A.; Atherton, P.; Seisler, D.; Qamar, R.; Lewis, G.C.; Grothey, A. Phase III randomized, placebo-controlled, double-blind study of intravenous calcium and magnesium to prevent oxaliplatin-induced sensory neurotoxicity (N08CB/Alliance). *J. Clin. Oncol.* **2014**, *32*, 997–1005. [CrossRef] [PubMed]

15. Ishibashi, K.; Okada, N.; Miyazaki, T.; Sano, M.; Ishida, H. Effect of calcium and magnesium on neurotoxicity and blood platinum concentrations in patients receiving mFOLFOX6 therapy: A prospective randomized study. *Int. J. Clin. Oncol.* **2010**, *15*, 82–87. [CrossRef] [PubMed]

16. Chay, W.-Y.; Tan, S.-H.; Lo, Y.-L.; Ong, S.Y.-K.; Ng, H.-C.; Gao, F.; Koo, W.-H.; Choo, S.-P. Use of calcium and magnesium infusions in prevention of oxaliplatin induced sensory neuropathy. *Asia Pac. J. Clin. Oncol.* **2010**, *6*, 270–277. [CrossRef] [PubMed]

17. Albers, J.W.; Chaudhry, V.; Cavaletti, G.; Donehower, R.C. Interventions for preventing neuropathy caused by cisplatin and related compounds. In *Cochrane Database of Systematic Reviews*; Albers, J.W., Ed.; John Wiley & Sons, Ltd.: Chichester, UK, 2014; p. CD005228.

18. Winkels, R.M.; Heine-Bröring, R.C.; van Zutphen, M.; van Harten-Gerritsen, S.; Kok, D.E.G.; van Duijnhoven, F.J.B.; Kampman, E. The COLON study: Colorectal cancer: Longitudinal, Observational study on Nutritional and lifestyle factors that may influence colorectal tumour recurrence, survival and quality of life. *BMC Cancer* **2014**, *14*, 374. [CrossRef] [PubMed]

19. Van Leersum, N.J.; Snijders, H.S.; Henneman, D.; Kolfschoten, N.E.; Gooiker, G.A.; ten Berge, M.G.; Eddes, E.H.; Wouters, M.W.J. M.; Tollenaar, R.A.E.M.; Bemelman, W.A.; et al. The Dutch Surgical Colorectal Audit. *Eur. J. Surg. Oncol.* **2013**, *39*, 1063–1070. [CrossRef] [PubMed]

20. Netherlands Nutrition Center: NEVO Nederlandse Voedingsmiddelen Tabel 2011 (In Englisch: Dutch Food Composition Table). Available online: http://nevo-online.rivm.nl/ (accessed on 10 May 2016).

21. Willett, W.C.; Howe, G.R.; Kushi, L.H. Adjustment for total energy intake in epidemiologic studies. *Am. J. Clin. Nutr.* **1997**, *65*, 1220S–1228S. [CrossRef] [PubMed]

22. Lavoie Smith, E.M.; Barton, D.L.; Qin, R.; Steen, P.D.; Aaronson, N.K.; Loprinzi, C.L. Assessing patient-reported peripheral neuropathy: The reliability and validity of the European Organization for Research and Treatment of Cancer QLQ-CIPN20 Questionnaire. *Qual. Life Res.* **2013**, *22*, 2787–2799. [CrossRef] [PubMed]

23. Mols, F.; van de Poll-Franse, L.V.; Vreugdenhil, G.; Beijers, A.J.; Kieffer, J.M.; Aaronson, N.K.; Husson, O. Reference data of the European Organisation for Research and Treatment of Cancer (EORTC) QLQ-CIPN20 Questionnaire in the general Dutch population. *Eur. J. Cancer* **2016**, *69*, 28–38. [CrossRef] [PubMed]

24. Roth, P.L. Missing Data in Multiple Item Scales: A Monte Carlo Analysis of Missing Data Techniques. *Organ. Res. Methods* **1999**, *2*, 211–232. [CrossRef]

25. Tamhane, A.R.; Westfall, A.O.; Burkholder, G.A.; Cutter, G.R. Prevalence odds ratio versus prevalence ratio: Choice comes with consequences. *Stat. Med.* **2016**, *35*, 5730–5735. [CrossRef] [PubMed]

26. Bewick, V.; Cheek, L.; Ball, J. Statistics review 8: Qualitative data—Tests of association. *Crit. Care* **2004**, *8*, 46–53. [CrossRef] [PubMed]

27. Institute of Medicine (US). Standing Committee on the Scientific Evaluation of Dietary Reference Intakes. Chapter 6 Magnesium; In *Dietary Reference Intakes for Calcium, Phosphorus, Magnesium, Vitamin D, and Fluoride*; National Academies Press US: Washington, DC, USA, 1997; pp. 71–145. ISBN 978-0-309-06403-3.

28. Institute of Medicine (US). Standing Committee on the Scientific Evaluation of Dietary Reference Intakes. Chapter 4 Calcium; In *Dietary Reference Intakes for Calcium, Phosphorus, Magnesium, Vitamin D, and Fluoride*; National Academies Press US: Washington, DC, USA, 1997; pp. 190–249. ISBN 978-0-309-06403-3.

29. Alberti, P.; Rossi, E.; Cornblath, D.R.; Merkies, I.S.J.; Postma, T.J.; Frigeni, B.; Bruna, J.; Velasco, R.; Argyriou, A.A.; Kalofonos, H.P.; et al. Physician-assessed and patient-reported outcome measures in chemotherapy-induced sensory peripheral neurotoxicity: Two sides of the same coin. *Ann. Oncol.* **2014**, *25*, 257–264. [CrossRef] [PubMed]

30. Le-Rademacher, J.; Kanwar, R.; Seisler, D.; Pachman, D.R.; Qin, R.; Abyzov, A.; Ruddy, K.J.; Banck, M.S.; Lavoie Smith, E.M.; Dorsey, S.G.; et al. Patient-reported (EORTC QLQ-CIPN20) versus physician-reported

(CTCAE) quantification of oxaliplatin- and paclitaxel/carboplatin-induced peripheral neuropathy in NCCTG/Alliance clinical trials. *Support. Care Cancer* **2017**, *25*, 3537–3544. [CrossRef] [PubMed]

31. Cavaletti, G.; Cornblath, D.R.; Merkies, I.S.J.; Postma, T.J.; Rossi, E.; Frigeni, B.; Alberti, P.; Bruna, J.; Velasco, R.; Argyriou, A.A.; et al. The chemotherapy-induced peripheral neuropathy outcome measures standardization study: From consensus to the first validity and reliability findings. *Ann. Oncol.* **2013**, *24*, 454–462. [CrossRef] [PubMed]

32. Hoenderop, J.G.J.; Bindels, R.J.M. Epithelial Ca^{2+} and Mg^{2+} Channels in Health and Disease. *J. Am. Soc. Nephrol.* **2004**, *16*, 15–26. [CrossRef] [PubMed]

33. Gamelin, E.; Gamelin, L.; Bossi, L.; Quasthoff, S. Clinical aspects and molecular basis of oxaliplatin neurotoxicity: Current management and development of preventive measures. *Semin. Oncol.* **2002**, *29*, 21–33. [CrossRef] [PubMed]

34. Bara, M.; Guiet-Bara, A.; Durlach, J. Regulation of sodium and potassium pathways by magnesium in cell membranes. *Magnes. Res.* **1993**, *6*, 167–177. [PubMed]

35. Miltenburg, N.C.; Boogerd, W. Chemotherapy-induced neuropathy: A comprehensive survey. *Cancer Treat. Rev.* **2014**, *40*, 872–882. [CrossRef] [PubMed]

36. De Baaij, J.H.F.; Hoenderop, J.G.J.; Bindels, R.J.M. Regulation of magnesium balance: Lessons learned from human genetic disease. *Clin. Kidney J.* **2012**, *5*, i15–i24. [CrossRef] [PubMed]

37. Elin, R.J. Magnesium: The Fifth but Forgotten Electrolyte. *Am. J. Clin. Pathol.* **1994**, *102*, 616–622. [CrossRef] [PubMed]

38. Leurs, J.L.; Schouten, L.J.; Mons, M.N.; Goldbohm, R.A.; van den Brandt, P. Relationship between Tap Water Hardness, Magnesium, and Calcium Concentration and Mortality Due to Ischemic Heart Disease or Stroke in the Netherlands. *Environ. Health Perspect.* **2010**, *118*, 414–420. [CrossRef] [PubMed]

39. Wolf, S.; Barton, D.; Kottschade, L.; Grothey, A.; Loprinzi, C. Chemotherapy-induced peripheral neuropathy: Prevention and treatment strategies. *Eur. J. Cancer* **2008**, *44*, 1507–1515. [CrossRef] [PubMed]

7

Serum Magnesium after Kidney Transplantation

Anne-Sophie Garnier [1,2], **Agnès Duveau** [1,2], **Martin Planchais** [1,2], **Jean-François Subra** [1,2,3], **Johnny Sayegh** [1,2] **and Jean-François Augusto** [1,2,3,*]

[1]   LUNAM Université, 49180 Angers, France; AnneSophie.Garnier@chu-angers.fr (A.-S.G.);
      agnes.duveau@chu-angers.fr (A.D.); martin.planchais@chu-angers.fr (M.P.); jfsubra@chu-angers.fr (J.-F.S.);
      josayegh@chu-angers.fr (J.S.)
[2]   Université Angers, CHU Angers, Service de Néphrologie-Dialyse-Transplantation, CHU d'Angers,
      49933 Angers CEDEX 9, France
[3]   CRCINA, INSERM, Université de Nantes, Université d'Angers, LabEx IGO Immunotherapy,
      Graft, Oncology, 44007 Angers, France
*   Correspondence: jfaugusto@chu-angers.fr

Abstract: Magnesium (Mg) status has recently drawn close attention in chronic kidney disease and in kidney transplant recipients. This review aims to evaluate the body of evidence linking hypomagnesemia to clinical consequences in these specific populations. After a brief summary of the main mechanisms involved in Mg regulation and of Mg status in end-stage renal disease, the review focuses on the relationship between hypomagnesemia and cardiovascular risk in kidney transplant recipients. A body of evidence in recent studies points to a negative impact of hypomagnesemia on post-transplant diabetes mellitus (PTDM) and cardiovascular risk, which currently represent the main threat for morbidity and mortality in kidney transplantation. Deleterious biological mechanisms induced by hypomagnesemia are also discussed. While data analysis enables us to conclude that hypomagnesemia is linked to the development of PTDM, studies prospectively evaluating the impact of hypomagnesemia correction after kidney transplantation are still lacking and needed.

Keywords: Magnesium-Kidney; transplantation-New-onset; diabetes after transplantation-cardiovascular risk

1. Magnesium: Physiology

Magnesium (Mg) is the fourth cation of the body and the second most prevalent intracellular cation [1]. Approximately half of total body Mg is located in bone [2], the remainder being contained in skeletal muscles and soft tissues [1]. Extracellular Mg represents only 1% of total body Mg [3] and is mostly found in serum with concentrations ranging between 0.65 to 1.05 mmol/L [4] and in red blood cells [3]. It is present in three different states: ionized Mg (55–70%), protein-bound Mg (20–30%), and Mg complexed with anions such as bicarbonate or phosphate (5–15%) [1].

Mg homeostasis is mainly dependent on intestinal absorption and renal excretion. In the intestine, absorption is modulated by luminal Mg concentration, at high concentrations, Mg is regulated by an active transcellular transport and passive paracellular diffusion; whereas in low concentrations, Mg is absorbed by an active transcellular pathway involving a Transient Receptor Potential Melastatin 6 (TRPM6) channel expressed on the small intestine cells [5].

In patients with normal kidney function, around 70 to 80% of plasma Mg is ultra-filtrable. About 40% of the filtered Mg is reabsorbed in the proximal tubule by paracellular uptake, while 50% is absorbed in the ascending limb of the loop of Henle and 5% is absorbed in the distal tubule by an active transport. Thus, only 5% of filtered Mg is excreted in final urine, but this excretion can vary widely from 0.5 to 70% to keep plasma Mg concentration within the normal range [6]. Figure 1 summarizes Mg exchange in nephron.

Hypomagnesemia is frequently associated with hypokalemia [7]. This is mainly due to common disorders leading to ion wasting, such as through diuretic intake or diarrhea.

However, reduction of intracellular Mg concentration induces a decline in ATP activity that in turn affects potassium ATP-dependent channels located in the ascending limb and cortical collecting tubule, leading to urinary potassium loss [8,9]. This mechanism may explain the common resistance to hypokalemia correction until hypomagnesemia is normalized.

Figure 1. Magnesium exchanges in nephron. PCT, proximal convoluted tubule; DCT, distal convoluted tubule.

2. Clinical Signs and Etiologies of Hypomagnesemia

Clinical manifestations of hypomagnesemia are quite unspecific. Early signs include nausea, vomiting, anorexia and weakness [1]. Neuromuscular signs can also be present, including numbness, tingling, cramps, fasciculation seizures and neuropsychological disorders [1]. Severe hypomagnesemia has been associated with cardiac arrhythmia and coronary spasm [10]. Mg depletion can induce changes in electrocardiogram readings from pointed T waves in mild hypomagnesemia to widening of the QRS complex, prolongation of the PR interval and ventricular arrhythmias in patients with severe Mg depletion. Arrhythmias are more frequently observed in the setting of an acute ischemic event [11], congestive heart failure—partly due to the administration of diuretics—or after a cardiopulmonary bypass [12]. Some authors showed that administration of magnesium after a cardiopulmonary bypass may prevent postoperative arrhythmias [13].

Hypomagnesemia results mainly from gastrointestinal and renal losses. Gastrointestinal losses can arise from diarrhea, malabsorption, steatorrhea, small bowel bypass surgery, acute pancreatitis and dietary deprivation [14]. Rarely, hypomagnesemia may occur due to a selective defect in the intestinal Mg absorption, also known as primary intestinal hypomagnesemia. Urinary Mg losses can be induced by loop or thiazide-type diuretics, volume expansion, alcohol, hypercalcemia, nephrotoxins such as aminoglycoside antibiotics, cisplatin or cyclosporine. Urinary Mg wasting can also be due to loop of Henle or distal tubule dysfunction, after acute tubular necrosis, post-obstructive diuresis or kidney transplantation [1,14]. Lastly, primary renal Mg wasting was observed in Bartter and Gitelman syndromes, in which hypomagnesemia is associated with hypercalciuria and hypocalciuria respectively [14].

3. Magnesium Status in CKD Patients

Chronic kidney disease (CKD) is frequently associated with hypermagnesaemia, which is usually mild or asymptomatic until end-stage renal disease (ESRD). In moderate CKD patients, increased fractional excretion of Mg compensates for a decline in renal function, providing a stable serum Mg within the normal range. However, in CKD stages IV-V, this compensatory mechanism becomes insufficient which results in hypermagnesaemia [6]. Thus, in this setting, dietary Mg intake and administration of Mg-containing drugs, such as laxatives or antacids, can more easily induce hypermagnesaemia [6]. Alternatively, Mg balance may be negative in some ESRD patients on high doses of diuretics, with reduced gastrointestinal uptake induced by severe metabolic acidosis or reduced albumin levels [5].

Dialysate Mg concentration has a significant impact on Mg balance in hemodialysis (HD) or peritoneal dialysis (PD) patients. Indeed, Mg has a significant diffusion across dialysis membranes and its elimination depends on ultrafiltration and the diffusible gradient between the serum and dialysate concentration. A significant reduction in serum Mg concentration has been observed in HD patients, probably due to the Gibbs–Donnan effect [15]. Conversely, mild hypermagnesemia is frequently observed in PD patients, because Mg concentration of PD "standard dialysate" is about 0.75 mmol/L [16]. Interestingly, bone appears as the greatest Mg reservoir in CKD patients. To support this, a 70% increase in both cortical and trabecular bone Mg content has been reported in uremic patients, compared to non-uremic patients, suggesting that dialysis induces positive net Mg balance in ESRD patients.

4. Magnesium and Cardiovascular Risk in CKD Patients

Several studies have shown an association between Mg status and survival in ESRD patients. Indeed, Ishimura et al. investigated the prognostic value of serum Mg concentration in 515 patients on maintenance hemodialysis (60 ± 12 years, 306 males and 209 females; 24% diabetics). Mortality was significantly higher in the lower Mg group (<2.77 mg/dL, i.e., <1.14 mmol/L, $n = 261$), compared to the higher Mg group ($\geq$2.77 mg/dL, $n = 254$) ($p < 0.001$). Thus, serum Mg was predictive of mortality (HR (per 1 mg/dL increase), 0.485 (95% CI, 0.241–0.975), $p = 0.0424$), particularly of non-cardiovascular mortality (HR 0.318 (95% CI, 0.132 to 0.769), $p = 0.0110$), after adjustment on confounding factors, including age, gender, hemodialysis duration and presence of diabetes [17]. Likewise, in a nationwide registry-based cohort of 142,555 hemodialysis patients, Sakaguchi et al. moreover observed a U-shaped relation with higher all-cause and cardiovascular mortality of patients in both the lowest Mg sextile (<0.95 mmol/L) and the highest (>1.27 mmol/L) [18].

Several studies maintain that the increased cardiovascular mortality in hypomagnaesemic ESRD patients may be related to accelerated atherosclerosis. In an observational study, PD patients who developed arterial calcifications had significantly lower serum Mg levels ($p < 0.001$) [19]. Similar results were found in a retrospective cohort of 390 non-diabetic and hemodialysis patients. Serum Mg was significantly lower in patients with vascular calcification than in those without (2.69 ± 0.28 vs. 2.78 ± 0.33 mg/dL, $p < 0.05$). Serum Mg concentration appeared as an independent risk factor of vascular calcification (OR 0.28, 95% CI 0.09–0.92/1 mg/dL increase in serum magnesium, $p = 0.036$) after adjustments for age, gender, duration of hemodialysis, calcium, phosphate and intact parathyroid hormone concentrations [20]. Given these observations, some authors investigated the effect of Mg supplementation in ESRD patients. In one study, 47 hemodialysis patients were randomized to one group receiving oral Mg citrate (610 mg per day) and oral calcium acetate, and the other oral calcium acetate and a placebo. After 2 months, patients receiving Mg had a significant decrease in intima-media thickness (0.70 vs. 0.97 mm, p = 0.001 and 0.78 vs. 0.95 mm, p = 0.002 for left and right carotid arteries respectively) [21]. In another work, hemodialysis patients were randomized to receive low (0.5 mmol/L) or high (0.75 mmol/L) dialysate Mg and were followed-up for 3 years. No difference was observed for all-cause mortality between groups, but an increase in cardiovascular mortality was observed after 3 years in the low dialysate Mg group (14.5% vs. 0%, p = 0.042) in HDM group [22].

5. Magnesium Status after Kidney Transplantation and Relation with Graft Function

Hypomagnesemia is frequently observed after kidney transplantation, in part to immunosuppressive regimens including calcineurin inhibitors (CNI) that induce Mg urinary waste. Hypomagnesemia was observed in 6.6% of patients treated with tacrolimus and in 1.5% of patients on cyclosporine [23]. The mechanisms leading to hypomagnesemia are not fully understood, but it has been shown that CNI induce a down-regulation of renal expression of the epidermal growth factor [24] and TRMP6 in the distal collecting tubule [25], leading to decreased Mg reabsorption. Sirolimus might induce hypomagnesemia through inhibition of Na-K-Cl co-transporter 2 expression in the thick ascending loop of Henle [26]. Renal Mg wasting has been shown to be similar between rats treated with sirolimus and those treated with cyclosporine or tacrolimus [27]. Many other factors influence Mg levels after kidney transplantation, such as post-transplantation volume expansion, metabolic acidosis, insulin resistance, decreased gastro-intestinal absorption due to diarrhea, low Mg intake and medication such as diuretics or proton pump inhibitors [28].

Hypomagnesemia was reported to develop frequently within the first few weeks following transplantation [29], with a serum Mg level nadir in the second month post-transplantation [30]. Hypomagnesemia may persist for several years after kidney transplantation. In a cohort of 49 kidney transplant recipients, 22.4% of patients had hypomagnesemia 6 years after transplantation [31]. As observed in the general population, serum Mg levels were inversely correlated with glomerular filtration rate [32].

The relationship between serum Mg and graft function has been poorly evaluated in literature. In a cohort study published in 2005, 320 kidney recipients were divided into two groups, based on median Mg level in the entire cohort: the low serum Mg group (n = 29, 0.74 (0.68–0.78) mmol/L) compared to the normal Mg group (n = 31, 0.9 (0.82–0.98) mmol/L, p < 0.05). The authors showed that hypomagnesemia was associated with a greater decline in allograft function and an increased risk of graft loss for patients with ciclosporine-induced nephropathy [33]. In animals studies, hypomagnesemia is associated with glomerular dysfunction and the development of chronic fibrotic lesions [34]. In mice treated with cyclosporine, Mg supplementation improved renal function and decreased kidney fibrotic lesions [35]. Likewise, Mg supplementation in cyclosporine-treated rats was associated with a reduction in tubular atrophy and interstitial fibrosis and prevented kidney function decline [34].

In murine studies, Mg supplementation has been shown to exert an effect using several mechanisms, including innate immune pathways. Indeed, Mg supplementation inhibits monocyte and macrophage recruitment, partly by abolishing expression of chemoattractant proteins (osteopontin and monocyte chemoattractant protein-1), fibrogenic molecules and extracellular matrix proteins [36]. Moreover, Mg induces down-regulation of endothelin-1 expression [36] and decreased nuclear factor kappa-light-chain-enhancer of activated B cells (NFkB) activation [37].

These data in human and mice converge to suggest that hypomagnesemia is not only associated with accelerated decline of graft function but is also an active contributor to renal lesions. Thus, prospective studies are needed to analyze the potential benefits of Mg supplements on graft function after kidney transplantation.

6. Serum Magnesium and New-Onset Diabetes Mellitus after Transplantation

6.1. Serum Magnesium and Diabetes Mellitus in the General Population

Hypomagnesemia has been reported to occur in 13.5 to 47.7% of non-hospitalized patients with type-2 diabetes [38]. Poor dietary Mg intake, glomerular hyperfiltration, osmotic diuresis, recurrent metabolic acidosis, hypophosphataemia and hypokalemia are all potential contributing factors for hypomagnesemia in diabetic patients [38,39]. A higher incidence of hypomagnesemia was reported in females as compared to males on a 2-to-1 ratio [40]. Several authors showed an inverse correlation between Mg intake and the risk of developing diabetes mellitus [41–44]. Moreover, in a study including 39,345 US women followed-up for 6 years, the protective role of high Mg intake was higher in the subgroup of overweight women [42]. In the Atherosclerosis Risk in Communities Study, low serum Mg level was an independent risk factor for incident diabetes mellitus [44].

The diabetogenic effects of hypomagnesemia are not yet well understood and have been attributed to several mechanisms. Data supporting the fact that hypomagnesemia may induce altered cellular glucose transport, reduced pancreatic insulin secretion, defective post-receptor insulin signaling and/or altered insulin–insulin receptor interactions have been reported. Dietary-induced Mg deficiency increased urinary thromboxane concentration and enhanced angiotensin-induced aldosterone synthesis, resulting in resistance to the effect of insulin [45]. This may be due to changes of tyrosine kinase expression on insulin receptor level and/or induction of inflammation and oxidative stress [46]. Conversely, it is interesting to note that oral Mg supplementation during a 16-week period showed an improvement in insulin sensitivity and a better metabolic control in type-2 diabetic patients [47].

6.2. Serum Magnesium and New-Onset Diabetes Mellitus after Transplantation

After transplantation, diabetes mellitus is frequently observed, with incidences ranging from 10 to 30%, depending on the criteria used for diagnosis and the length of follow-up [48,49]. Post-transplant diabetes mellitus (PTDM) affects both patient and graft survival [50], highlighting the importance of identifying potentially modifiable risk factors. Several risk factors for PTDM have already been identified, such as older age, male gender, ethnicity, acute rejection, hepatitis C, higher body mass index, higher pre-transplant glucose levels and higher trough tacrolimus levels [51–53], some of them being common risk factors for type-2 diabetes in the general population. Hypomagnesemia has recently been identified as an independent risk factor for PTDM, however with some conflicting data in literature. Van Laecke et al., in a retrospective study, were the first to identify a relationship between PTDM and post-transplant Mg level in a cohort of 254 kidney transplant recipients. Serum Mg values were recorded at months 1 and 2 after transplantation. 29.5% of recipients developed PTDM after a mean time of 90 ± 80 days post-transplantation. Patients with PTDM had significantly lower Mg levels compared to those without ($p < 0.001$). Post-transplant Mg appeared as an independent predictor of PTDM after adjustment on classical risk factors and on CNI use. Moreover, the association between the use of CNI and PTDM disappeared after adjustments to Mg levels in the multivariate analysis, suggesting that the diabetogenic effect of CNI may be more related to hypomagnesemia itself than to CNI [53]. In another study recently published, the association between serum Mg level and PTDM was examined in a retrospective cohort study of 948 non-diabetic kidney transplant recipients. The authors used multivariable Cox proportional hazards models to evaluate the risk of PTDM as a function of baseline (at 1 month post-transplantation), time-varying (every 3 months) and rolling-average (mean for 3 months moving at 3-month intervals). Hypomagnesemia, defined as a serum Mg concentration below 0.74 mmol/L, was significantly associated with an increased risk of PTDM in baseline (HR, 1.58; 95% CI, 1.07 to 2.34; $p = 0.02$), time-varying (HR, 1.78; 95% CI, 1.29 to 2.45; $p = 0.001$) and rolling-average models (HR, 1.83; 95% CI, 1.30 to 2.57; $p = 0.001$) [54].

The association between hypomagnesemia and PTDM was also studied in pediatric kidney recipients. In a retrospective cohort of 173 young recipients with a median age of 7 years at transplantation, 20 patients developed PTDM at 9 days post transplantation on average. Hypomagnesemia and high tacrolimus levels were significant and independent risk factors for PTDM ($p = 0.01$ and $p < 0.001$, respectively). No association between hypomagnesemia and tacrolimus levels was observed, suggesting that both risk factors were independent from each other [55]. Conversely, in a cohort study of 451 pediatric solid organ transplant recipients, Chanchlani et al. failed to identify an association between hypomagnesemia and PTDM. However, lack of close Mg monitoring and frequent Mg supplementation in their cohort (75% of children) make the study difficult to interpret [56]. Two other studies failed to demonstrate a significant difference in Mg levels between PTDM and non-PTDM adult recipients [57,58]. Osorio et al. analyzed 589 kidney recipients and did not identify a relationship between Mg levels and occurrence of PTDM in patients receiving CNI treatment [57]. Santos et al. observed similar results in a cohort of 205 kidney recipients [58]. However, again, in these studies, no information was given about immunosuppressive regimens, which also limits their interpretation.

In order to minimize the possible effect of post-transplant confounders, our group evaluated the relationship between pre-transplant hypomagnesemia and the risk of PTDM in a cohort of 154 kidney transplant recipients. 28 patients (18.2%) developed a PTDM within the first year of transplantation, and in most patients within the first 2 months. Patients who developed PTDM were older, had a higher body mass index and a higher pre-transplant glucose level, compared to patients without PTDM. The pre-transplant Mg level was significantly lower in patients that developed PTDM ($p = 0.014$). Moreover, a pre-transplant Mg level <2 mg/dL compared to >2.3 mg/dL was associated with a higher risk of PTDM within the first year of transplantation (HR, 2.99; 95% CI, 1.07–8.37, $p = 0.037$) [49]. In the field of liver transplantation, a retrospective cohort of 169 patients showed that both pre-transplant and month 1 post-transplant Mg levels were independent risk factors for PTDM [59]. In these studies, patients were free of diabetes mellitus at inclusion, thus hypomagnesemia was not the result of Mg wasting induced by diabetes.

Based on these observations, Van Laecke et al. investigated the effect of Mg supplementation on post-transplant glucose metabolism [60,61]. In a single-center parallel group study, 54 patients with serum Mg level ≤1.7 mg/dL were randomized to receive 450 mg oral Mg oxide (MgO) one to three times daily, aiming for an Mg concentration of >1.9 mg/dL ($n = 27$) or no treatment ($n = 27$). The primary outcome was a fasting serum glucose concentration at 3 months post-transplantation. Secondary outcomes were the 2 h area under the curve (AUC) for glycaemia and insulin resistance, assessed by a homeostasis model assessment-estimated insulin-resistance index (HOMA_IR) at month 3 post-transplantation. Six patients in the control group received MgO (450 mg daily) as serum Mg concentration dropped below to 1.2 mg/dL. Fasting serum glucose concentration was lower in the Mg group compared to the control group (95% CI; 1.7–21.3; $p = 0.02$), even after adjustment on tacrolimus concentrations. No differences were observed between groups for 2 h-AUC glucose and HOMA-IR. The authors suggest that a disparity in the timing of supplementation and consequent drug exposure along with the use of tacrolimus versus cyclosporine can explain the smaller effect of their intervention compared with other trials [60]. Similar results were observed in another study including 52 renal transplant recipients on tacrolimus with chronic hypomagnesemia. Recipients were randomized to the Mg group ($n = 26$), with a similar Mg supplementation as previously described, or the control group ($n = 26$). No differences between the groups were observed in first-phase insulin release, in second-phase insulin release, HbA1c and HOMA-IR index at month 6 post-transplantation [61]. The main limitation of this study was that oral Mg supplementation failed to increase both serum and intracellular Mg significantly over the concentrations observed in the control group. Thus, it was impossible to draw conclusions on the effects of Mg supplementation on insulin resistance and glucose metabolism.

While most studies converge to confirm that hypomagnesemia is an independent risk factor for PTDM, the impact of hypomagnesemia correction after kidney transplantation has not yet been fully explored. Literature analysis also highlights the need for studies in order to determine the best routes for Mg supplementation, formulations and doses to achieve normal serum Mg concentration in these patients.

An important issue is the impact of immunosuppressive regimen according to diabetes risk and their impact on post-transplant Mg status. As underline above, CNI induce renal Mg wasting which contributes to hypomagnesemia. In the study from Van Laecke et al., the association between CNI and PTDM disappeared after adjustment on Mg levels, suggesting that the diabetogenic effect of CNI was at least partially related to CNI-induced hypomagnesemia [53]. The switch from CNI to mTOR inhibitors has been shown to result in serum Mg increase [62]. Thus, the early use of mTOR inhibitors soon after transplantation could be an interesting approach to decrease PTDM risk. However, several reports have shown a diabetogenic effect of mTOR inhibitors, and in the study from Van Laecke et al., sirolimus appeared as an independent risk factor of PTDM [53,63]. Moreover, the use of mTOR inhibitors soon after kidney transplantation has been shown to be associated with a higher risk of allograft rejection [64]. For these reasons, mTOR inhibitor in replacement of CNI may not be an interesting approach to reduce PTDM risk.

7. Magnesium Status and Cardiovascular Risk before and after Kidney Transplantation

PTDM-associated mortality is mainly related to cardiovascular events, which are today the main causes of death in kidney transplant patients [65]. Hypomagnesemia has been shown to play a role in the pathogenesis of arterial hypertension, endothelial dysfunction, dyslipidemia and inflammation, with all these factors contributing to coronary heart disease (CHD).

In vitro, exposure of endothelial cells to low Mg concentrations reversibly inhibits endothelial proliferation and was associated with an up-regulation of interleukin-1, Vascular Cell Adhesion Molecule-1 and Plasminogen Activator Inhibitor-1 [66]. In vivo, hypomagnesemia is associated with increased CRP levels, leukocyte and macrophage activation, NFKB/cytokines activation and platelet aggregation. Furthermore, inbred mice with low intracellular Mg levels have significantly impaired endothelial function together with decreased endothelial NO synthase expression [67].

The relationship between CHD and serum Mg concentrations was studied in a cohort of 13,922 middle-age adults. In this study, after adjustment, the relative risk of CHD across quartiles of serum Mg was 1.00, 0.92, 0.48, and 0.44 (p for trend = 0.009) among women and 1.00, 1.32, 0.95, and 0.73 (p for trend = 0.07) among men. Moreover, patients who developed CHD had a lower serum Mg concentration than the controls, suggesting that low serum Mg was an independent risk factor for CHD [68].

In a Japanese cohort of 728 subjects, lower serum Mg was significantly and independently associated with mean intima-media thickness (p = 0.004) and risk of $\geq$2 carotid plaques (p = 0.03) [69]. Hypomagnesemia was also reported to directly or indirectly affect vascular stiffness in the general population [70]. In another study, Mg supplementation improved endothelial dysfunction in patients with CHD [71]. In parallel, hypomagnesemia may play a role in the promotion and progression of vascular calcification as underlined earlier. Indeed, Mg is known to prevent tissue calcification by increasing natural inhibitors of calcification such as fetuin A, carboxylated matrix Gla protein (MGP), osteopontin and the inorganic inhibitory compound pyrophosphate [72].

Few studies investigated the association between Mg levels and cardiovascular risk after kidney transplantation. In a small crossover trial published in 1998, 15 renal transplant patients were randomized in a 6-week treatment period with either placebo or Mg oxide (MgO) 2 g per os with a 2-week washout interval, then 6-weeks of the alternative agent (placebo or MgO). There was no reduction in systolic or diastolic blood pressure in either cholesterol or triglyceride level with magnesium supplementation [73].

Finally, the association between serum Mg level and cardiovascular risk after kidney transplantation has been poorly studied. A small crossover trial, including 15 kidney transplant patients randomized in a 6-week treatment period with either the placebo or Mg oxide (MgO) 2 g per os with a 2-week washout interval, then 6-weeks of the alternative agent (placebo or MgO), was published 1998. No change in metabolic profile, including systolic or diastolic blood pressure control, or cholesterol or triglyceride levels was observed with Mg supplementation [73]. The relationship between hypomagnesemia and vascular stiffness was investigated in a study published in 2011. An evaluation was conducted in 512 renal transplant recipients, by determination of carotid-femoral pulse wave velocity. Serum Mg was an independent risk factor for arterial stiffness, but this association was attenuated after adjustment on the use of sirolimus ($p = 0.054$). After stratification according to the median age of 55 years and adjustment with covariates, Mg remained an independent predictor of pulse wave velocity ($p = 0.024$) [74].

8. Conclusions

Despite relying on retrospective studies, a body of evidence links hypomagnesemia to PTDM and cardiovascular risk in kidney transplant patients (Figure 2). Given the frequency of PTDM and its relationship with cardiovascular risk, correcting hypomagnesemia soon after transplantation could translate into a significant decrease in vascular disease, which today is the primary cause of death in kidney transplant recipients. Thus, prospective studies to evaluate the impact of hypomagnesemia correction after kidney transplantation, as well as the best ways of achieving correction are needed.

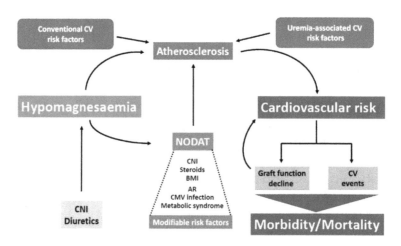

Figure 2. Deleterious effects of hypomagnesaemia after kidney transplantation. Several studies support that posttransplant hypomagnesaemia increases cardiovascular (CV) risk by increasing the risk of post-transplant diabetes mellitus (PTDM) development and by favoring accelerated atherosclerosis, along with other more conventional risk factors. We suggest that hypomagnesaemia correction soon after kidney transplantation may allow to decrease CV risk and result in less CV-related morbidity and mortality in kidney transplant recipients.

Author Contributions: A.-S.G., wrote and revised the manuscript. A.D., revised the manuscript. M.P., revised the manuscript. J.-F.S., revised the manuscript. J.S., revised the manuscript. J.-F.A., corresponding author wrote and revised the manuscript.

Abbreviations

AUC	Area under the curve
CKD	Chronic kidney disease
CNI	Calcineurin inhibitors
ESRD	End-stage renal disease
HD	Hemodialysis
HOMA_IR	Homeostasis model assessment-estimated insulin-resistance index
Mg	Magnesium
PD	Peritoneal dialysis
PTDM	Post-transplant diabetes mellitus
TRPM6	Transient Receptor Potential Melastatin 6

References

1. Jahnen-Dechent, W.; Ketteler, M. Magnesium basics. *Clin. Kidney J.* **2012**, *5*, i3–i14. [CrossRef] [PubMed]
2. Weisinger, J.R.; Bellorín-Font, E. Magnesium and phosphorus. *Lancet* **1998**, *352*, 391–396. [CrossRef]
3. Fawcett, W.J.; Haxby, E.J.; Male, D.A. Magnesium: Physiology and pharmacology. *Br. J. Anaesth.* **1999**, *83*, 302–320. [CrossRef] [PubMed]
4. Tietz, N.W.; Rinker, A.D.; Morrison, S.R. When is a serum iron really a serum iron? The status of serum iron measurements. *Clin. Chem.* **1994**, *40*, 546–551. [PubMed]
5. Kanbay, M.; Goldsmith, D.; Uyar, M.E.; Turgut, F.; Covic, A. Magnesium in chronic kidney disease: Challenges and opportunities. *Blood Purif.* **2010**, *29*, 280–292. [CrossRef] [PubMed]
6. Cunningham, J.; Rodríguez, M.; Messa, P. Magnesium in chronic kidney disease Stages 3 and 4 and in dialysis patients. *Clin. Kidney J.* **2012**, *5*, i39–i51. [CrossRef] [PubMed]
7. Whang, R.; Ryder, K.W. Frequency of hypomagnesemia and hypermagnesemia. Requested vs. routine. *JAMA* **1990**, *263*, 3063–3064. [CrossRef] [PubMed]
8. Nichols, C.G.; Ho, K.; Hebert, S. Mg(2+)-dependent inward rectification of ROMK1 potassium channels expressed in Xenopus oocytes. *J. Physiol. (Lond.)* **1994**, *476*, 399–409. [CrossRef]
9. Agus, Z.S.; Kelepouris, E.; Dukes, I.; Morad, M. Cytosolic magnesium modulates calcium channel activity in mammalian ventricular cells. *Am. J. Physiol.* **1989**, *256*, C452–C455. [CrossRef] [PubMed]
10. Hashizume, N.; Mori, M. An analysis of hypermagnesemia and hypomagnesemia. *Jpn. J. Med.* **1990**, *29*, 368–372. [CrossRef] [PubMed]
11. Kafka, H.; Langevin, L.; Armstrong, P.W. Serum magnesium and potassium in acute myocardial infarction. Influence on ventricular arrhythmias. *Arch. Intern. Med.* **1987**, *147*, 465–469. [CrossRef] [PubMed]
12. Aglio, L.S.; Stanford, G.G.; Maddi, R.; Boyd, J.L.; Nussbaum, S.; Chernow, B. Hypomagnesemia is common following cardiac surgery. *J. Cardiothorac. Vasc. Anesth.* **1991**, *5*, 201–208. [CrossRef]
13. England, M.R.; Gordon, G.; Salem, M.; Chernow, B. Magnesium administration and dysrhythmias after cardiac surgery. A placebo-controlled, double-blind, randomized trial. *JAMA* **1992**, *268*, 2395–2402. [CrossRef] [PubMed]
14. Agus, Z.S. Hypomagnesemia. *J. Am. Soc. Nephrol.* **1999**, *10*, 1616–1622. [PubMed]
15. Truttmann, A.C.; Faraone, R.; Von Vigier, R.O.; Nuoffer, J.M.; Pfister, R.; Bianchetti, M.G. Maintenance hemodialysis and circulating ionized magnesium. *Nephron* **2002**, *92*, 616–621. [CrossRef] [PubMed]
16. Blumenkrantz, M.J.; Kopple, J.D.; Moran, J.K.; Coburn, J.W. Metabolic balance studies and dietary protein requirements in patients undergoing continuous ambulatory peritoneal dialysis. *Kidney Int.* **1982**, *21*, 849–861. [CrossRef] [PubMed]
17. Ishimura, E.; Okuno, S.; Yamakawa, T.; Inaba, M.; Nishizawa, Y. Serum magnesium concentration is a significant predictor of mortality in maintenance hemodialysis patients. *Magnes. Res.* **2007**, *20*, 237–244. [PubMed]
18. Sakaguchi, Y.; Fujii, N.; Shoji, T.; Hayashi, T.; Rakugi, H.; Isaka, Y. Hypomagnesemia is a significant predictor of cardiovascular and non-cardiovascular mortality in patients undergoing hemodialysis. *Kidney Int.* **2014**, *85*, 174–181. [CrossRef] [PubMed]
19. Meema, H.E.; Oreopoulos, D.G.; Rapoport, A. Serum magnesium level and arterial calcification in end-stage renal disease. *Kidney Int.* **1987**, *32*, 388–394. [CrossRef] [PubMed]
20. Ishimura, E.; Okuno, S.; Kitatani, K.; Tsuchida, T.; Yamakawa, T.; Shioi, A.; Inaba, M.; Nishizawa, Y. Significant association between the presence of peripheral vascular calcification and lower serum magnesium in hemodialysis patients. *Clin. Nephrol.* **2007**, *68*, 222–227. [CrossRef] [PubMed]
21. Turgut, F.; Kanbay, M.; Metin, M.R.; Uz, E.; Akcay, A.; Covic, A. Magnesium supplementation helps to improve carotid intima media thickness in patients on hemodialysis. *Int. Urol. Nephrol.* **2008**, *40*, 1075–1082. [CrossRef] [PubMed]
22. Schmaderer, C.; Braunisch, M.C.; Suttmann, Y.; Lorenz, G.; Pham, D.; Haller, B.; Angermann, S.; Matschkal, J.; Renders, L.; Baumann, M.; et al. Reduced Mortality in Maintenance Haemodialysis Patients on High versus Low Dialysate Magnesium: A Pilot Study. *Nutrients* **2017**, *9*, 926. [CrossRef] [PubMed]
23. Margreiter, R. European Tacrolimus vs. Ciclosporin Microemulsion Renal Transplantation Study Group Efficacy and safety of tacrolimus compared with ciclosporin microemulsion in renal transplantation: A randomised multicentre study. *Lancet* **2002**, *359*, 741–746. [CrossRef]

24. Ledeganck, K.J.; De Winter, B.Y.; Van den Driessche, A.; Jürgens, A.; Bosmans, J.-L.; Couttenye, M.M.; Verpooten, G.A. Magnesium loss in cyclosporine-treated patients is related to renal epidermal growth factor downregulation. *Nephrol. Dial. Transplant.* **2014**, *29*, 1097–1102. [CrossRef] [PubMed]

25. Nijenhuis, T.; Hoenderop, J.G.J.; Bindels, R.J.M. Downregulation of Ca(2+) and Mg(2+) transport proteins in the kidney explains tacrolimus (FK506)-induced hypercalciuria and hypomagnesemia. *J. Am. Soc. Nephrol.* **2004**, *15*, 549–557. [CrossRef] [PubMed]

26. Da Silva, C.A.; de Bragança, A.C.; Shimizu, M.H.M.; Sanches, T.R.; Fortes, M.A.Z.; Giorgi, R.R.; Andrade, L.; Seguro, A.C. Rosiglitazone prevents sirolimus-induced hypomagnesemia, hypokalemia, and downregulation of NKCC2 protein expression. *Am. J. Physiol. Renal Physiol.* **2009**, *297*, F916–F922. [PubMed]

27. Andoh, T.F.; Burdmann, E.A.; Fransechini, N.; Houghton, D.C.; Bennett, W.M. Comparison of acute rapamycin nephrotoxicity with cyclosporine and FK506. *Kidney Int.* **1996**, *50*, 1110–1117. [CrossRef] [PubMed]

28. Van Laecke, S.; Van Biesen, W. Hypomagnesaemia in kidney transplantation. *Transplant. Rev.* **2015**, *29*, 154–160. [CrossRef] [PubMed]

29. Barton, C.H.; Vaziri, N.D.; Martin, D.C.; Choi, S.; Alikhani, S. Hypomagnesemia and renal magnesium wasting in renal transplant recipients receiving cyclosporine. *Am. J. Med.* **1987**, *83*, 693–699. [CrossRef]

30. Stevens, R.B.; Lane, J.T.; Boerner, B.P.; Miles, C.D.; Rigley, T.H.; Sandoz, J.P.; Nielsen, K.J.; Skorupa, J.Y.; Skorupa, A.J.; Kaplan, B.; Wrenshall, L.E. Single-dose rATG induction at renal transplantation: Superior renal function and glucoregulation with less hypomagnesemia: RATGS minimizes glucose dysregulation. *Clin. Transplant.* **2012**, *26*, 123–132. [CrossRef] [PubMed]

31. Van de Cauter, J.; Sennesael, J.; Haentjens, P. Long-term evolution of the mineral metabolism after renal transplantation: A prospective, single-center cohort study. *Transplant. Proc.* **2011**, *43*, 3470–3475. [CrossRef] [PubMed]

32. Rodrigues, N.; Santana, A.; Guerra, J.; Neves, M.; Nascimento, C.; Gonçalves, J.; da Costa, A.G. Serum Magnesium and Related Factors in Long-Term Renal Transplant Recipients: An Observational Study. *Transplant. Proc.* **2017**, *49*, 799–802. [CrossRef] [PubMed]

33. Holzmacher, R.; Kendziorski, C.; Michael Hofman, R.; Jaffery, J.; Becker, B.; Djamali, A. Low serum magnesium is associated with decreased graft survival in patients with chronic cyclosporin nephrotoxicity. *Nephrol. Dial. Transplant.* **2005**, *20*, 1456–1462. [CrossRef] [PubMed]

34. Miura, K.; Nakatani, T.; Asai, T.; Yamanaka, S.; Tamada, S.; Tashiro, K.; Kim, S.; Okamura, M.; Iwao, H. Role of hypomagnesemia in chronic cyclosporine nephropathy. *Transplantation* **2002**, *73*, 340–347. [CrossRef] [PubMed]

35. Yuan, J.; Zhou, J.; Chen, B.C.; Zhang, X.; Zhou, H.M.; Du, D.F.; Chang, S.; Chen, Z.K. Magnesium supplementation prevents chronic cyclosporine nephrotoxicity via adjusting nitric oxide synthase activity. *Transplant. Proc.* **2005**, *37*, 1892–1895. [CrossRef] [PubMed]

36. Asai, T.; Nakatani, T.; Yamanaka, S.; Tamada, S.; Kishimoto, T.; Tashiro, K.; Nakao, T.; Okamura, M.; Kim, S.; Iwao, H.; et al. Magnesium supplementation prevents experimental chronic cyclosporine a nephrotoxicity via renin-angiotensin system independent mechanism. *Transplantation* **2002**, *74*, 784–791. [CrossRef] [PubMed]

37. Asai, T.; Nakatani, T.; Tamada, S.; Kuwabara, N.; Yamanaka, S.; Tashiro, K.; Nakao, T.; Komiya, T.; Okamura, M.; Kim, S.; et al. Activation of transcription factors AP-1 and NF-kappaB in chronic cyclosporine A nephrotoxicity: Role in beneficial effects of magnesium supplementation. *Transplantation* **2003**, *75*, 1040–1044. [CrossRef] [PubMed]

38. Pham, P.-C.T.; Pham, P.-M.T.; Pham, S.V.; Miller, J.M.; Pham, P.-T.T. Hypomagnesemia in Patients with Type 2 Diabetes. *Clin. J. Am. Soc. Nephrol.* **2007**, *2*, 366–373. [CrossRef] [PubMed]

39. Geiger, H.; Wanner, C. Magnesium in disease. *Clin. Kidney J.* **2012**, *5*, i25–i38. [CrossRef] [PubMed]

40. Pham, P.C.T.; Pham, P.M.T.; Pham, P.a.T.; Pham, S.V.; Pham, H.V.; Miller, J.M.; Yanagawa, N.; Pham, P.T.T. Lower serum magnesium levels are associated with more rapid decline of renal function in patients with diabetes mellitus type 2. *Clin. Nephrol.* **2005**, *63*, 429–436. [CrossRef] [PubMed]

41. Lopez-Ridaura, R.; Willett, W.C.; Rimm, E.B.; Liu, S.; Stampfer, M.J.; Manson, J.E.; Hu, F.B. Magnesium intake and risk of type 2 diabetes in men and women. *Diabetes Care* **2004**, *27*, 134–140. [CrossRef] [PubMed]

42. Song, Y.; Manson, J.E.; Buring, J.E.; Liu, S. Dietary magnesium intake in relation to plasma insulin levels and risk of type 2 diabetes in women. *Diabetes Care* **2004**, *27*, 59–65. [CrossRef] [PubMed]

43. Fang, X.; Wang, K.; Han, D.; He, X.; Wei, J.; Zhao, L.; Imam, M.U.; Ping, Z.; Li, Y.; Xu, Y.; et al. Dietary magnesium intake and the risk of cardiovascular disease, type 2 diabetes, and all-cause mortality: A dose-response meta-analysis of prospective cohort studies. *BMC Med.* **2016**, *14*, 210. [CrossRef] [PubMed]

44. Kao, W.H.; Folsom, A.R.; Nieto, F.J.; Mo, J.P.; Watson, R.L.; Brancati, F.L. Serum and dietary magnesium and the risk for type 2 diabetes mellitus: The Atherosclerosis Risk in Communities Study. *Arch. Intern. Med.* **1999**, *159*, 2151–2159. [CrossRef] [PubMed]

45. Nadler, J.L.; Buchanan, T.; Natarajan, R.; Antonipillai, I.; Bergman, R.; Rude, R. Magnesium deficiency produces insulin resistance and increased thromboxane synthesis. *Hypertension* **1993**, *21*, 1024–1029. [CrossRef] [PubMed]

46. Van Laecke, S.; Van Biesen, W.; Vanholder, R. Hypomagnesaemia, the kidney and the vessels. *Nephrol. Dial. Transplant.* **2012**, *27*, 4003–4010. [CrossRef] [PubMed]

47. Rodriguez-Moran, M.; Guerrero-Romero, F. Oral Magnesium Supplementation Improves Insulin Sensitivity and Metabolic Control in Type 2 Diabetic Subjects: A randomized double-blind controlled trial. *Diabetes Care* **2003**, *26*, 1147–1152. [CrossRef] [PubMed]

48. Kasiske, B.L.; Snyder, J.J.; Gilbertson, D.; Matas, A.J. Diabetes mellitus after kidney transplantation in the United States. *Am. J. Transplant.* **2003**, *3*, 178–185. [CrossRef] [PubMed]

49. Augusto, J.-F.; Subra, J.-F.; Duveau, A.; Rakotonjanahary, J.; Dussaussoy, C.; Picquet, J.; Croue, A.; Villemain, F.; Onno, C.; Sayegh, J. Relation between Pretransplant Magnesemia and the Risk of New Onset Diabetes After Transplantation within the First Year of Kidney Transplantation. *Transplantation* **2014**, *97*, 1155–1160. [CrossRef] [PubMed]

50. Yates, C.J.; Fourlanos, S.; Hjelmesaeth, J.; Colman, P.G.; Cohney, S.J. New-onset diabetes after kidney transplantation-changes and challenges. *Am. J. Transplant.* **2012**, *12*, 820–828. [CrossRef] [PubMed]

51. Mazali, F.C.; Lalli, C.A.; Alves-Filho, G.; Mazzali, M. Posttransplant diabetes mellitus: Incidence and risk factors. *Transplant. Proc.* **2008**, *40*, 764–766. [CrossRef] [PubMed]

52. Maes, B.D.; Kuypers, D.; Messiaen, T.; Evenepoel, P.; Mathieu, C.; Coosemans, W.; Pirenne, J.; Vanrenterghem, Y.F.C. Posttransplantation Diabetes Mellitus in Fk-506-Treated Renal Transplant Recipients: Analysis of Incidence and Risk Factors. *Transplantation* **2001**, *72*, 1655–1661. [CrossRef] [PubMed]

53. Van Laecke, S.; Van Biesen, W.; Verbeke, F.; De Bacquer, D.; Peeters, P.; Vanholder, R. Posttransplantation hypomagnesemia and its relation with immunosuppression as predictors of new-onset diabetes after transplantation. *Am. J. Transplant.* **2009**, *9*, 2140–2149. [CrossRef] [PubMed]

54. Huang, J.W.; Famure, O.; Li, Y.; Kim, S.J. Hypomagnesemia and the Risk of New-Onset Diabetes Mellitus after Kidney Transplantation. *J. Am. Soc. Nephrol.* **2016**, *27*, 1793–1800. [CrossRef] [PubMed]

55. Hayes, W.; Boyle, S.; Carroll, A.; Bockenhauer, D.; Marks, S.D. Hypomagnesemia and increased risk of new-onset diabetes mellitus after transplantation in pediatric renal transplant recipients. *Pediatr. Nephrol.* **2017**, *32*, 879–884. [CrossRef] [PubMed]

56. Chanchlani, R.; Joseph Kim, S.; Kim, E.D.; Banh, T.; Borges, K.; Vasilevska-Ristovska, J.; Li, Y.; Ng, V.; Dipchand, A.I.; Solomon, M.; et al. Incidence of hyperglycemia and diabetes and association with electrolyte abnormalities in pediatric solid organ transplant recipients. *Nephrol. Dial. Transplant.* **2017**, *32*, 1579–1586. [CrossRef] [PubMed]

57. Osorio, J.M.; Bravo, J.; Pérez, A.; Ferreyra, C.; Osuna, A. Magnesemia in Renal Transplant Recipients: Relation With Immunosuppression and Posttransplant Diabetes. *Transplant. Proc.* **2010**, *42*, 2910–2913. [CrossRef] [PubMed]

58. Santos, L.; Rodrigo, E.; Piñera, C.; Robledo, C.; Palomar, R.; Gómez Alamillo, C.; González-Cotorruelo, J.; Arias, M. Elevated serum gamma-glutamyltransferase and hypomagnesemia are not related with new-onset diabetes after transplantation. *Transplant. Proc.* **2010**, *42*, 2914–2916. [CrossRef] [PubMed]

59. Van Laecke, S.; Desideri, F.; Geerts, A.; Van Vlierberghe, H.; Berrevoet, F.; Rogiers, X.; Troisi, R.; de Hemptinne, B.; Vanholder, R.; Colle, I. Hypomagnesemia and the risk of new-onset diabetes after liver transplantation. *Liver Transplant.* **2010**, *16*, 1278–1287. [CrossRef] [PubMed]

60. Van Laecke, S.; Nagler, E.V.; Taes, Y.; Van Biesen, W.; Peeters, P.; Vanholder, R. The effect of magnesium supplements on early post-transplantation glucose metabolism: A randomized controlled trial. *Transpl. Int.* **2014**, *27*, 895–902. [CrossRef] [PubMed]

61. Van Laecke, S.; Caluwe, R.; Huybrechts, I.; Nagler, E.V.; Vanholder, R.; Peeters, P.; Van Vlem, B.; Van Biesen, W. Effect of Magnesium Supplements on Insulin Secretion After Kidney Transplantation: A Randomized Controlled Trial. *Ann. Transplant.* **2017**, *22*, 524–531. [CrossRef] [PubMed]

62. Sánchez-Fructuoso, A.I.; Santín Cantero, J.M.; Pérez Flores, I.; Valero San Cecilio, R.; Calvo Romero, N.; Vilalta Casas, R. Changes in magnesium and potassium homeostasis after conversion from a calcineurin inhibitor regimen to an mTOR inhibitor-based regimen. *Transplant. Proc.* **2010**, *42*, 3047–3049. [CrossRef] [PubMed]

63. Murakami, N.; Riella, L.V.; Funakoshi, T. Risk of metabolic complications in kidney transplantation after conversion to mTOR inhibitor: A systematic review and meta-analysis. *Am. J. Transplant.* **2014**, *14*, 2317–2327. [CrossRef] [PubMed]

64. Grimbert, P.; Thaunat, O. mTOR inhibitors and risk of chronic antibody-mediated rejection after kidney transplantation: Where are we now? *Transpl. Int.* **2017**, *30*, 647–657. [CrossRef] [PubMed]

65. Zhang, R.; Kumar, P.; Reisin, E.; Ramcharan, T. Kidney Transplantation: The Evolving Challenges. *Am. J. Med. Sci.* **2004**, *328*, 156–161. [CrossRef] [PubMed]

66. Maier, J.A.M.; Malpuech-Brugère, C.; Zimowska, W.; Rayssiguier, Y.; Mazur, A. Low magnesium promotes endothelial cell dysfunction: Implications for atherosclerosis, inflammation and thrombosis. *Biochim. Biophys. Acta* **2004**, *1689*, 13–21. [CrossRef] [PubMed]

67. Paravicini, T.M.; Yogi, A.; Mazur, A.; Touyz, R.M. Dysregulation of Vascular TRPM7 and Annexin-1 is Associated with Endothelial Dysfunction in Inherited Hypomagnesemia. *Hypertension* **2009**, *53*, 423–429. [CrossRef] [PubMed]

68. Liao, F.; Folsom, A.R.; Brancati, F.L. Is low magnesium concentration a risk factor for coronary heart disease? The Atherosclerosis Risk in Communities (ARIC) Study. *Am. Heart J.* **1998**, *136*, 480–490. [CrossRef]

69. Hashimoto, T.; Hara, A.; Ohkubo, T.; Kikuya, M.; Shintani, Y.; Metoki, H.; Inoue, R.; Asayama, K.; Kanno, A.; Nakashita, M.; et al. Serum Magnesium, Ambulatory Blood Pressure, and Carotid Artery Alteration: The Ohasama Study. *Am. J. Hypertens.* **2010**, *23*, 1292–1298. [CrossRef] [PubMed]

70. Kisters, K.; Gremmler, B.; Hausberg, M. Magnesium and arterial stiffness. *Hypertension* **2006**, *47*, e3. [CrossRef] [PubMed]

71. Shechter, M.; Sharir, M.; Labrador, M.J.; Forrester, J.; Silver, B.; Bairey Merz, C.N. Oral magnesium therapy improves endothelial function in patients with coronary artery disease. *Circulation* **2000**, *102*, 2353–2358. [CrossRef] [PubMed]

72. Massy, Z.A.; Drüeke, T.B. Magnesium and outcomes in patients with chronic kidney disease: Focus on vascular calcification, atherosclerosis and survival. *Clin. Kidney J.* **2012**, *5*, i52–i61. [CrossRef] [PubMed]

73. Nguyen, T.; Steiner, R.W. A trial of oral magnesium supplementation in renal transplant recipients receiving cyclosporine. *Transplant. Proc.* **1998**, *30*, 4317–4319. [CrossRef]

74. Van Laecke, S.; Maréchal, C.; Verbeke, F.; Peeters, P.; Van Biesen, W.; Devuyst, O.; Jadoul, M.; Vanholder, R. The relation between hypomagnesaemia and vascular stiffness in renal transplant recipients. *Nephrol. Dial. Transplant.* **2011**, *26*, 2362–2369. [CrossRef] [PubMed]

8

Magnesium Absorption in Intestinal Cells: Evidence of Cross-Talk between EGF and TRPM6 and Novel Implications for Cetuximab Therapy

Giuseppe Pietropaolo [1,†], Daniela Pugliese [2], Alessandro Armuzzi [2]●, Luisa Guidi [2], Antonio Gasbarrini [2], Gian Lodovico Rapaccini [2], Federica I. Wolf [1,*] and Valentina Trapani [1,*]●

[1] Sezione di Patologia Generale, Dipartimento di Medicina e Chirurgia Traslazionale, Fondazione Policlinico Universitario A. Gemelli IRCCS—Università Cattolica del Sacro Cuore, 00168 Rome, Italy; giuseppe.pietropaolo@uniroma1.it

[2] UOC Medicina Interna e Gastroenterologia, Dipartimento di Medicina e Chirurgia Traslazionale, Fondazione Policlinico Universitario A. Gemelli IRCCS—Università Cattolica del Sacro Cuore, 00168 Rome, Italy; daniela.pugliese@policlinicogemelli.it (D.P.); alessandro.armuzzi@unicatt.it (A.A.); luisa.guidi@unicatt.it (L.G.); antonio.gasbarrini@unicatt.it (A.G.); gianludovico.rapaccini@policlinicogemelli.it (G.L.R.)

[*] Correspondence: federica.wolf@unicatt.it (F.I.W.); valentina.trapani@unicatt.it (V.T.)

[†] Current address: Dipartimento di Medicina Molecolare, laboratory affiliated to Istituto Pasteur Italia-Fondazione Cenci Bolognetti, Sapienza Università di Roma, 00161 Rome, Italy.

Abstract: Hypomagnesemia is very commonly observed in cancer patients, most frequently in association with therapy with cetuximab (CTX), a monoclonal antibody targeting the epithelial growth factor receptor (EGFR). CTX-induced hypomagnesemia has been ascribed to renal magnesium (Mg) wasting. Here, we sought to clarify whether CTX may also influence intestinal Mg absorption and if Mg supplementation may interfere with CTX activity. We used human colon carcinoma CaCo-2 cells as an in vitro model to study the mechanisms underlying Mg transport and CTX activity. Our findings demonstrate that TRPM6 is the key channel that mediates Mg influx in intestinal cells and that EGF stimulates such influx; consequently, CTX downregulates TRPM6-mediated Mg influx by interfering with EGF signaling. Moreover, we show that Mg supplementation does not modify either the CTX IC50 or CTX-dependent inhibition of ERK1/2 phosphorylation. Our results suggest that reduced Mg absorption in the intestine may contribute to the severe hypomagnesemia that occurs in CTX-treated patients, and Mg supplementation may represent a safe and effective nutritional intervention to restore Mg status without impairing the CTX efficacy.

Keywords: biomarker; colorectal cancer; EGFR; hypomagnesemia; magnesium supplementation; monoclonal antibodies; targeted therapy

1. Introduction

Nutritional deficits, defined as an imbalance between intake and metabolic requirements, are very common in cancer patients and may be caused by both the tumor itself and its treatment [1]. Appropriate nutritional interventions that correct such an imbalance reduce the risk of interruption or discontinuous treatment and improve quality of life [2]. Hypomagnesemia is frequent in oncologic patients, especially in those subjected to cisplatin-based therapies [3]. More recently, hypomagnesemia has emerged as the most notable adverse effect of the anti-EGFR monoclonal antibody cetuximab (CTX), which is widely used for advanced colorectal cancer (CRC) [4]. Several meta-analyses have shown that the incidence of all-grade hypomagnesemia in CTX-treated patients could be as high as about 35%; in about 5% of cases, hypomagnesemia can be severe (grade 3–4) and cause symptoms that require magnesium (Mg) supplementation [5–8]. On the other hand, early hypomagnesemia seems to act as a good predictor of the efficacy and outcome of CTX in *KRAS* wild-type CRC patients [9]. Although opposing results have also been reported [10], a recent meta-analysis confirmed that hypomagnesemia is associated with better progression-free survival, overall survival, and overall relative risk in CTX-treated *KRAS* wild-type CRC patients [11]. In addition to the clinical relevance of these findings, Vincenzi et al. [12] went as far as proposing that reduced serum Mg levels might potentiate the chemotherapeutic effects of CTX, which raised an intense debate among the scientific community [13,14].

Mg is a micronutrient involved in a plethora of cell functions, acting as a cofactor for a multitude of enzymes [15]. Systemic Mg homeostasis depends on the concomitant action of the intestine, responsible for Mg uptake from food, and the kidneys, which regulate Mg excretion. Magnesium is absorbed through different mechanisms, including passive paracellular transport, which is driven by the electrochemical gradient, and active transcellular transport, which is mediated by two highly homologous Mg channels—transient receptor potential melastatin (TRPM) channels type 6 and 7. TRPM7 is ubiquitously expressed, while TRPM6 is mainly expressed in the kidneys, the distal small intestine, and the colon [16]. Although the distal convoluted tubule of the kidney has long been considered the key gatekeeper of systemic Mg, the latest findings challenged such a view and suggested that intestinal Mg uptake might be of primary relevance [17]. Recent results corroborate the view that TRPM6, rather than TRPM7, modulates magnesium homeostasis in the colon. Ferioli et al. reported that TRPM6 function cannot be replaced by other channels [18]. Likewise, our group demonstrated that, in colon mucosa, TRPM6 is responsible for Mg influx and cell proliferation leading to mucosal healing [19,20].

The present view is that CTX-induced hypomagnesemia originates from molecular cross-talk between the EGF pathway and the regulatory mechanism for systemic Mg homeostasis in the kidneys. Such interaction was elucidated through the discovery of a mutation in the *EGF* gene in a rare genetic condition characterized by renal Mg wasting [21] and the following molecular characterization [22]. It was demonstrated that EGF acts as a magnesiotropic hormone by stimulating the surface expression and activity of the TRPM6 channel on the apical membrane of kidney epithelial cells, which in turn mediates Mg uptake. Therefore, by antagonizing EGF, ultimately CTX inhibits renal Mg reabsorption by TRPM6 and alters the whole-body Mg balance.

In addition to its well-established role in tumor growth and progression, EGF is also an important actor in intestinal development and mucosal repair [23]. Furthermore, EGF has been shown to be an important regulator of the expression, trafficking, and activity of epithelial transport proteins in the intestine [24]. However, despite the current emphasis on the importance of gut absorption for Mg homeostasis, the molecular cross-talk between EGF and TRPM6 has never been investigated in intestinal epithelial cells so far, nor is it known whether CTX can also affect the intestinal Mg absorption. Moreover, evidence that hypomagnesemia may serve as a positive prognostic factor in CTX-treated patients strongly contrasts with the fact that hypomagnesemia may cause severe discomfort and may even pose a serious threat to their lives. In this context, a crucial issue remains unanswered regarding the possibility that Mg supplementation may interfere with CTX efficacy. In the present paper, we sought to clarify two pressing issues that might have important clinical implications for CTX therapy: (1) the role of altered intestinal Mg absorption in the development of CTX-induced hypomagnesaemia; (2) the effect of Mg supplementation on the efficacy of CTX treatment.

2. Materials and Methods

2.1. Cell Culture

The constitutive activation of the MAPK pathway may limit the effectiveness of CTX treatment [25]. We screened different colon cancer cell lines and chose human colon carcinoma CaCo-2 cells, which harbor wild-type forms of critical genes, such as *KRAS*, *BRAF*, *PI3K3CA*, and *PTEN* [26]. CaCo-2 cells also express EGFR [27]. Cells were routinely grown in Dulbecco's modified Eagle's medium (DMEM) supplemented with 20% fetal bovine serum (FBS), 2mM of glutamine, 100 U/mL of penicillin, and 100 μg/mL of streptomycin in a 5% CO_2 humidified atmosphere at 37 °C. The reagents for cell culture were from Euroclone (Pero, Milan, Italy). Recombinant EGF was purchased from PeproTech (London, UK) and used at a concentration of 10 ng/mL, as previously reported [28]. Before EGF stimulation, the cells were starved in FBS-free medium for 24 h. Cetuximab was kindly provided by the Oncology Pharmacy Unit, "Agostino Gemelli" University Hospital, and used at an optimal concentration of 70 μg/mL, as inferred from cytotoxicity assays (see Sections 2.2 and 3.1). To obtain a transient downregulation of TRPM6, predesigned siRNA against human *TRPM6* was purchased from Qiagen. Specific siRNAs were transfected into cells (1300 ng per 400,000 cells) using HiPerFect Transfection Reagent (Qiagen, Milan, Italy) following the manufacturer's protocol (https://www.qiagen.com/it/transfectionprotocols/transfectionprotocol/). Non-silencing scrambled sequences were used as controls.

2.2. MTT Cytotoxicity Assay

Cells were seeded in 24-well plates at a density of 40,000 cells/well and allowed to adhere for 24 h before drug treatment. CTX (concentration range: 7.5 μg/mL to 240 μg/mL) was added to the culture medium in triplicates. After 24 h, the culture medium was replaced with serum-free medium containing 3-[4,5-dimethylthiazol-2-yl]-2,5-diphenyltetrazolium bromide (MTT, 1 mg/mL), and cells were incubated for 90 min at 37 °C. Finally, formazan crystals were dissolved in acidified isopropanol (0.04 N HCl in isopropanol), and the absorbance was read at $\lambda = 565$ nm. Data were analyzed using Prism software (version 5.01, GraphPad Software Inc., La Jolla, CA, USA) and dose–response curves were obtained by nonlinear regression (sigmoidal curve, variable slope).

2.3. Western Blotting

Cells were lysed in RIPA buffer (50 mM of Tris, pH 8, 150 mM of NaCl, 1 mM of EDTA, 1% NP-40, 0.05% sodium deoxycholate, 0.1% SDS) supplemented with protease and phosphatase inhibitors (Halt™ inhibitor cocktail, ThermoFisher Scientific, Milan, Italy). Protein concentrations were determined using the Bradford protein assay (Bio-Rad). Cell extracts were resolved by SDS-PAGE; transferred to PVDF membranes; and probed with rabbit polyclonal anti-TRPM6 (1:500, Biorbyt), anti-ERK1/2 (1:1000, Cell Signaling Technology), anti phospho-ERK1/2 (1:1000, Cell Signaling Technology), or anti-β-actin (1:1000, Sigma-Aldrich) primary antibodies. Horseradish peroxidase-conjugated secondary antibodies (GE Healthcare) were detected by the ECL Prime Western Blotting Detection Reagent (GE Healthcare) and the ChemiDoc XRS system (Bio-Rad). Densitometric analysis was performed by the ImageJ software (NIH, http://imagej.nih.gov/ij/).

2.4. Mg Influx Measurements

Subconfluent cells grown on 35 mm microscopy dishes (μ-dish, ibidi GmbH) were loaded with 3 μM of Mag-Fluo-4-AM (ThermoFisher Scientific), and imaged in a Na^+, Ca^{2+}, and Mg^{2+}-free buffer at a confocal laser scanning microscope (Nikon A1 MP), as previously described [28]. Cytosolic fluorescence signals were recorded as time series at a sampling frequency of 30 frames/min. The baseline was monitored for 30 s, then $MgSO_4$ was added drop-wise to a final concentration of 5 mM. Changes in the intracellular Mg levels at the single-cell level were estimated by the mean fluorescent increment $\Delta F/F$ [29]. Image analysis was performed by the NIS-Elements Confocal Software on 10 representative cells in each microscopic field, and experiments were repeated independently at least three times.

2.5. Statistical Analyses

All the experiments were repeated independently three times. The Prism software (version 5.01, GraphPad Software Inc., La Jolla, CA, USA) was used for all the statistical analyses. Statistical significance was evaluated using Student's t-test, when comparing two groups; one-way ANOVA, when comparing more groups in relation to only one variable; and two-way ANOVA, when comparing more groups in relation to two variables. ANOVA was followed by Bonferroni's test. Differences were considered statistically significant for p-values < 0.05, and significance levels were assigned as follows: * for $p < 0.05$, ** for $p < 0.01$.

3. Results

3.1. TRPM6 Mediates Mg Influx in CTX-Sensitive CaCo-2 Cells

First, we assessed the sensitivity of CaCo-2 cells to CTX with an MTT assay. The IC50 at 24h was (66 ± 16) µg/mL; therefore, in the following experiments, a CTX dose of 70 µg/mL was used. Next, we characterized the basal Mg influx capacity by the live imaging of CaCo-2 cells loaded with the Mg-specific fluorescent probe Mag-Fluo-4. The addition of 5 mM of $MgSO_4$ to the extracellular medium induced a rapid increase in fluorescence (i.e., intracellular Mg concentration) up to about 10% of the basal level; the fluorescence then gradually decreased to basal levels within about 3 min (Figure 1a, solid circles). CaCo-2 cells express the TRPM6 channel [19]. To determine whether the detected Mg influx is mediated by TRPM6, we repeated the same experiment in *TRPM6*-silenced CaCo-2 cells. Silencing by transient siRNA transfection significantly decreased the TRPM6 protein levels, as assessed by Western blot analysis at 48h (Figure 1b,c). After 48 h from siRNA transfection, the Mg influx upon the addition of extracellular $MgSO_4$ was nearly abolished in *TRPM6*-silenced cells in comparison with the control cells (Figure 1a, open circles). These results prove that TRPM6 is the key channel that mediates the Mg influx in CaCo-2 cells.

3.2. Cetuximab and EGF Modulate Mg Influx

Molecular crosstalk between the EFGR pathway and TRPM6 has been described in kidney epithelial cells [21,22]. We sought to assess whether the same mechanisms may modulate the Mg influx in intestinal epithelial cells. As shown in Figure 2a, EGF stimulation (10 ng/mL, 24 h) induced an increase in the basal Mg influx capacity of CaCo-2 cells (open circles vs. open squares), while CTX reduced the EGF-dependent increase in Mg influx (solid circles vs. open circles) and completely abrogated the basal Mg influx (solid squares vs. open squares). Western blot analysis proved that 24h of treatment with EGF (10 ng/mL) upregulated the TRPM6 expression, while concomitant exposure to CTX (70 µg/mL) resulted in TRPM6 levels comparable to the basal expression (Figure 2b,c). We conclude that EGF signaling leads to increased levels of the TRPM6 channel in intestinal cells, and CTX, by interfering with this signaling, downregulates the TRPM6-mediated Mg influx.

Figure 1. The TRPM6 channel mediates the Mg influx in human colon carcinoma cells. CaCo-2 cells were transiently silenced for *TRPM6* and assessed 48h after transfection. (**a**) Mg influx capacity in *TRPM6*-silenced (open circles) vs. control cells (solid circles), as assessed by the live imaging of Mag-Fluo-4-loaded cells; a representative experiment is shown. (**b**) TRPM6 protein expression in *TRPM6*-silenced and control cells, as evaluated by Western blot analysis; a representative blot is shown. (**c**) Quantification of TRPM6 protein expression by Western blot densitometry normalized to β-actin levels ($n = 3$, mean ± SD) in *TRPM6*-silenced (white bar) and control (black bar) cells. ** $p < 0.01$ by paired Student's t-test. Full scans of original blots are available in Figure S1.

Figure 2. Epidermal growth factor (EGF) stimulates TRPM6 channel expression and Mg influx in human colon carcinoma cells. CaCo-2 cells were serum-starved for 24 h and exposed to EGF (10 ng/mL) and cetuximab (CTX, 70 µg/mL), either alone or in combination, for a further 24h. (**a**) Mg influx capacity, as assessed by the live imaging of Mag-Fluo-4-loaded cells; a representative experiment is shown. (**b**) TRPM6 protein expression, as evaluated by Western blot analysis; a representative blot is shown. (**c**) Quantification of TRPM6 protein expression by Western blot densitometry normalized to β-actin levels ($n = 3$, mean ± SD). Data sharing the same letter are not significantly different ($p > 0.05$) according to one-way ANOVA, followed by Bonferroni's test. Full scans of original blots are available in Figure S2.

3.3. Mg Supplementation Does Not Affect Cetuximab Efficacy

To evaluate whether the extracellular Mg availability may alter sensitivity to the growth inhibitory effects of CTX, we challenged CaCo-2 cells with CTX in Mg-supplemented (5 mM of $MgSO_4$) medium. As shown in Figure 3a, the IC50 for CTX at 24h did not change significantly in the Mg-supplemented cells in comparison to the control cells (50 ± 10 vs. 66 ± 16 µg/mL, respectively). CTX prevents the dimerization of the EGFR and the activation of downstream pathways; primary or acquired resistance to CTX is mainly due to the constitutive activation of MEK signaling with subsequent MAPK activation [30]. Therefore, we also assessed whether Mg supplementation could interfere with the CTX-dependent inhibition of ERK1/2 phosphorylation. Western blot analysis showed that the presence of 5 mM of $MgSO_4$ did not substantially change the amount of phospho-ERK1/2 in CTX-treated cells (Figure 3b); two-way ANOVA confirmed that the Mg supplementation had no effect ($p = 0.70$), while CTX treatment had a very significant effect ($p < 0.001$, Figure 3c) on the ERK1/2 phosphorylation.

Figure 3. Mg supplementation does not affect cancer cell sensitivity to CTX. (**a**) A representative dose-response curve of CaCo-2 cells exposed to CTX (24 h) in control medium (0.8 mM of $MgSO_4$, solid line and circles) or Mg-supplemented medium (5 mM of $MgSO_4$, dotted line and open circles). (**b**) Phosphorylation of extracellular signal-regulated kinase (ERK) 1/2 in CaCo2 cells challenged for 24h with EGF (10 ng/mL) with or without CTX (70 µg/mL) in control (0.8 mM of $MgSO_4$) or Mg-supplemented (5 mM of $MgSO_4$) medium, as assessed by Western blot analysis; a representative blot is shown. (**c**) Quantification of ERK1/2 phosphorylation by Western blot densitometry, normalized to total ERK1/2 levels ($n = 3$, mean ± SD). Two-way ANOVA indicated a very significant effect ($p < 0.001$) of EGF/CTX treatment, while Mg concentration had no significant effect ($p = 0.70$). The effect of CTX on unstimulated cells in control or Mg-supplemented medium is reported in Figure S3.

4. Discussion

Cancer-associated hypomagnesemia has long been recognized, and was originally attributed to the metabolic demands of tumor growth; now, it has become clear that also cancer therapies play an important role [13,14]. In contrast to cisplatin, which damages renal tubules and hence causes a generalized electrolyte wasting [3], CTX induces hypomagnesemia by a specific antagonistic effect on renal Mg reabsorption. However, the interference between the mode of action of CTX and the homeostatic mechanisms of Mg has not received the deserved attention to its clinical implications. In this paper, we provide evidence supporting two relevant issues: (1) CTX-induced hypomagnesemia is not just due to renal wasting, but also to impaired intestinal absorption; (2) Mg supplementation does not modify CTX cytotoxicity.

Until recently, renal Mg reabsorption was thought to play a pivotal role in maintaining systemic Mg homeostasis [16]. However, conditional knockout murine models have proved that wild-type kidneys are not able to compensate for the ablation of intestinal TRPM6 and have pointed to an indispensable function of gut Mg absorption in the maintenance of proper Mg status [17]. The data we present here are in line with this view, confirming that cross-talk between EGF and TRPM6 occurs also in intestinal cells. In our work, we focus on the pathological setting of colon cancer and the mechanisms of CTX-induced hypomagnesemia. We are aware that our results do not conclusively prove that the activation of the EGFR pathway regulates the TRPM6-mediated intestinal Mg absorption in a more physiological context; future studies in more appropriate models will address this issue. On the other hand, it could be speculated that, in cancer cells, autocrine signaling by EGF may potentiate the TRPM6-mediated magnesium influx or compete with CTX. However, the EGF production by CaCo-2 cells does not undermine the value of our results, since in our model CTX does inhibit cellular growth as well as both basal and EGF-stimulated magnesium influx.

We propose that the impaired Mg absorption in the intestine heavily contributes to the severe hypomagnesemia that occurs in many CTX-treated patients. In the kidneys, the EGF-dependent modulation of TRPM6 has been ascribed to two different mechanisms: (1) the altered endomembrane trafficking of TRPM6, which results in increased TRPM6 channel activity on the cell surface [22], and (2) a transcriptional effect on the *TRPM6* mRNA expression via the MAPK/ERK pathway [31]. In our colon cellular model, we confirm that EGF increases the TRPM6 protein expression, while we have no evidence that acute EGF stimulation affects the number of recycling channels in favor of increased plasma membrane expression. We are aware of the limitations of our approach resulting from analyzing the TRPM6 protein expression by Western blot. However, the mRNA expression levels might not necessarily translate into a functional channel protein. Indeed, post-translational modifications may affect the protein levels, regardless of (or in addition to) transcriptional events; for example, this has been demonstrated for the sister channel TRPM7 [32]. On the other hand, ion channels are notoriously challenging to study for two main reasons: (a) the paucity of channel molecules per cell—a rough estimate obtained by electrophysiological studies is about 70 molecules/cell (Prof. Andrea Fleig, personal communication); (b) the difficulty of producing specific antibodies, due to structural constraints and sequence similarity. The commercial anti-TRPM6 antibody that we use is the only known antibody that does not display cross-reactivity with TRPM7 [19]. Ultimately, we are interested in the functional effects of cross-talk between EGF and TRPM6; in this respect, by using a functional assay we provide definitive proof that, in intestinal cells, (a) TRPM6 is indispensable for mediating the Mg influx (Figure 1a), and (b) CTX modulates the TRPM6-mediated Mg influx (Figure 2a).

The symptoms of hypomagnesemia range from depression and muscle spasms to arrhythmias and seizures, and significantly worsen the quality of life of patients [16]. Severe hypomagnesemia warrants treatment by intravenous and/or oral magnesium supplementation for the duration of CTX therapy, and cases of CTX dose reduction and discontinuation have been documented [33]. No evidence-based guidelines have currently been developed for the management of hypomagnesaemia in the context of CTX cancer therapy [33]. We demonstrate that CTX inhibits the TRPM6-mediated transcellular Mg transport. However, oral Mg supplementation, by increasing the intraluminal Mg concentration and thus favoring the paracellular route, may represent an effective strategy to restore the Mg status in CTX-treated patients, even in the presence of limited renal transcellular reabsorption. Most importantly, such approach would be feasible on an outpatient basis.

Although most medical oncologists agree on the necessity of restoring the Mg status in symptomatic patients [31], the relationship between Mg and cancer remains highly controversial [34]. Early reports found that, in murine models, a low Mg availability resulted in the inhibition of primary tumor growth, but at the same time enhanced metastasis formation [35,36]. On the other hand, more recently Mg status was reported to have no influence on tumor progression in two different animal models [37,38]. Notably, Mg supplementation protected against cisplatin-induced acute kidney injury without compromising the cisplatin-mediated killing of an ovarian tumor xenograft in mice [37]. Despite the limitations of an in vitro model, our data oppose the view that the effect of Mg deficiency on cell proliferation is synergistic with that of CTX: Mg supplementation did not significantly affect cell growth (Figure S4), nor did it alter the effect of CTX inhibitory activity on cell growth or on MAPK signaling (Figure 3).

In conclusion, we present evidence that Mg supplementation does not compromise CTX efficacy, and suggest that nutritional intervention may be a safe and cost-effective approach by which to maximize patient wellbeing and improve CRC management. Further preclinical and clinical research will be necessary to clarify the relationship between Mg and CTX in various experimental tumor models and the potential of Mg supplementation in CTX-treated patients.

Author Contributions: Conceptualization, F.I.W. and V.T.; formal analysis, G.P. and V.T.; investigation, G.P., D.P. and V.T.; resources, A.A. and L.G.; writing—original draft preparation, V.T.; writing—review and editing, G.P., D.P., A.A., L.G., A.G., G.L.R., F.I.W. and V.T.; supervision, F.I.W. and V.T.; funding acquisition, F.I.W. All authors have read and agreed to the published version of the manuscript.

Acknowledgments: Confocal imaging was performed at the LABCEMI (Laboratorio Centralizzato di Microscopia Ottica ed Elettronica), Università Cattolica del Sacro Cuore, Fondazione Policlinico Universitario "Agostino Gemelli" IRCCS, Rome, Italy.

References

1. Martin, L.; Senesse, P.; Gioulbasanis, I.; Antoun, S.; Bozzetti, F.; Deans, C.; Strasser, F.; Thoresen, L.; Jagoe, R.T.; Chasen, M.; et al. Diagnostic criteria for the classification of cancer-associated weight loss. *J. Clin. Oncol.* **2015**, *33*, 90–99. [CrossRef] [PubMed]

2. Arends, J.; Bachmann, P.; Baracos, V.; Barthelemy, N.; Bertz, H.; Bozzetti, F.; Fearon, K.; Hütterer, E.; Isenring, E.; Kaasa, S.; et al. ESPEN guidelines on nutrition in cancer patients. *Clin. Nutr.* **2017**, *36*, 11–48. [CrossRef] [PubMed]

3. Finkel, M.; Goldstein, A.; Steinberg, Y.; Granowetter, L.; Trachtman, H. Cisplatinum nephrotoxicity in oncology therapeutics: Retrospective review of patients treated between 2005 and 2012. *Pediatr. Nephrol.* **2014**, *29*, 2421–2424. [CrossRef] [PubMed]

4. Hofheinz, R.D.; Segaert, S.; Safont, M.J.; Demonty, G.; Prenen, H. Management of adverse events during treatment of gastrointestinal cancers with epidermal growth factor inhibitors. *Crit. Rev. Oncol. Hematol.* **2017**, *114*, 102–113. [CrossRef]

5. Cao, Y.; Liao, C.; Tan, A.; Liu, L.; Gao, F. Meta-analysis of incidence and risk of hypomagnesemia with cetuximab for advanced cancer. *Chemotherapy* **2010**, *56*, 459–465. [CrossRef]

6. Petrelli, F.; Borgonovo, K.; Cabiddu, M.; Ghilardi, M.; Barni, S. Risk of anti-EGFR monoclonal antibody-related hypomagnesemia: Systematic review and pooled analysis of randomized studies. *Expert Opin. Drug Saf.* **2012**, *11*, S9–S19. [CrossRef]

7. Chen, P.; Wang, L.; Li, H.; Liu, B.; Zou, Z. Incidence and risk of hypomagnesemia in advanced cancer patients treated with cetuximab: A meta-analysis. *Oncol. Lett.* **2013**, *5*, 1915–1920. [CrossRef]

8. Wang, Q.; Qi, Y.; Zhang, D.; Gong, C.; Yao, A.; Xiao, Y.; Yang, J.; Zhou, F.; Zhou, Y. Electrolyte disorders assessment in solid tumor patients treated with anti-EGFR monoclonal antibodies: A pooled analysis of 25 randomized clinical trials. *Tumour Biol.* **2015**, *36*, 3471–3482. [CrossRef]

9. Vincenzi, B.; Galluzzo, S.; Santini, D.; Rocci, L.; Loupakis, F.; Correale, P.; Addeo, R.; Zoccoli, A.; Napolitano, A.; Graziano, F.; et al. Early magnesium modifications as a surrogate marker of efficacy of cetuximab-based anticancer treatment in KRAS wild-type advanced colorectal cancer patients. *Ann. Oncol.* **2011**, *22*, 1141–1146. [CrossRef]

10. Vickers, M.M.; Karapetis, C.S.; Tu, D.; O'Callaghan, C.J.; Price, T.J.; Tebbutt, N.C.; Van Hazel, G.; Shapiro, J.D.; Pavlakis, N.; Gibbs, P.; et al. Association of hypomagnesemia with inferior survival in a phase III, randomized study of cetuximab plus best supportive care versus best supportive care alone: NCIC CTG/AGITG CO.17. *Ann. Oncol.* **2013**, *24*, 953–960. [CrossRef]

11. Hsieh, M.C.; Wu, C.F.; Chen, C.W.; Shi, C.S.; Huang, W.S.; Kuan, F.C. Hypomagnesemia and clinical benefits of anti-EGFR monoclonal antibodies in wild-type KRAS metastatic colorectal cancer: A systematic review and meta-analysis. *Sci. Rep.* **2018**, *8*, 2047. [CrossRef] [PubMed]

12. Vincenzi, B.; Santini, D.; Tonini, G. Biological interaction between anti-epidermal growth factor receptor agent cetuximab and magnesium. *Exp. Opin. Pharmacother.* **2008**, *9*, 1267–1269. [CrossRef] [PubMed]

13. Wolf, F.I.; Trapani, V.; Cittadini, A.; Maier, J.A. Hypomagnesaemia in oncologic patients: To treat or not to treat? *Magnes. Res.* **2009**, *22*, 5–9. [CrossRef] [PubMed]

14. Wolf, F.I.; Cittadini, A.R.; Maier, J.A. Magnesium and tumors: Ally or foe? *Cancer Treat. Rev.* **2009**, *35*, 378–382. [CrossRef]

15. Bairoch, A. The ENZYME database in 2000. *Nucleic Acids Res.* **2000**, *28*, 304–305. [CrossRef]

16. de Baaij, J.H.; Hoenderop, J.G.; Bindels, R.J. Magnesium in man: Implications for health and disease. *Physiol. Rev.* **2015**, *95*, 1–46. [CrossRef]

17. Chubanov, V.; Ferioli, S.; Wisnowsky, A.; Simmons, D.G.; Leitzinger, C.; Einer, C.; Jonas, W.; Shymkiv, Y.; Bartsch, H.; Braun, A.; et al. Epithelial magnesium transport by TRPM6 is essential for prenatal development and adult survival. *Elife* **2016**, *5*, e20914. [CrossRef]

18. Ferioli, S.; Zierler, S.; Zaißerer, J.; Schredelseker, J.; Gudermann, T.; Chubanov, V. TRPM6 and TRPM7 differentially contribute to the relief of heteromeric TRPM6/7 channels from inhibition by cytosolic Mg^{2+} and Mg•ATP. *Sci. Rep.* **2017**, *7*, 8806. [CrossRef]

19. Luongo, F.; Pietropaolo, G.; Gautier, M.; Dhennin-Duthille, I.; Ouadid-Ahidouch, H.; Wolf, F.I.; Trapani, V. TRPM6 is Essential for Magnesium Uptake and Epithelial Cell Function in the Colon. *Nutrients* **2018**, *10*, 784. [CrossRef]

20. Trapani, V.; Petito, V.; Di Agostini, A.; Arduini, D.; Hamersma, W.; Pietropaolo, G.; Luongo, F.; Arena, V.; Stigliano, E.; Lopetuso, L.R.; et al. Dietary Magnesium Alleviates Experimental Murine Colitis Through Upregulation of the Transient Receptor Potential Melastatin 6 Channel. *Inflamm. Bowel Dis.* **2018**, *24*, 2198–2210. [CrossRef]

21. Groenestege, W.M.; Thébault, S.; van der Wijst, J.; van den Berg, D.; Janssen, R.; Tejpar, S.; van den Heuvel, L.P.; van Cutsem, E.; Hoenderop, J.G.; Knoers, N.V.; et al. Impaired basolateral sorting of pro-EGF causes isolated recessive renal hypomagnesemia. *J. Clin. Invest.* **2007**, *117*, 2260–2267. [CrossRef]

22. Thebault, S.; Alexander, R.T.; Tiel Groenestege, W.M.; Hoenderop, J.G.; Bindels, R.J. EGF increases TRPM6 activity and surface expression. *J. Am. Soc. Nephrol.* **2009**, *20*, 78–85. [CrossRef] [PubMed]

23. Tang, X.; Liu, H.; Yang, S.; Li, Z.; Zhong, J.; Fang, R. Epidermal Growth Factor and Intestinal Barrier Function. *Med. Inflamm.* **2016**, *2016*, 1927348. [CrossRef]

24. Mroz, M.S.; Keely, S.J. Epidermal growth factor chronically upregulates Ca^{2+}-dependent Cl⁻ conductance and TMEM16A expression in intestinal epithelial cells. *J. Physiol.* **2012**, *590*, 1907–1920. [CrossRef]

25. Parseghian, C.M.; Napolitano, S.; Loree, J.M.; Kopetz, S. Mechanisms of Innate and Acquired Resistance to Anti-EGFR Therapy: A Review of Current Knowledge with a Focus on Rechallenge Therapies. *Clin. Cancer Res.* **2019**, *25*, 6899–6908. [CrossRef]

26. Ahmed, D.; Eide, P.W.; Eilertsen, I.A.; Danielsen, S.A.; Eknæs, M.; Hektoen, M.; Lind, G.E.; Lothe, R.A. Epigenetic and genetic features of 24 colon cancer cell lines. *Oncogenesis* **2013**, *2*, e71. [CrossRef] [PubMed]

27. Shigeta, K.; Hayashida, T.; Hoshino, Y.; Okabayashi, K.; Endo, T.; Ishii, Y.; Hasegawa, H.; Kitagawa, Y. Expression of Epidermal Growth Factor Receptor Detected by Cetuximab Indicates Its Efficacy to Inhibit In Vitro and In Vivo Proliferation of Colorectal Cancer Cells. *PLoS ONE* **2013**, *8*, e66302. [CrossRef]

28. Trapani, V.; Arduini, D.; Luongo, F.; Wolf, F.I. EGF stimulates Mg^{2+} influx in mammary epithelial cells. *Biochem. Biophys. Res. Commun.* **2014**, *454*, 572–575. [CrossRef] [PubMed]

29. Trapani, V.; Schweigel-Röntgen, M.; Cittadini, A.; Wolf, F.I. Intracellular magnesium detection by fluorescent indicators. *Methods Enzymol.* **2012**, *505*, 421–444.

30. Troiani, T.; Napolitano, S.; Vitagliano, D.; Morgillo, F.; Capasso, A.; Sforza, V.; Nappi, A.; Ciardiello, D.; Ciardiello, F.; Martinelli, E. Primary and acquired resistance of colorectal cancer cells to anti-EGFR antibodies converge on MEK/ERK pathway activation and can be overcome by combined MEK/EGFR inhibition. *Clin. Cancer Res.* **2014**, *20*, 3775–3786. [CrossRef]

31. Ikari, A.; Sanada, A.; Okude, C.; Sawada, H.; Yamazaki, Y.; Sugatani, J.; Miwa, M. Up-regulation of TRPM6 transcriptional activity by AP-1 in renal epithelial cells. *J. Cell. Physiol.* **2010**, *222*, 481–487. [CrossRef] [PubMed]

32. Castiglioni, S.; Cazzaniga, A.; Trapani, V.; Cappadone, C.; Farruggia, G.; Merolle, L.; Wolf, F.I.; Iotti, S.; Maier, J. Magnesium homeostasis in colon carcinoma LoVo cells sensitive or resistant to doxorubicin. *Sci. Rep.* **2015** *5*, 16538. [CrossRef] [PubMed]

33. Thangarasa, T.; Gotfrit, J.; Goodwin, R.A.; Tang, P.A.; Clemons, M.; Imbulgoda, A.; Vickers, M.M. Epidermal growth factor receptor inhibitor-induced hypomagnesemia: A survey of practice patterns among Canadian gastrointestinal medical oncologists. *Curr. Oncol.* **2019**, *26*, e162–e166. [CrossRef]

34. Trapani, V.; Wolf, F.I. Dysregulation of Mg^{2+} homeostasis contributes to acquisition of cancer hallmarks. *Cell Calcium.* **2019**, *83*, 102078. [CrossRef]

35. Maier, J.A.; Nasulewicz-Goldeman, A.; Simonacci, M.; Boninsegna, A.; Mazur, A.; Wolf, F.I. Insights into the mechanisms involved in magnesium-dependent inhibition of primary tumor growth. *Nutr. Cancer.* **2007**, *59*, 192–198. [CrossRef] [PubMed]

36. Nasulewicz, A.; Wietrzyk, J.; Wolf, F.I.; Dzimira, S.; Madej, J.; Maier, J.A.; Rayssiguier, Y.; Mazur, A.; Opolski, A. Magnesium deficiency inhibits primary tumor growth but favors metastasis in mice. *Biochim. Biophys. Acta.* **2004**, *1739*, 26–32. [CrossRef]

37. Solanki, M.H.; Chatterjee, P.K.; Xue, X.; Gupta, M.; Rosales, I.; Yeboah, M.M.; Kohn, N.; Metz, C.N. Magnesium protects against cisplatin-induced acute kidney injury without compromising cisplatin-mediated killing of an ovarian tumor xenograft in mice. *Am. J. Physiol. Renal Physiol.* **2015**, *309*, F35–F47. [CrossRef]

38. Huang, J.; Furuya, H.; Faouzi, M.; Zhang, Z.; Monteilh-Zoller, M.; Kawabata, K.G.; Horgen, F.D.; Kawamori, T.; Penner, R.; Fleig, A. Inhibition of TRPM7 suppresses cell proliferation of colon adenocarcinoma in vitro and induces hypomagnesemia in vivo without affecting azoxymethane-induced early colon cancer in mice. *Cell Commun. Signal.* **2017**, *15*, 30. [CrossRef]

9

Effects of Magnesium Supplementation on Unipolar Depression: A Placebo-Controlled Study and Review of the Importance of Dosing and Magnesium Status in the Therapeutic Response

Beata Ryszewska-Pokraśniewicz [1], Anna Mach [2,*], Michał Skalski [2], Piotr Januszko [2], Zbigniew M. Wawrzyniak [3], Ewa Poleszak [4], Gabriel Nowak [5,†], Andrzej Pilc [5] and Maria Radziwoń-Zaleska [2,†]

[1] Nowowiejski Hospital, 00-685 Warsaw, Poland; beataryszewska@wp.pl
[2] Department of Psychiatry, Medical University of Warsaw, 00-685 Warsaw, Poland; michal.skalski@wum.edu.pl (M.S.); piotr.januszko@wp.pl (P.J.); mariar@wum.edu.pl (M.R.-Z.)
[3] Faculty of Electronics and Information Technology, Warsaw University of Technology, 00-685 Warsaw, Poland; z.wawrzyniak@ise.pw.edu.pl
[4] Faculty of Pharmacy, Medical University of Lublin, 20-093 Lublin, Poland; ewa.poleszak@umlub.pl
[5] Institute of Pharmacology, Polish Academy of Sciences, 31-343 Kraków, Poland; nowak@if-pan.krakow.pl (G.N.); nfpilc@cyf-kr.edu.pl (A.P.)
* Correspondence: anna.mach@wum.edu.pl
† These authors equally contributed to this study.

Abstract: Animal studies using tests and models have demonstrated that magnesium exerts an antidepressant effect. The literature contains few studies in humans involving attempts to augment antidepressant therapy with magnesium ions. The purpose of our study was to assess the efficacy and safety of antidepressant treatment, in combination with magnesium ions. A total of 37 participants with recurrent depressive disorder who developed a depressive episode were included in this study. As part of this double-blind study, treatment with the antidepressant fluoxetine was accompanied with either magnesium ions (120 mg/day as magnesium aspartate) or placebo. During an 8-week treatment period, each patient was monitored for any clinical abnormalities. Moreover, serum fluoxetine and magnesium levels were measured, and pharmaco-electroencephalography was performed. The fluoxetine + magnesium and fluoxetine + placebo groups showed no significant differences in either Hamilton Depression Rating Scale (HDRS) scores or serum magnesium levels at any stage of treatment. Multivariate statistical analysis of the whole investigated group showed that the following parameters increased the odds of effective treatment: lower baseline HDRS scores, female gender, smoking, and treatment augmentation with magnesium. The parameters that increased the odds of remission were lower baseline HDRS scores, shorter history of disease, the presence of antidepressant-induced changes in the pharmaco-EEG profile at 6 h after treatment, and the fact of receiving treatment augmented with magnesium ions. The limitation of this study is a small sample size.

Keywords: unipolar depression; magnesium; pharmaco-electroencephalography; efficacy; remission

1. Introduction

According to the recent data from the World Health Organization, depression affects over 300 million people worldwide. By 2030, recurrent unipolar depressive disorders are projected to become the leading cause of the burden of disease worldwide, as calculated on the basis of Disability-Adjusted Life Years (DALYs) [1].

Despite having been studied for years, the etiology of depression is yet to be fully understood. More and more animal and clinical studies have suggested a role of the N-methyl-D-aspartate (NMDA) receptor complex and NMDA-mediated excitatory amino acid neurotransmission both in the pathophysiology and treatment of depression [2–5]. This concept seems to be confirmed by evidence of glutamate system abnormalities detected in the blood [6], cerebrospinal fluid [7], and brain tissue [8] of patients with depressive disorders. Modifying glutamatergic transmission by means of NMDA receptors is currently a promising target of antidepressant treatment [9].

The NMDA receptor complex is modified by multiple ligand binding sites. Recent years saw a number of experimental studies that confirmed an antidepressant effect of various NMDA receptor antagonists, such as ketamine, memantine, dextromethorphan, or MK-0657 [9]. However, the risk of severe side effects limits the use of these agents as antidepressant drugs [10].

One of the natural, inorganic modulators of the NMDA receptor complex are magnesium ions. They inhibit voltage-gated NMDA receptor channels at the same time inhibiting the flow of calcium ions. Moreover, they increase the expression of the GluN2B subunit of the NMDA receptor complex [11]. In the hippocampus, low magnesium levels in combination with high calcium and glutamate levels are believed to potentially cause functional changes in synapses, leading to the development of mood disorders, including depression [11,12]. There are several mechanisms responsible for antidepressant effects of magnesium. Apart from their direct NMDA-receptor antagonism, magnesium ions interact with other factors crucial in depression pathophysiology. Magnesium ions suppress hippocampal kindling and modulate protein kinase C [13]. Moreover, they affect P-glycoprotein (a protein responsible for blood-brain barrier permeability to glucocorticoids and other molecules), which alters the hypothalamic-pituitary-adrenal axis and damages the hippocampus [14]. Magnesium also plays a role in serotoninergic, noradrenergic, and dopaminergic neurotransmission [15] and it has an anti-inflammatory effect [16], which additionally increases its antidepressant potential.

Antidepressant properties of magnesium have been demonstrated in animal preclinical screen tests and models. Magnesium salts are active in the forced swim test (FST) as well as in olfactory bulbectomy and chronic mild stress models [17–20]. Furthermore, this bio-metal enhances antidepressant activity of standard antidepressants in the FST [15,21,22]. On the other hand, magnesium deficiency (induced by low-magnesium diet in laboratory animals) is related to depression-like behavior [23].

Multiple studies have demonstrated a relationship between depressive disorders and magnesium intake [24–27]. However, the data on the changes in magnesium levels in patients with depression are inconclusive. Some authors showed a positive correlation between magnesium levels and depression [28], whereas others showed a negative correlation [29]. Similar discrepancies were observed in the case of the severity of depression symptoms [30]. Nonetheless, Camardese et al. concluded that serum magnesium levels correlate with the response to treatment [31].

We would like to emphasize that the main goal in the treatment of a depressive episode is first to achieve a full therapeutic response and remission, followed by recurrence prevention, and ensuring the patient's return to normal functioning [32]. One of the major problems in treating depression is the effectiveness of therapy. Some patients fail to achieve a satisfactory response to treatment. Initial antidepressant treatment, with adequate dosing and treatment duration, leads to remission only in 50% of patients [33]. Moreover, 20–30% of patients achieve incomplete remission, with some depressive symptoms persisting for a long time. Another therapeutic problem is a delay in therapeutic effects. All currently approved monoaminergic antidepressants exhibit latency in the therapeutic response, which considerably increases the risk of suicide and self-harm. Thus, there are unceasing attempts to potentiate and speed up the therapeutic effect [32].

Due to the limited effectiveness of antidepressant treatment, there is a great need for developing novel, satisfactory therapies. To date, there have been few clinical studies on magnesium supplementation in depressive disorders, and their findings have been inconclusive [34–36]. Therefore, the purpose of our study was to assess the efficacy and safety of antidepressant treatment accompanied with magnesium supplements.

2. Materials and Methods

Our 8-week study included 37 patients (admitted either to the Department of Psychiatry, Medical University of Warsaw or to Nowowiejski Hospital in Warsaw) who met the inclusion criterion of an ICD-10-codable depressive episode or major depression as defined in DSM-IV. The exclusion criteria were delusional disorders, organic disorders, high risk of suicide requiring electroconvulsive therapy, absolute contraindications for selective serotonin re-uptake inhibitors (SSRIs), absolute contraindications for magnesium ions, alcohol and substance abuse, and baseline pharmaco-EEG abnormalities. Patients with severe depression (more than 19 points in the HDRS) were included in the study. Patients were recruited without age or gender restrictions—adults over 18 years old.

All patients received fluoxetine at a daily dose of 20–40 mg. This standard treatment was augmented, in a double-blind manner, with either placebo or magnesium. The magnesium supplements used in this study were 40-mg magnesium effervescent tablets or powder containing 40 mg of magnesium (equivalent to 3.30 mEq of magnesium aspartate) administered 3 times per day.

The study was conducted in accordance with the Declaration of Helsinki. The protocol was approved by the Institutional Review Board and Bioethics Committee at the Medical University of Warsaw (KB/96/2006; KB/227/2012). All participants gave informed written consent prior to participating in this study.

Study participants were recruited based on baseline assessments, which included a physical examination (conducted by the same psychiatrist as those conducted later, throughout the study), psychometric scale score, and pharmaco-electroencephalography. Individuals who qualified to take part in the study underwent a one-week wash-out period (except in cases of previous SSRI treatment, where wash-out was extended to 6 weeks).

All study group patients were examined by the same physician at pre-defined time points: prior to treatment initiation (time 0), 6 h after the first dose of the drug (maximum serum concentration of the drug), and subsequently at 24 h, 2 weeks, 4 weeks, 6 weeks, and 8 weeks after treatment initiation [37].

The psychometric scales used in this study were the 21-item Hamilton Depression Rating Scale (HDRS), Hamilton Anxiety Rating Scale (HARS), and Clinical Global Impression Scale (CGIS). Treatment was considered effective when there was a 50% reduction in the baseline HDRS score. The cut-off HDRS score that defined remission was 6 or less [38].

The presence and severity of side effects were assessed based on history-taking, changes in Side Effect Rating Scale (SERS) scores as compared to baseline, and laboratory assessments, which were conducted at the same time as psychometric assessments. Any drugs that could affect the levels of the antidepressant were avoided during the study. When necessary, zopiclone (7.5 mg) or zolpidem (10 mg) was allowed every other day.

A high-performance liquid chromatography (HPLC) system (Shimadzu Corporation, Analytical Instruments Division, Kyoto, Japan) was used in this study to measure serum fluoxetine (FLU) and norfluoxetine (NFLU) levels. The measurement method was based on the reports by El-Yazigi and Raines [39], Aymard [40], Meineke [41], and Komorowska [42].

The following therapeutic ranges were adopted [42,43]: fluoxetine 50–450 ng/mL, norfluoxetine 50–350 ng/mL, fluoxetine and norfluoxetine 50–550 ng/mL. Serum fluoxetine levels were measured at the Psychopharmacology Laboratory of the Department of Psychiatry, WUM. Serum magnesium levels were measured by ALAB Laboratories and analyzed with the use of Hulanicki's method [44]. The established ALAB reference range for serum magnesium levels (1.7–2.5 mg/dL) was adopted for this study. This was a double-blind study—with the principal investigator blinded to the magnesium levels in individual participants before study completion, as the laboratory reported only abnormalities in magnesium levels.

Pharmaco-EEG examinations were conducted prior to, and 6 and 24 h after, treatment initiation, and then at 2, 4, 6, and 8 weeks of treatment. The electroencephalograph used in this study was DigiTrack, version DTW (Elmico). Subsequently, EEG relative power spectra were calculated with NeuroGuide software using the fast Fourier transformation (FFT) algorithm. Adopting a 0.5-Hz resolution, we calculated the power spectra in delta (1.5–5.0 Hz), theta (5.5–8.0 Hz), alpha 1 (8.5–10.0 Hz), alpha 2 (10.5–12.0 Hz), beta 1 (12.5–18.5 Hz), beta 2 (19.0–20.5 Hz), and beta 3 (21.0–29.5 Hz) frequency bands. Arranged chronologically, t-test values for the individual bands formed a profile of EEG power spectrum changes over the treatment period.

Each of the graphs was classified by an expert, based on the presence or absence of an antidepressant-induced pharmaco-EEG profile. The following pharmaco-EEG profile, typical for tricyclic antidepressants (TCAs), was considered positive in fluoxetine-treated patients: an increase in high frequency beta waves (beta 3) [37,45,46].

All EEG examinations were performed at the Clinical Electroencephalography and Neurophysiology Laboratory of the Department of Psychiatry, WUM.

In the statistical analysis of our results, the Wilcoxon Rank-Sum Test for independent samples was used for the comparison of groups. Moreover, we used descriptive statistics and multivariate logistic regression models (GLIMMIX procedure), which allowed us to assess the odds ratios for an ineffective treatment and lack of remission with respect to each of the evaluated factors. The level of statistical significance was set at $p < 0.05$. All calculations were conducted with SAS 14.1.

3. Results

Seventeen (11 women [65%] and 6 men [35%]) out of the 37 participants included in the study received fluoxetine and magnesium, whereas 20 (10 women [50%] and 10 men [50%]) received fluoxetine and placebo. The mean age in the magnesium group ($n = 17$, group I) was 48.1 ± 15.5 years; the median age was 50 years; the age range was from 23 to 71 years, with 5 participants (29%) 60 years old or older. Body weight in this group ranged from 50.0 to 110.0 kg, with the mean of 71.2 ± 15.0 kg and median 70.0 kg. The mean height was 169.9 ± 10.0 cm (with the median of 168.0 cm and range of 158.0–192.0 cm). Mean disease duration at baseline was 5.6 ± 5.8 years (with the median of 4.0 years and range of 0.3–20.0 years). The mean age in the placebo group ($n = 20$, group II) was 49.7 ± 12.3 years; the median age was 52 years; the age range was from 24 to 65 years, with 6 participants (30%) 60 years old or older. The mean body weight in this group was 76.2 ± 16.1 kg (median 75.0 kg, range 48.0–112.0 kg). The mean height in this group was 171.9 ± 7.7 cm (median 173.5 cm, range 156.0–187.0 cm). Mean disease duration at baseline was 3.8 ± 4.5 years (median 2.0 years, range 0.4–16.0 years).

In group I, 10 participants (60%) were hospitalized once, 4 participants (23.5%) were hospitalized twice, one participant (5.9%) was hospitalized 3 times, one (5.9%) 4 times, and one participant (5.9%) was hospitalized more than 5 times. In group II, 15 participants (75.0%) were hospitalized once, 4 participants (20.0%) were hospitalized 2 times, one participant (5.0%) was hospitalized 5 times, and there were no participants hospitalized more than 5 times.

There were 2 non-smokers (11.8%) and 15 smokers (88.2%) in group I. The mean BMI in this group was 24.6 kg/m^2 (median 24.2 kg/m^2, range 19.1–35.5 kg/m^2). There were 5 non-smokers (25.0%) and 15 smokers (75.0%) in group II. The mean BMI in this group was 25.8 kg/m^2 (median 24.8 kg/m^2, range 17.6–37.4 kg/m^2).

Prior to treatment initiation, the mean HDRS score in group I (fluoxetine and magnesium) was 30.5 ± 6.0 (median 29; range 21–44) (Table 1). Other scales used in this study yielded the following scores prior to treatment initiation: HARS (mean score 20.1 ± 4.8, median 19, range 13–28), CGI (mean score 2.9 ± 0.7, median 3, range 2–4), and SERS (mean score 10.5 ± 3.4, median 10, range 6–18).

Table 1. Effect of magnesium or placebo supplementation on Hamilton Depression Rating Scale (HDRS) scores in patients treated with fluoxetine.

Variable	Group I: Magnesium						Group II: Placebo						
	N	Mean	SD	Med	Min	Max	N	Mean	SD	Med	Min	Max	*p*-Value
HDRS_0	17	30.5	6	29	21	44	20	27.5	5.5	28	18	38	0.1120
HDRS_6H	17	30.4	5.8	29	21	43	20	27.5	5.5	28	18	38	0.1197
HDRS_24H	17	30.4	5.8	29	21	43	20	27.4	5.4	28	18	38	0.1059
HDRS_2W	17	24.5	5.6	24	13	36	20	21.8	7.5	23	9	36	0.2237
HDRS_4W	17	18.5	5.9	17	10	31	17	17.2	6.4	17	5	28	0.5605
HDRS_6W	17	14.6	6.9	13	5	29	16	13.4	6.6	14	2	28	0.6100
HDRS_8W	17	10.7	7.9	8	1	29	15	10.4	6.8	10	1	28	0.9080

N—number of patients; SD—standard deviation; Med—Median; Min—minimum; Max—maximum HDRS: Hamilton Depression Rating Scale; HDRS_0—scores before treatment; H—hours; W—week. The Wilcoxon Rank-Sum Test for independent samples was used for the comparison of groups.

Prior to treatment initiation, the mean HDRS score in group II (fluoxetine and placebo) was 27.5 ± 5.5 (median 28; range 18–38) (Table 1). Other scales yielded the following scores at baseline: HARS scores: mean 18.5 ± 3.8, median 19, range 8–25; CGI scores: mean 3.1 ± 0.7, median 3, range 2–5; SERS scores: mean 11.3 ± 3.5, median 11, range 5–20.

There were no differences between groups at each examined time points in either HDRS (Table 1) or in CGI, HARS, and SERS scores (data not shown).

After 8 weeks of treatment, there was a 50% improvement in HDRS scores in 15 participants (88%) from group I and in 11 participants (73%) from group II. There was no significant difference between the groups in terms of treatment efficacy.

Remission, which had been pre-defined as HDRS score reduction to 6 points or less, was achieved in 6 participants (35%) from group I and in 4 participants (27%) from group II. There was no significant difference between the groups in terms of remission rates.

The two study groups (I and II) showed no significant differences in terms of HDRS score changes during treatment (Figure 1). The two study groups (I and II) showed no significant differences in terms of serum magnesium levels during treatment (Figure 2).

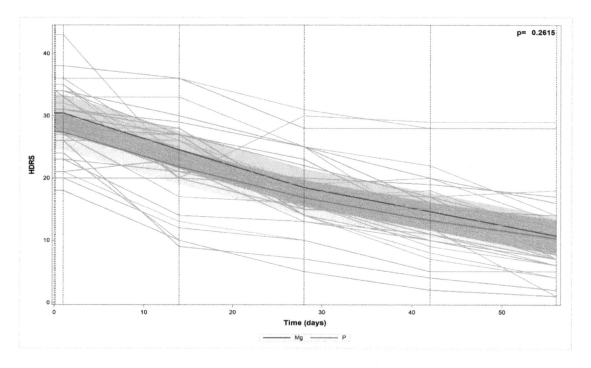

Figure 1. Hamilton Depression Rating Scale (HDRS) scores over time—the measured data and trend.

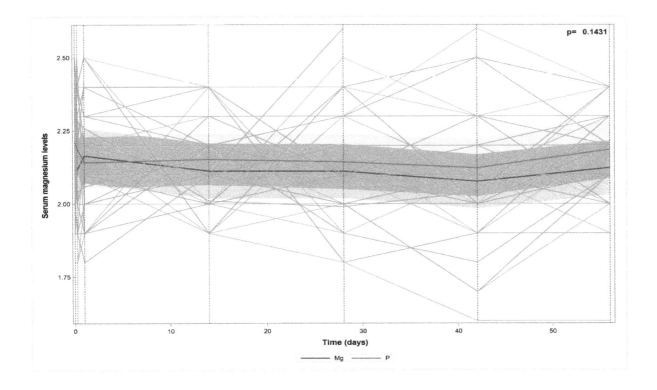

Figure 2. Serum magnesium levels over time—the measured data and trend.

Models of multivariate analysis were used to calculate odds ratios for both remission (model 1) and treatment efficacy (model 2) using the compared values of each evaluated parameter.

Model 1 (Table 2), which was used to analyze the odds of remission, included the following parameters: the baseline HDRS score; disease duration; pharmaco-EEG profile (obtained 6 h after treatment initiation) showing evidence of TCA use (yes vs. no); and the type of treatment (magnesium vs. placebo).

Table 2. Odds ratio values for the parameters evaluated in this model—the odds ratio for remission.

Parameter	Values	Odds Ratio	95% LCL	95% UCL	p-Value
HDRS-0	$[x + 1]$ vs. $[x]$	0.8982	0.7503	1.0752	0.2422
Duration of disease	$[x + 1]$ vs. $[x]$	0.8001	0.5842	1.0956	0.1643
PROF-1	0 vs. 1	0.4151	0.1637	1.0527	0.0641
Mg-P	Mg vs. P	1.5545	0.6206	3.8938	0.3464

LCL lower confidence limit; UCL upper confidence limit.

Figure 3 shows the odds ratios (ORs) for remission (with 95% confidence intervals) for the individual parameters. A statistically significant parameter would have its OR = 1.0 value positioned completely beyond the confidence interval. An odds ratio equal to 1.0 means that both compared values of the given parameter yield identical odds of remission.

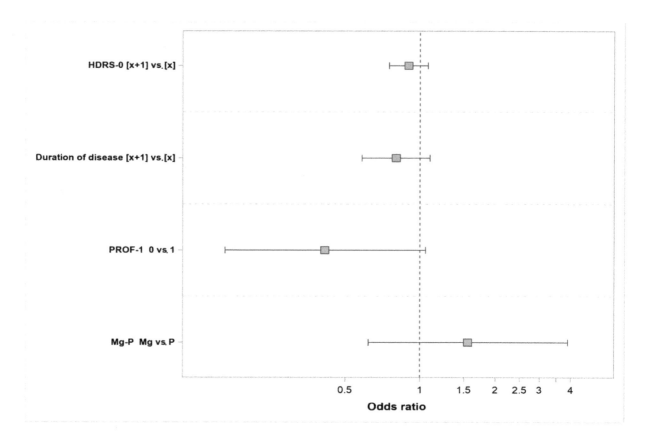

Figure 3. Odds ratio values for remission.

We found that an increase in the HDRS score by 1 point as compared to baseline, disease duration longer by 1 year, and a lack of antidepressant-induced changes in the pharmaco-EEG profile at 6 h after treatment decrease the odds of remission. The use of magnesium to augment the effect of treatment increases the odds of remission.

Model 2 (Table 3)—which was used to analyze treatment efficacy, included the following parameters: the baseline HDRS score; the patients' gender; smoking status; and the type of treatment (magnesium vs. placebo). Figure 4 shows the increase in the baseline HDRS score by 1 point and being a non-smoker ($p = 0.0034$) reduced the odds of effective treatment. The female sex and the use of magnesium to potentialize the effect of fluoxetine increased the odds of effective treatment.

Table 3. Odds ratio values for the parameters evaluated in this model—the odds of achieving 50% improvement in HDRS scores (efficacy).

Parameter	Values	Odds Ratio	95% LCL	95% UCL	*p*-Value
HDRS-0	$[x + 1]$ vs. $[x]$	0.8614	0.7093	1.0461	0.1321
Gender	F vs. M	2.1942	0.6840	7.0392	0.1864
Smoking status	0 vs. 1	0.1242	0.0181	0.8530	0.0339
Mg-P	Mg vs. P	2.5869	0.7510	8.9111	0.1320

LCL, lower confidence limit; UCL, upper confidence limit.

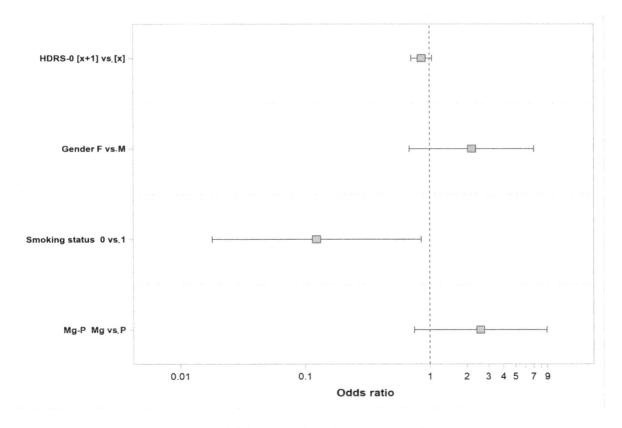

Figure 4. Odds ratio values for treatment efficacy.

4. Discussion

Our study evaluated the efficacy and safety of antidepressant treatment augmented with magnesium. Despite the fact that the fluoxetine-and-magnesium group showed higher rates of 50% improvement in HDRS scores at week 8 than the fluoxetine-and-placebo group, the difference was not statistically significant. Similar, though also non-significant, results were obtained while evaluating remission. Moreover, the magnesium and placebo groups showed no significant differences in terms of the efficacy and safety of treatment at any evaluated time point.

Our findings are unlike those reported in some earlier studies. Tarleton et al. demonstrated a decrease in depression symptoms already after a two-week period of magnesium supplementation at 248 mg per day. Their study employed the PHQ-9 for the diagnosis of depression [47], with 126 participants with mild-to-moderate depression symptoms included in the study. Their results showed no relationship with the participants' age, gender, baseline disease severity, or antidepressant treatment [48]. Earlier reports by Tarleton et al. also showed a relationship between low magnesium intake (<184 mg/day) and depression [26]. This observation was also supported by a Finnish study including exclusively males (2320 participants). That study demonstrated that adequate magnesium intake may prevent depression [27]. In light of the available studies, the reports of major depression cases described by Eby et al. seem very interesting, as they showed a rapid (within under 7 days) recovery in response to treatment with magnesium (in the form of glycinate and taurinate) at 125–300-mg administered with every meal and before sleep [35]. Moreover, another two-week randomized study in a group of 23 elderly patients with newly diagnosed depression, associated with type 2 diabetes and hypomagnesemia, showed treatment with magnesium chloride (450 mg/day) to be equally effective as that with imipramine (50 mg/day) [49].

Nonetheless, our findings were consistent with those of some other authors. Mehdi et al. observed no changes in HDRS scores following magnesium supplementation in a group of participants (n = 12) with mild-to-moderate treatment-resistant depression [50]. Similar results were observed in a randomized clinical study in a group of female patients with postpartum depression, where an 8-week treatment with magnesium at 320 mg/day failed to reduce the symptoms of depression evaluated with the Edinburgh Postnatal Depression Scale [51]. Moreover, a large Spanish study conducted in a Mediterranean population (15,836 participants) showed no conclusive evidence to support the claim that an increased magnesium intake might be associated with a lower risk of developing depression [52]. Due to these conflicting findings, the efficacy of magnesium in antidepressant treatment is still unknown.

Table 4 presents a compilation of clinical studies on the use of magnesium in the treatment of depressive disorders as well as data on the study methods used.

Table 4. Effect of magnesium (Mg) supplementation in human depression.

Depression Type	Type of Study	N	Dose of Mg^{+2} mg/day p.o.	Salt	Effect	References
Major depression	Case	4	125–300	Glycinate taurinate	+	[28]
Depression (early, type 2 diabetes, hypomagnesemia)	Randomized Mg vs. IMI	23	450	Chloride	+	[42]
Depression Gitelman's syndrome, (hypomagnesemia)	Case	1	300–900 plus intravenous 1200	Oxide sulfate	+	[46]
Major depression (hypomagnesemia)	Placebo	60	300	Oxide	+	[47]
Major depression	Placebo cross-over	112	248	Chloride	+	[41]
Postpartum depression	Placebo	66	87	Sulfate	−	[44]
Major depression	Placebo	37	120	Aspartate	−	present study
Major depression (TRD)	Monotherapy	12	Intravenous 1000	Sulfate	−	[43]

N—number of patients; + positive effect of Mg supplementation; − no effect of Mg supplementation.

We would like to emphasize the fact that the tools for assessing depression symptoms which were used in the studies cited above were non-uniform, with the following being the most commonly used questionnaires: the Human Population Laboratory (HPL) Depression Scale [27], Patient Health Questionnaire (PHQ-9), Yasavage and Brink Scale [49], and Hamilton Depression Rating Scale (HDRS) [50]. It seems obvious that these psychometric instruments differ in terms of accuracy, reliability, or standardization. Therefore, the selection of an appropriate questionnaire may determine the study findings. Consistent with our observations, a study by Mehdi et al. showed no significant changes in HDRS scores following magnesium supplementation; however, increased serum magnesium levels correlated with a clinical improvement measured with the PHQ-9 [50]. The questionnaire used in our study is currently considered to be the gold standard among psychometric tools used to assess the severity of depression. Additionally, it helps precisely monitor the patient's condition during antidepressant treatment. The HDRS is an observer-rated instrument, which means that the assessment is conducted by an experienced physician who knows the standards in symptom severity assessment. Unlike self-administered questionnaires used by other investigators, the HDRS is considered to be a more objective and accurate tool. The methods of assessing a response to treatment in our study additionally included looking for antidepressant-induced changes in pharmaco-EEG profiles at various time points. Our results showed no statistically significant differences between the study groups. The discrepancies between our findings and the ones reported by other authors may be also due to a varied duration of magnesium supplementation and different assessment time points.

Other factors that may affect treatment efficacy include both the dosage and form of magnesium supplements. In all the studies mentioned above where oral magnesium supplementation was shown to decrease depression symptoms magnesium doses ranged from 125 to 900 mg/day. In all these cases the dosage was higher than that used in our study. Currently, there are a number of available magnesium formulations. The key criterion that makes these formulations different is their bioavailability. Due to the fact that only some (30–40%) of the ingested magnesium is absorbed by the body, it is very important to conduct magnesium supplementation using formulations characterized by better absorption. Magnesium aspartate, citrate, lactate, and chloride are considered to have a higher bioavailability in comparison with that of either magnesium oxide or sulfate [11]. In the present study dose of magnesium (120 mg Mg^{2+}/day) was chosen as the acceptable (and widely applied) in Poland (indicated by Pharmindex—polish drug encyclopedia). Despite the fact that we used magnesium aspartate characterized by high bioavailability and a structure similar to that of magnesium compounds found in a normal diet, we observed no significant improvement in depression symptoms. Moreover, since our study was conducted exclusively in a Polish population, we cannot exclude the potential effects of genetic and environmental factors.

Despite the well-documented relationship between magnesium and depression, its mechanisms are still unknown. Thus, the role of magnesium in antidepressant treatment augmentation is difficult to elucidate. A study by Camardese et al. demonstrated a more pronounced response to antidepressant treatment in patients with higher magnesium levels [31]. Another study showed a marked increase in intracellular magnesium levels following treatment with either amitriptyline or sertraline. It is precisely this increase in intracellular magnesium levels that has been suggested to be partially responsible for the effect of antidepressant drugs [53].

Experimental pre-clinical studies on animal models demonstrated that the antidepressant effect of magnesium is a result of its role in serotoninergic neurotransmission [54]. The potential synergism between magnesium and antidepressants warrants further studies on antidepressant treatment potentialization.

Further studies are necessary to discover whether magnesium supplementation can justify the use of antidepressants at lower doses or help avoid the necessity of combination regimens.

We would like to emphasize our multivariate analysis results that identified the parameters that increased the odds of remission and treatment efficacy. The parameters increasing the odds of remission (i.e., HDRS score of <6) included lower baseline HDRS scores, shorter history of disease, the presence of antidepressant-induced pharmaco-EEG profile at 6 h after drug administration, and treatment augmentation with magnesium ions. The parameters increasing the odds of treatment efficacy were lower baseline HDRS scores, female gender, being a smoker, and treatment augmentation with magnesium ions. It seems obvious that an earlier diagnosis and lower symptom severity are favorable prognostic factors. The benefits of magnesium supplementation have been widely discussed. One of the arguments explaining the better treatment efficacy in females observed in our study may be other authors' reports of generally lower magnesium levels in females [55,56]. Pregnancy and chronic use of oral contraceptives are known to lead to hypomagnesemia [57]. Moreover, magnesium supplementation has been shown to prevent the development of postpartum depression [35].

We would like to emphasize that one of the parameters shown to significantly increase the odds of effective treatment was the fact of being a smoker. Nicotine is known to directly affect mood in humans. The relationship between depression and smoking has been extensively studied, and the findings demonstrated antidepressant properties of nicotine [58–60]. Smokers with a history of depression who refrain from smoking have a higher risk of developing another depressive episode [61]. Salin-Pascual et al. observed an improvement in the mood of non-smoking participants with major depression following the use of nicotine patches [62]. This effect is most likely associated with dopaminergic reward system activation [63] and serotoninergic neurotransmission [60]. The results of our study demonstrate potentially antidepressant effects of nicotine. However, our findings need to be confirmed in a larger number of patients.

Despite the fact that our study did not conclusively demonstrate an increased efficacy of antidepressant treatment augmented with magnesium, magnesium supplementation helped predict treatment efficacy and remission. Further studies are necessary to assess whether magnesium supplementation may be a valuable complement to standard antidepressant treatments.

5. Conclusions

The magnesium and placebo groups showed no statistically significant differences in terms of HDRS scores, serum magnesium levels, treatment safety and efficacy, or pharmaco-EEG profiles. Nonetheless, supplementation with magnesium ions is one of the parameters that help increase the chances of treatment efficacy and remission. The limitation of this study is the small sample size.

Author Contributions: M.S., G.N. and M.R.-Z. conceived and designed the experiments; B.R.-P., A.M., P.J. and M.R.-Z. performed the experiments; A.M., M.S., Z.M.W., E.P., G.N., A.P. and M.R.-Z. analyzed the data; P.J., A.M. and M.S. contributed reagents/materials/analysis tools; B.R.-P., A.M., G.N. and M.R.-Z. wrote the paper.

References

1.   World Health Organization. Available online: http://www.who.int/en/news-room/fact-sheets/detail/depression (accessed on 15 May 2018).
2.   Deutschenbaur, L.; Beck, J.; Kiyhankhadiv, A.; Mühlhauser, M.; Borgwardt, S.; Walter, M.; Hasler, G.; Sollberger, D.; Lang, U.E. Role of calcium, glutamate and NMDA in major depression and therapeutic application. *Prog. Neuro-Psychopharmacol. Biol. Psychiatry* **2016**, *64*, 325–333. [CrossRef] [PubMed]
3.   Poleszak, E.; Wlaź, P.; Socała, K.; Wrobel, A.; Szewczyk, B.; Kasperek, R.; Nowak, G. Interaction of glycine/NMDA receptor ligands and antidepressant drugs in the forced swim test. *Pharmacol. Rep.* **2010**, *62*, 58. [CrossRef]
4.   Nowak, G.; Papp, M.; Paul, I.A. The NMDA receptor complex and the action of antidepressant drugs in the CMS model of depression. *Eur. J. Pharm. Sci.* **1996**, *4*, S53. [CrossRef]
5.   Wlaź, P.; Kasperek, R.; Wlaź, A.; Szumiło, M.; Wróbel, A.; Nowak, G.; Poleszak, E. NMDA and AMPA receptors are involved in the antidepressant-like activity of tianeptine in the forced swim test in mice. *Pharmacol. Rep.* **2011**, *63*, 1526–1532. [PubMed]
6.   Küçükibrahimoğlu, E.; Saygin, M.Z.; Calişkan, M.; Kaplan, O.K.; Unsal, C.; Gören, M.Z. The change in plasma GABA, glutamine and glutamate levels in fluoxetine- or S-citalopram-treated female patients with major depression. *Eur. J. Clin. Pharmacol.* **2009**, *65*, 571–577. [CrossRef] [PubMed]
7.   Frye, M.A.; Tsai, G.E.; Huggins, T.; Coyle, J.T.; Post, R.M. Low Cerebrospinal Fluid Glutamate and Glycine in Refractory Affective Disorder. *Biol. Psychiatry* **2007**, *61*, 162–166. [CrossRef] [PubMed]
8.   Hashimoto, K.; Sawa, A.; Iyo, M. Increased Levels of Glutamate in Brains from Patients with Mood Disorders. *Biol. Psychiatry* **2007**, *62*, 1310–1316. [CrossRef] [PubMed]
9.   Machado-Vieira, R.; Henter, I.D.; Zarate, C.A., Jr. New targets for rapid antidepressant action. *Prog. Neurobiol.* **2017**, *152*, 21–37. [CrossRef] [PubMed]
10.   Sanacora, G.; Wilkinson, S.; Schalkwyk, G.V. 201. Measuring Dissociative Effects of NMDA Receptor Antagonists in the Treatment of Depression. *Biol. Psychiatry* **2017**, *81*, S83. [CrossRef]
11.   Serefko, A.; Szopa, A.; Poleszak, E. Magnesium and depression. *Magnes. Res.* **2016**, *29*, 112–119. [CrossRef]
12.   Poleszak, E.; Wlaz, P.; Kedzierska, E.; Nieoczym, D.; Wrobel, A.; Fidecka, S.; Pilc, A.; Nowak, G. NMDA/glutamate mechanism of antidepressant-like action of magnesium in forced swim test in mice. *Pharmacol. Biochem. Behav.* **2007**, *88*, 158–164. [CrossRef] [PubMed]
13.   Murck, H. Ketamine, magnesium and major depression—From pharmacology to pathophysiology and back. *J. Psychiatr. Res.* **2013**, *47*, 955–965. [CrossRef] [PubMed]
14.   Gould, T.D.; Manji, H.K. Glycogen synthase kinase-3: A putative molecular target for lithium mimetic drugs. *Neuropsychopharmacol. Off. Publ. Am. Coll. Neuropsychopharmacol.* **2005**, *30*, 1223–1237. [CrossRef] [PubMed]
15.   Cardoso, C.C.; Lobato, K.R.; Binfare, R.W.; Ferreira, P.K.; Rosa, A.O.; Santos, A.R.; Rodrigues, A.L. Evidence for the involvement of the monoaminergic system in the antidepressant-like effect of magnesium. *Prog. Neuro-Psychopharmacol. Biol. Psychiatry* **2009**, *33*, 235–242. [CrossRef] [PubMed]
16.   King, D.E.; Mainous, A.G., 3rd; Geesey, M.E.; Ellis, T. Magnesium intake and serum C-reactive protein levels in children. *Magnes. Res.* **2007**, *20*, 32–36. [PubMed]
17.   Decollogne, S.; Tomas, A.; Lecerf, C.; Adamowicz, E.; Seman, M. NMDA receptor complex blockade by oral

administration of magnesium: Comparison with MK-801. *Pharmacol. Biochem. Behav.* **1997**, *58*, 261–268. [CrossRef]

18. Poleszak, E.; Szewczyk, B.; Kedzierska, E.; Wlaz, P.; Pilc, A.; Nowak, G. Antidepressant- and anxiolytic-like activity of magnesium in mice. *Pharmacol. Biochem. Behav.* **2004**, *78*, 7–12. [CrossRef] [PubMed]

19. Pochwat, B.; Szewczyk, B.; Sowa-Kucma, M.; Siwek, A.; Doboszewska, U.; Piekoszewski, W.; Gruca, P.; Papp, M.; Nowak, G. Antidepressant-like activity of magnesium in the chronic mild stress model in rats: Alterations in the NMDA receptor subunits. *Int. J. Neuropsychopharmacol.* **2014**, *17*, 393–405. [CrossRef] [PubMed]

20. Pochwat, B.; Sowa-Kucma, M.; Kotarska, K.; Misztak, P.; Nowak, G.; Szewczyk, B. Antidepressant-like activity of magnesium in the olfactory bulbectomy model is associated with the AMPA/BDNF pathway. *Psychopharmacology* **2015**, *232*, 355–367. [CrossRef] [PubMed]

21. Poleszak, E.; Wlaz, P.; Szewczyk, B.; Kedzierska, E.; Wyska, E.; Librowski, T.; Szymura-Oleksiak, J.; Fidecka, S.; Pilc, A.; Nowak, G. Enhancement of antidepressant-like activity by joint administration of imipramine and magnesium in the forced swim test: Behavioral and pharmacokinetic studies in mice. *Pharmacol. Biochem. Behav.* **2005**, *81*, 524–529. [CrossRef] [PubMed]

22. Serefko, A.; Szopa, A.; Wlaź, P.; Nowak, G.; Radziwoń-Zaleska, M.; Skalski, M.; Poleszak, E. Magnesium in depression. *Pharmacol. Rep.* **2013**, *65*, 547–554. [CrossRef]

23. Singewald, N.; Sinner, C.; Hetzenauer, A.; Sartori, S.B.; Murck, H. Magnesium-deficient diet alters depression- and anxiety-related behavior in mice—Influence of desipramine and Hypericum perforatum extract. *Neuropharmacology* **2004**, *47*, 1189–1197. [CrossRef] [PubMed]

24. Jacka, F.N.; Overland, S.; Stewart, R.; Tell, G.S.; Bjelland, I.; Mykletun, A. Association between magnesium intake and depression and anxiety in community-dwelling adults: The Hordaland Health Study. *Aust. N. Z. J. Psychiatry* **2009**, *43*, 45–52. [CrossRef] [PubMed]

25. Huang, J.H.; Lu, Y.F.; Cheng, F.C.; Lee, J.N.; Tsai, L.C. Correlation of magnesium intake with metabolic parameters, depression and physical activity in elderly type 2 diabetes patients: A cross-sectional study. *Nutr. J.* **2012**, *11*, 41. [CrossRef] [PubMed]

26. Tarleton, E.K.; Littenberg, B. Magnesium intake and depression in adults. *J. Am. Board Fam. Med.* **2015**, *28*, 249–256. [CrossRef] [PubMed]

27. Yary, T.; Lehto, S.M.; Tolmunen, T.; Tuomainen, T.P.; Kauhanen, J.; Voutilainen, S.; Ruusunen, A. Dietary magnesium intake and the incidence of depression: A 20-year follow-up study. *J. Affect Disord.* **2016**, *193*, 94–98. [CrossRef] [PubMed]

28. Linder, J.; Brismar, K.; Beck-Friis, J.; Saaf, J.; Wetterberg, L. Calcium and magnesium concentrations in affective disorder: Difference between plasma and serum in relation to symptoms. *Acta Psychiatr. Scand.* **1989**, *80*, 527–537. [CrossRef] [PubMed]

29. Barragan-Rodriguez, L.; Rodriguez-Moran, M.; Guerrero-Romero, F. Depressive symptoms and hypomagnesemia in older diabetic subjects. *Arch. Med. Res.* **2007**, *38*, 752–756. [CrossRef] [PubMed]

30. Derom, M.-L.; Sayón-Orea, C.; Martínez-Ortega, J.M.; Martínez-González, M.A. Magnesium and depression: A systematic review. *Nutr. Neurosci.* **2013**, *16*, 191–206. [CrossRef] [PubMed]

31. Camardese, G.; De Risio, L.; Pizi, G.; Mattioli, B.; Buccelletti, F.; Serrani, R.; Leone, B.; Sgambato, A.; Bria, P.; Janiri, L. Plasma magnesium levels and treatment outcome in depressed patients. *Nutr. Neurosci.* **2012**, *15*, 78–84. [CrossRef] [PubMed]

32. Bauer, M.; Bschor, T.; Pfennig, A.; Whybrow, P.C.; Angst, J.; Versiani, M.; Möller, H.-J. World Federation of Societies of Biological Psychiatry (WFSBP) Guidelines for Biological Treatment of Unipolar Depressive Disorders in Primary Care. *World J. Biol. Psychiatry Off. J. World Fed. Soc. Biol. Psychiatry* **2007**, *8*, 67–104. [CrossRef] [PubMed]

33. Trevino, K.; McClintock, S.M.; McDonald Fischer, N.; Vora, A.; Husain, M.M. Defining treatment-resistant depression: A comprehensive review of the literature. *Ann. Clin. Psychiatry Off. J. Am. Acad. Clin. Psychiatr.* **2014**, *26*, 222–232.

34. Radziwoń-Zaleska, M.; Ryszewska-Pokraśniewicz, B.; Skalski, M.; Skrzeszewski, J.; Drozdowicz, E.; Nowak, G.; Pilc, A.; Bałkowiec-Iskra, E. Therapeutic drug monitoring of depression—Amplification by magnesium ions. *Pharmacol. Rep.* **2015**, *67*, 36. [CrossRef]

35. Eby, G.A.; Eby, K.L. Rapid recovery from major depression using magnesium treatment. *Med. Hypotheses* **2006**, *67*, 362–370. [CrossRef] [PubMed]

36. Derom, M.L.; Martinez-Gonzalez, M.A.; Sayon-Orea Mdel, C.; Bes-Rastrollo, M.; Beunza, J.J.; Sanchez-Villegas, A. Magnesium intake is not related to depression risk in Spanish university graduates. *J. Nutr.* **2012**, *142*, 1053–1059. [CrossRef] [PubMed]

37. Radziwoń-Zaleska, M.; Matsumoto, H.; Skalski, M.; Androsiuk, W.; Dziklińska, A.; Grobel, I.; Kunicki, P. Monitored therapy of depression. *Farmakoterapia w Psychiatrii i Neurologii* **1998**, *3*, 5–12.

38. Hamilton, M. A rating scale for depression. *J. Neurol. Neurosurg. Psychiatry* **1960**, *23*, 56–62. [CrossRef] [PubMed]

39. El-Yazigi, A.; Raines, D.A. Concurrent liquid chromatographic measurement of fluoxetine, amitryptyline, imipramine, and their active metabolites norfluoxetine, nortyptyline, and desipramine in plasma. *Ther. Drug. Monit.* **1993**, *15*, 305–309. [CrossRef] [PubMed]

40. Aymard, G.; Livi, P.; Pham, Y.T.; Diquet, B. Sensitive and rapid method for the simultaneous quantification of five antidepressants with their respective metabolites in plasma using high-performance liquid chromatography with diode-array detection. *J. Chromatogr. B Biomed. Sci. Appl.* **1997**, *700*, 183–189. [CrossRef]

41. Meineke, I.; Schreeb, K.; Kress, I.; Gundert-Remy, U. Routine measurement of fluoxetine and norfluoxetine by high-performance liquid chromatography with ultraviolet detection in patients under concomitant treatment with tricyclic antidepressants. *Ther. Drug Monit.* **1998**, *20*, 14–19. [CrossRef] [PubMed]

42. Komorowska, E. *Walidacja i Zastosowanie Metody Oznaczania Fluoksetyny Techniką HPLC*; Akademia Medyczna w Warszawie, Wydział Farmaceutyczny: Warszawa, Poland, 2002.

43. Baldessarini, R.J. Drugs and treatment of psychiatric disorders: Depression and mania. W. In *Goodman & Gilman's The Pharmacological Basis of Therapeutic*; McGraw-Hills Co.: New York, NY, USA, 1996; pp. 431–461.

44. Hulanicki, A.; Lewenstam, A.; Maj-Żurawska, M. *Magnesium; Clinical Significance and Analytical Determination*; Reviews on Analytical Chemistry, Euroanalysis VIII; Littlejohn, D., Thorburn Burns, D., Eds.; RSC: Cambridge, CA, USA, 1994; pp. 317–325.

45. Szelenberger, W. Farmakoelektroencefalografia: Aktualny stan wiedzy i perspektywy. *Psychiatr. Polska* **1990**, *24*, 52–57.

46. Skalski, M.; Szelenberger, W.; Radziwoń-Zaleska, M.; Matsumoto, H. Zastosowanie metody farmakoelektroencefalografii (farmako—EEG) w monitorowaniu terapii depresji. *Farmakoterapia w Psychiatrii i Neurologii* **1995**, *4*, 60–70.

47. Kroenke, K.; Spitzer, R.L.; Williams, J.B. The PHQ-9: Validity of a brief depression severity measure. *J. Gen. Intern. Med.* **2001**, *16*, 606–613. [CrossRef] [PubMed]

48. Tarleton, E.K.; Littenberg, B.; MacLean, C.D.; Kennedy, A.G.; Daley, C. Role of magnesium supplementation in the treatment of depression: A randomized clinical trial. *PLoS ONE* **2017**, *12*, e0180067. [CrossRef] [PubMed]

49. Barragan-Rodriguez, L.; Rodriguez-Moran, M.; Guerrero-Romero, F. Efficacy and safety of oral magnesium supplementation in the treatment of depression in the elderly with type 2 diabetes: A randomized, equivalent trial. *Magnes. Res.* **2008**, *21*, 218–223. [PubMed]

50. Mehdi, S.M.; Atlas, S.E.; Qadir, S.; Musselman, D.; Goldberg, S.; Woolger, J.M.; Corredor, R.; Abbas, M.H.; Arosemena, L.; Caccamo, S.; et al. Double-blind, randomized crossover study of intravenous infusion of magnesium sulfate versus 5% dextrose on depressive symptoms in adults with treatment-resistant depression. *Psychiatry Clin. Neurosci.* **2017**, *71*, 204–211. [CrossRef] [PubMed]

51. Fard, F.E.; Mirghafourvand, M.; Mohammad-Alizadeh Charandabi, S.; Farshbaf-Khalili, A.; Javadzadeh, Y.; Asgharian, H. Effects of zinc and magnesium supplements on postpartum depression and anxiety: A randomized controlled clinical trial. *Women Health* **2017**, *57*, 1115–1128. [CrossRef] [PubMed]

52. Martínez-González, M.Á.; Sánchez-Villegas, A. Magnesium intake and depression: The SUN cohort. *Magnes. Res.* **2016**, *29*, 102–111. [PubMed]

53. Nechifor, M. Magnesium in major depression. *Magnes. Res.* **2009**, *22*, 163s–166s. [PubMed]

54. Poleszak, E. Modulation of antidepressant-like activity of magnesium by serotonergic system. *J. Neural Transm.* **2007**, *114*, 1129–1134. [CrossRef] [PubMed]

55. George, M.S.; Rosenstein, D.; Rubinow, D.R.; Kling, M.A.; Post, R.M. CSF magnesium in affective disorder: Lack of correlation with clinical course of treatment. *Psychiatry Res.* **1994**, *51*, 139–146. [CrossRef]

56. Herzberg, L.; Bold, A.M. Sex difference in mean serum-magnesium levels in depression. *Lancet* **1972**, *1*, 1128–1129. [CrossRef]

57. Stanton, M.F.; Lowenstein, F.W. Serum magnesium in women during pregnancy, while taking contraceptives, and after menopause. *J. Am. Coll. Nutr.* **1987**, *6*, 313–319. [CrossRef] [PubMed]

58. Brown, R.A.; Abrantes, A.M.; Strong, D.R.; Niaura, R.; Kahler, C.W.; Miller, I.W.; Price, L.H. Efficacy of sequential use of fluoxetine for smoking cessation in elevated depressive symptom smokers. *Nicotine Tob. Res. Off. J. Soc. Res. Nicotine Tob.* **2014**, *16*, 197–207. [CrossRef] [PubMed]

59. Kenney, B.A.; Holahan, C.J.; North, R.J.; Holahan, C.K. Depressive symptoms and cigarette smoking in American workers. *Am. J. Health Promot. AJHP* **2006**, *20*, 179–182. [CrossRef] [PubMed]

60. Vázquez-Palacios, G.; Bonilla-Jaime, H.; Velázquez-Moctezuma, J. Antidepressant effects of nicotine and fluoxetine in an animal model of depression induced by neonatal treatment with clomipramine. *Prog. Neuro-Psychopharmacol. Biol. Psychiatry* **2005**, *29*, 39–46. [CrossRef] [PubMed]

61. Glassman, A.H.; Covey, L.S.; Stetner, F.; Rivelli, S. Smoking cessation and the course of major depression: A follow-up study. *Lancet* **2001**, *357*, 1929–1932. [CrossRef]

62. Salín-Pascual, R.J.; Galicia-Polo, L.; Drucker-Colín, R.; de la Fuente, J.R.; Drucker-Colín, R.; Salín-Pascual, R.J. Effects of transderman nicotine on mood and sleep in nonsmoking major depresssed patients. *Psychopharmacology* **1995**, *121*, 476–479. [CrossRef] [PubMed]

63. Cosci, F.; Nardi, A.E.; Griez, E.J. Nicotine effects on human affective functions: A systematic review of the literature on a controversial issue. *CNS Neurol. Disord. Drug Targets* **2014**, *13*, 981–991. [CrossRef] [PubMed]

10

A Pilot Randomized Trial of Oral Magnesium Supplementation on Supraventricular Arrhythmias

Pamela L. Lutsey [1,*], Lin Y. Chen [2], Anne Eaton [3], Melanie Jaeb [1], Kyle D. Rudser [3], James D. Neaton [3] and Alvaro Alonso [4]

[1] Division of Epidemiology & Community Health, School of Public Health, University of Minnesota, 1300 South 2nd Street, Suite 300, Minneapolis, MN 55454, USA; jaebx008@umn.edu
[2] Cardiovascular Division, Department of Medicine, University of Minnesota, Minneapolis, MN 55455, USA; chenx484@umn.edu
[3] Division of Biostatistics, School of Public Health, University of Minnesota, Minneapolis, MN 55455, USA; eato0055@umn.edu (A.E.); rudser@umn.edu (K.D.R.); jim@ccbr.umn.edu (J.D.N.)
[4] Department of Epidemiology, Rollins School of Public Health, Emory University, Atlanta, GA 30322, USA; alvaro.alonso@emory.edu
* Correspondence: Lutsey@umn.edu

Abstract: Low magnesium may increase the risk of atrial fibrillation. We conducted a double-blind pilot randomized trial to assess adherence to oral magnesium supplementation (400 mg of magnesium oxide daily) and a matching placebo, estimate the effect on circulating magnesium concentrations, and evaluate the feasibility of using an ambulatory heart rhythm monitoring device (ZioPatch) for assessing premature atrial contractions. A total of 59 participants were randomized; 73% were women, and the mean age was 62 years. A total of 98% of the participants completed the follow-up. In the magnesium supplement group, 75% of pills were taken, and in the placebo group, 83% were taken. The change in magnesium concentrations was significantly greater for those given the magnesium supplements than for those given the placebo (0.07; 95% confidence interval: 0.03, 0.12 mEq/L; $p = 0.002$). The ZioPatch wear time was approximately 13 of the requested 14 days at baseline and follow-up. There was no difference by intervention assignment in the change in log premature atrial contractions burden, glucose, or blood pressure. Gastrointestinal changes were more common among the participants assigned magnesium (50%) than among those assigned the placebo (7%), but only one person discontinued participation. In sum, compliance with the oral magnesium supplementation was very good, and acceptance of the ZioPatch monitoring was excellent. These findings support the feasibility of a larger trial for atrial fibrillation (AF) prevention with oral magnesium supplementation.

Keywords: magnesium; atrial fibrillation; glucose; randomized controlled trial

1. Introduction

Atrial fibrillation (AF) is a common cardiac arrhythmia characterized by irregular atrial electrical activity. In the United States (US), more than 3 million individuals had AF in 2010, and this figure is expected to more than double by 2050 [1–3]. Current AF treatments, including antiarrhythmic drugs and catheter ablation for rhythm restoration and oral anticoagulation for the prevention of thromboembolism, have suboptimal efficacy and carry significant risks [4]. The limitations of the available therapeutic approaches highlight the need for primary prevention interventions [5,6]. As highlighted in a 2009 National Heart, Lung, and Blood Institute (NHLBI) report [5] and stressed in a more recent Heart Rhythm Society-sponsored whitepaper [6], there is an urgent need to identify new and effective strategies for the primary prevention of AF.

Compelling evidence from numerous lines of inquiry suggests that low concentrations of serum magnesium may be causally associated with AF risk. First, magnesium supplementation is recommended as prophylaxis for the prevention of AF in patients undergoing cardiac surgery. A recent Cochrane systematic review and meta-analysis of randomized trials assessing the efficacy of magnesium supplementation for AF prevention in heart surgery reported an odds ratio of 0.55 (95% CI: 0.41, 0.73) for AF or supraventricular arrhythmia, comparing the magnesium intervention to the control [7]. Second, indirect evidence from three prospective epidemiologic studies provides some support for such intervention; each reported that individuals in the lowest versus the highest quantile of serum magnesium were 35–50% more likely to develop incident AF, after multivariable adjustment [8–10]. Finally, additional evidence for the effect of magnesium on the risk of arrhythmias is provided by a study of dietary magnesium restriction, in which 3 out of 14 women fed a low-magnesium diet developed AF, which resolved quickly after magnesium repletion [11].

Whether magnesium supplementation could have a role in the prevention of AF in the community has not been tested. Were magnesium supplementation shown to prevent AF and be safe over the long-term, it would be an ideal intervention for primary prevention, as it is easy to implement, inexpensive, and low concentrations are common. The population prevalence of low magnesium is not known but is believed to be high. Individuals at particularly high risk of hypomagnesemia are alcoholics, those who take certain diuretics, those with poorly controlled diabetes [12], and the elderly. In a study of nursing home residents, 33% were clinically deficient [13]. Intake of magnesium in the US population is also low, to the extent that the 2015 Dietary Guidelines Advisory Committee classified magnesium as a "shortfall nutrient", based on the finding that approximately 50% of Americans consume less than the estimated average requirement [14]. However, dietary magnesium intake and serum magnesium are poorly correlated; in the community-based Atherosclerosis Risk in Communities (ARIC) study, the Pearson's correlation coefficient was only 0.04 [9].

As part of the planning effort for a large randomized trial to prevent AF with magnesium supplementation, we conducted a double-blind, placebo-controlled randomized clinical trial of oral magnesium supplementation to assess supplement adherence, the side effects, the effect on serum magnesium concentration, and the feasibility of using an ambulatory monitoring device for the identification of arrhythmias.

2. Materials and Methods

The study was registered at Clinicaltrials.gov (# NCT02837328). The study protocol was approved by the University of Minnesota Institutional Review Board, and all participants provided written informed consent.

2.1. Study Participants

Participants of 55 years of age or older were recruited using fliers, the University of Minnesota StudyFinder website, invitations to individuals enrolled in the ResearchMatch research volunteer database, and invitations to University of Minnesota School of Public Health employees. The exclusion criteria included a prior history of heart disease (coronary heart disease, heart failure, AF), stroke, or known kidney disease; the use of type I or III antiarrhythmic drugs or digoxin; the current use of magnesium supplements; any prior history of allergy or intolerance to magnesium; lactose intolerance; and a prior history of inflammatory bowel disease or any severe gastrointestinal disorder. The use of multivitamins was allowable, because these typically contain relatively low dosages of Magnesium (e.g., 50 mg).

The eligible participants attended a baseline visit where measurements were conducted and a Zio® XT Patch (ZioPatch; iRhythm Technologies, Inc., San Francisco, CA, USA) heart rhythm monitor was applied by trained staff. After wearing the ZioPatch for 2 weeks, the participants were randomized 1:1 to either 400 mg of magnesium oxide or a placebo using block randomization within two strata of age (younger than 65 and 65 and older). The randomization was carried out separately for the two randomization strata. In each group, a randomization schedule was generated using randomly permuted blocks of random sizes. Block sizes of 2, 4, or 6 were permitted. The randomization was implemented using the blockrand package in R.

Following randomization, the participants were mailed the study intervention, which they took for a total of 12 weeks. Then, 10 weeks after beginning the study intervention, the participants took part in a follow-up clinic visit, and a second ZioPatch was applied. The participants continued the study intervention until the second ZioPatch was removed (2 weeks after the follow-up clinic visit). A participant flow diagram is provided in Figure 1.

Participant Flow Diagram

Figure 1. * Due to missing data on individual items, the total numbers of observations included in the linear models are 57, 57, 54, 54, 58, and 58 for the outcomes log premature atrial contraction (PAC) burden, PAC burden, serum magnesium, serum glucose, systolic blood pressure, and diastolic blood pressure, respectively.

2.2. Study Intervention and Blinding

The University of Minnesota Institute for Therapeutics Discovery and Drug Development produced the active study intervention (400 mg of magnesium oxide) and the matched placebo (lactose) according to Good Manufacturing Practices. The University of Minnesota Investigational Drug Service managed the bottling per the randomization scheme. The study participants and all the study staff were blinded to the treatment given.

2.3. Measurements

At the baseline and follow-up clinic visits, the participants completed questionnaires, and trained study staff conducted physiological measurements (i.e., anthropometry, blood pressure), phlebotomy, and applied the ZioPatch device. Treatment compliance was assessed by a pill count at the follow-up visit. At intervention days 21, 42, and 80, the participants were also emailed unique links to online questionnaires, administered via REDCap [15], which queried compliance and asked the following open-ended question about adverse effects: "Since starting the study, have you experienced anything out of the ordinary?" Participant blinding was also assessed on intervention day 80, the last day of the study.

The ZioPatch was used to identify premature atrial contractions (PACs). PACs are supraventricular arrhythmias associated with the future risk of AF [6,16,17] and are considered an intermediate phenotype of the arrhythmia, reflecting the underlying cardiac substrate that facilitates the development of AF [18]. The participants were asked to wear the ZioPatches for 2 weeks after each clinic visit. The information obtained from the ZioPatch devices was processed by the ZEUS algorithm, a comprehensive system that analyzes electrocardiographic data received from the device [19]. We counted as PACs isolated supraventricular ectopic beats, supraventricular ectopic couplet total count, and supraventricular ectopic triplet total count. The total PACs were then divided by the number of hours the ZioPatch recorded analyzable data, which yielded PACs per hour.

The participants were asked to fast for 8 h prior to blood draws. Serum magnesium and glucose were measured using the Roche Cobas 6000 at the University of Minnesota Advanced Research and Diagnostic Laboratory. Blood pressure was measured with the participant sitting, after a 5 min rest, with a random zero sphygmomanometer (Omron Digital Blood Pressure Monitor HEM-907XL; Omron Healthcare Inc., Kyoto, Japan). Three measurements were taken; all three measurements were averaged for use in analyses. Height and weight were measured with the participants in light clothing and shoes removed. Height was measured with a research stadiometer and weight with a scale.

2.4. Statistical Analysis

The goal of the pilot study was to assess adherence to the magnesium supplement and the feasibility of using the ZioPatch and to collect preliminary data on PACs, a predictor of AF. The targeted sample size of 60 was determined to detect a difference in the change in log PACs (follow-up minus baseline) between treatment groups of 0.79 standard deviation units with 80% power and 5% type I error (2-sided), assuming five participants would not complete the follow-up.

All analyses were intent-to-treat. Descriptive statistics are provided according to treatment assignment for baseline characteristics, adherence, magnesium concentrations, and other outcomes. The differences in baseline characteristics between groups were assessed using t-tests for continuous variables and Fisher's exact tests for categorical variables. Linear regression was used to evaluate whether change in outcomes differed according to treatment assignment, adjusting for the randomization stratification factor (age $\geq$65 vs. <65) and the baseline value of the outcome with robust variance estimates for confidence intervals and p-values. Post-hoc sensitivity analyses further adjusted for sex. As PAC burden is highly skewed, we pre-specified using log PAC burden for analysis and reported the ratio of geometric means. Pre-specified subgroup analyses were also performed, stratified by baseline magnesium concentration (< vs. $\geq$median). A two-sided p-value of <0.05 was used to indicate statistical significance. The analyses were conducted using R [20] version 3.4.0 (R Foundation, Vienna, Austria).

3. Results

3.1. Study Participants

Between March and June 2017, 59 participants were randomized: 29 were assigned to the magnesium supplement and 30 to the matching placebo. The participant characteristics were generally similar by treatment group, with the notable exception of sex; 86.2% of the participants in the treatment group were women, while in the placebo group, 60.0% were female (Table 1). The mean age of the participants was 61.5 ± 5.2 years. The baseline serum magnesium concentration was 1.74 ± 0.11 mEq/L in the participants assigned the magnesium supplements and 1.71 ± 0.10 in those assigned the placebo; 6.9% had magnesium concentrations below the threshold for clinical deficiency (<1.5 mEq/L), while 37.9% had concentrations below the threshold for subclinical deficiency (<1.7 mEq/L).

Table 1. Baseline participant characteristics * overall and stratified by intervention status.

	Overall	Magnesium (400 mg Daily)	Placebo	p-Value
N	59	29	30	
Demographics				
Age, years	61.5 ± 5.2	61.3 ± 5.3	61.6 ± 5.2	0.814
Age category				0.761
≥65 years	14 (23.7)	6 (20.7)	8 (26.7)	
<65 years	45 (76.3)	23 (79.3)	22 (73.3)	
Sex				0.039
Female	43 (72.9)	25 (86.2)	18 (60.0)	
Male	16 (27.1)	4 (13.8)	12 (40)	
Race				0.612
White	56 (94.9)	27 (93.1)	29 (96.7)	
Nonwhite	3 (5.1)	2 (6.9)	1 (3.3)	
Educational attainment				0.279
High school graduate or GED	1 (1.7)	0 (0)	1 (3.3)	
Some college	10 (16.9)	6 (20.7)	4 (13.3)	
College graduate	26 (44.1)	10 (34.5)	16 (53.3)	
Graduate school or professional school	22 (37.3)	13 (44.8)	9 (30)	
Physiologic characteristics				
Height, cm	167.9 (9.2)	167.1 (8.1)	168.7 (10.3)	0.491
Weight, kg	79.2 (18.2)	78.0 (18.0)	80.5 (18.7)	0.603
BMI, kg/m^2	27.9 ± 4.6	27.7 ± 4.9	28.0 ± 4.5	0.804
Serum magnesium, mEq/L	1.72 ± 0.11	1.74 ± 0.12	1.71 ± 0.10	0.308
Systolic blood pressure, mmHg	119 ± 16	119 ± 14	119 ± 18	0.933
Diastolic blood pressure, mmHg	71 ± 9	72 ± 9	71 ± 10	0.627
Antihypertensive medication	14 (24)	9 (31)	5 (17)	0.233
Serum glucose, mg/dL	98.9 ± 29.9	94.2 ± 10.6	103.2 ± 40.2	0.242
Sensitivity analysis **	95.2 ± 11.1	94.2 ± 10.6	96.2 ± 11.6	0.494
Glucose lowering medication	2 (3.4)	0 (0)	2 (6.7)	0.492
PAC burden, episodes/h	14.5 ± 58	8.5 ± 14	20.2 ± 80	0.437
Median (25th, 75th percentiles)	2.28 (1.22, 6.86)	3.64 (1.31, 7.57)	1.75 (1.12, 4.01)	
Log PAC burden, log(episodes/h)	1.15 ± 1.42	1.26 ± 1.35	1.04 ± 1.49	0.566
Median (25th, 75th percentiles)	0.82 (0.20, 1.92)	1.29 (0.27, 2.02)	0.55 (0.11, 1.39)	

GED, general education diploma; BMI, body mass index; PAC, premature atrial contractions; and SD, standard deviation. * mean ± SD or *n* (%). ** Omission of one participant with a baseline glucose value of 307 mg/dL.

Log PAC burden (episodes per hour) at baseline was 1.26 ± 1.35 in the treatment group and 1.15 ± 1.42 in the placebo group. At baseline, the average ZioPatch analyzable time in the intervention and placebo groups were 13.1 ± 1.7 and 12.9 ± 2.6 days, respectively, with 93.1% assigned to magnesium and 90.0% assigned to placebo wearing ≥12 days.

3.2. Follow-Up

A total of two participants, both in the intervention group, were missing ZioPatch information at follow-up; one participant dropped out of the study, and one was missing information due to a device malfunction.

3.3. Adherence and Magnesium Concentrations

Based on pill count, the participants in the magnesium group took 75.1% ± 17.8% of tablets, whereas those in the placebo group took 83.4% ± 5.9%. Self-reported information about the percent of missing pills and the reasons for missing pills is provided in Table 2. Of the participants, 60% in the Magnesium group reported missing at least 1 pill, as did 52% in the placebo group. The most common reason for missing pills was forgetting. However, five individuals in the Magnesium group marked the response "makes me sick" as the reason for not taking a pill, whereas no individuals in the placebo group reported missing pills for that reason.

Table 2. Self-reported compliance.

Compliance	% Reporting Missing Pills			Reason for Missing Pills, N			
				Forgot	Too Busy	Makes Me Sick	Other
Ever reported *							
Magnesium	60%			7	0	5	2
Placebo	52%			11	2	0	3
	% Reporting Missing Pills in:			Reason for Missing Pills, N			
Reported at Specific Follow-Up Visits **	Last 3 Days	Last 1 Week	Last 2 Weeks				
Intervention Day 21							
Magnesium	8%	12%	20%	2	0	2	1
Placebo	0%	7%	24%	7	1	0	0
Intervention Day 42							
Magnesium	22%	33%	39%	5	0	5	1
Placebo	15%	22%	31%	6	2	0	2
Intervention Day 80							
Magnesium	14%	27%	40%	5	0	1	0
Placebo	12%	23%	28%	6	1	0	1

* Over any time frame (i.e., last 3 days, last 1 week, last 2 weeks). ** Responses not mutually exclusive (e.g., the same individual could have reported forgetting to take pills at intervention days 21, 42, 80).

Over the 12-week follow-up period, those assigned magnesium supplementation had a significant increase in serum magnesium concentration as compared with those assigned the placebo (0.07 mEq/L; 95% CI: 0.03, 0.12; $p = 0.002$) (Table 3). In subgroup analyses, the change in magnesium concentration did not vary by baseline magnesium concentration (Table 4; p-interaction 0.24). Specifically, among the participants who at baseline were below the median serum magnesium concentration (i.e., 1.74 mEq/L), the effect of the magnesium versus the placebo on the change in the serum magnesium concentration was 0.05 (95% CI: 0.00, 0.10), whereas among those at or above the median at baseline, the effect was 0.12 (95% CI: 0.04, 0.20).

Table 3. Change in PACs and secondary endpoints (i.e., systolic blood pressure (SBP), diastolic blood pressure (DBP), serum glucose, serum magnesium) according to treatment group.

	Magnesium (400 mg Daily) Mean (SD)	Placebo Mean (SD)	Intervention Effect Coefficient * (95% CI)	p-Value
Primary outcome (episodes/h)				
Log PAC burden			0.94 (0.69, 1.3) **	0.73
Baseline	1.26 (1.4)	1.04 (1.49)		
Follow-up †	1.16 (1.41)	1.09 (1.53)		
Change	−0.06 (0.68)	0.05 (0.75)		
PAC burden			0.44 (−2.58, 3.46)	
Baseline	8.5 ± 14	20.2 ± 80		
Follow-up †	8.1 ± 12	14.6 ± 48		
Change	−0.6 ± 7	−5.6 ± 33		
Secondary outcomes				
Serum magnesium, mEq/L			0.07 (0.03, 0.12)	0.002
Baseline	1.74 (0.12)	1.71 (0.1)		
Follow-up ‡	1.8 (0.13)	1.71 (0.11)		
Change	0.07 (0.09)	0 (0.1)		
Serum glucose, mg/dL			2.4 (−3.0, 7.7)	0.39
Baseline	94.2 (10.6)	103.2 (40.2)		
Follow-up ‡	96.3 (12.2)	96.2 (13.7)		
Change	1.8 (7.5)	−7.1 (32.8)		
Serum glucose ¥, mg/dL			2.8 (−0.9, 6.4)	0.14
Baseline	94.2 (10.6)	96.2 (11.6)		
Follow-up ‡	96.3 (12.2)	95 (12.4)		
Change	1.75 (7.5)	−1.21 (6.7)		
Systolic blood pressure, mmHg			2.9 (−1.8, 7.2)	0.18
Baseline	119 (14)	119 (18)		
Follow-up ‡	118 (14)	115 (14)		
Change	−1 (10)	−4 (10)		
Diastolic blood pressure, mmHg			−0.5 (−3.5, 2.5)	0.74
Baseline	71.8 (8. 7)	70.6 (10.3)		
Follow-up ‡	71.0 (8.8)	70.8 (8.7)		
Change	−0.5 (7.1)	0.2 (6.1)		

CI, confidence Interval; DBP, diastolic blood pressure; PAC, premature atrial contractions; SD, standard deviation; and SBP, systolic blood pressure. * Adjusted for age (≥65 or <65), and baseline concentration (e.g., when change in glucose is the outcome, models were adjusted for baseline glucose). The numbers of observations included in linear models are 57, 57, 54, 54, 53, 58, and 58 for the outcomes log PAC burden, PAC burden, serum magnesium, serum glucose, serum glucose excluding outlier, systolic blood pressure and diastolic blood pressure, respectively. ** Presented as a ratio of geometric means (i.e., exp(coefficient)). † ZioPatch was worn for a 2-week period, from the follow-up clinic visit (intervention week 10) through the end of the study (intervention week 12). ‡ Follow-up information obtained at clinic visit (intervention week 10). ¥ Outlier removed.

Table 4. Change in PACs and secondary endpoints (i.e., SBP, DBP, serum glucose, serum magnesium) according to treatment group, stratified by baseline serum magnesium concentration.

Primary Outcome	Baseline Serum Magnesium Concentration				p-Interaction
	<Median		≥Median		
	Intervention Effect Coefficient * (95% CI)	p-Value	Intervention Effect Coefficient * (95% CI)	p-Value	
Log PAC burden	0.89 (0.51, 1.54) **	0.67	0.91 (0.61, 1.35) **	0.64	0.88
Serum magnesium, mEq/L	0.05 (0, 0.10)	0.04	0.12 (0.04,0.20)	0.004	0.24
Serum glucose, magnesium/dL	−4.7 (−13.3, 4.0)	0.29	6.0 (2.0, 10.0)	0.03	0.06
Serum glucose, magnesium/dL ¥	−3.2 (−9.0, 2.6)	0.28	6.0 (2.0, 10.0)	0.03	0.01
Systolic blood pressure, mmHg	4.8 (1.0, 8.5)	0.01	3.8 (−2.5, 10.2)	0.24	0.96
Diastolic blood pressure, mmHg	5.5 (0.6, 10.4)	0.03	2.4 (−5.6, 0.8)	0.14	0.009

CI, confidence Interval; DBP, diastolic blood pressure; PAC, premature atrial contractions; and SBP, systolic blood pressure. * Adjusted for age (≥65 or <65) and baseline concentration (e.g., when change in glucose is the outcome, models were adjusted for baseline glucose). ¥ Outlier removed. ** Ratio of geometric means.

3.4. Effect of Magnesium Supplementation on Trial Outcomes

Table 3 presents the study outcome values at baseline and follow-up, as well as age- and baseline value-adjusted differences in change according to intervention assignment. Spaghetti plots depicting individual change over the intervention period are provided in Figure 2. At follow-up, the ZioPatch average wear times were similar to the baseline, with 13.0 ± 1.8 days for the intervention group, 12.7 ± 2.3 days for the placebo group, and 92.6% assigned to magnesium and 73.3% assigned to placebo wearing ≥ 12 days. For the primary outcome, log PAC burden (episodes per hour), change over the intervention period was -0.06 (95% confidence interval (CI): $-0.33, 0.20$) for those randomized to the magnesium supplement and 0.05 (95% CI: $-0.23, 0.33$) for those randomized to the placebo. In the multivariable-adjusted models, there was no evidence of an intervention effect; the ratio of geometric means was 0.94 ($0.69, 1.3$), p-value = 0.73. Similarly, in subgroup analyses, the effect did not differ according to baseline magnesium concentration above versus below the median (Table 4; p-interaction = 0.88).

Magnesium supplementation was not significantly associated with change in serum glucose (2.4 (95% CI: $-3.0, 7.7$) mg/dL; $p = 0.39$). The lack of association remained in sensitivity analyses, excluding one participant with extremely high baseline glucose (2.8 (95% CI: $-0.9, 6.4$) mg/dL) and one participant who reported changing his/her diabetes medication status during the follow-up (2.0 (95%: $-3.6, 7.5$) mg/dL). The intervention was also not significantly associated with change in systolic or diastolic blood pressure overall (2.9 (95%: $-1.4, 7.2$) mmHg and -0.5 (95%: $-3.5, 2.5$) mmHg, respectively) or after excluding two participants who changed their blood pressure medication status between the baseline and follow-up visits.

In post-hoc analyses, where we additionally adjusted for sex, the results were similar. Also, no meaningful patterns emerged in additional subgroup analyses by age category and sex.

3.5. Safety and Tolerability of the Intervention

When asked an open-ended question about adverse events, the most commonly reported responses were related to gastrointestinal (GI) symptoms. Of the intervention group, 32% commented on GI changes at intervention day 21, 30% at day 42, and 33% at day 80. In the placebo group 7% commented on GI changes at intervention day 21, 4% at day 42, and 0% at day 80. When considering unique individuals, 50% assigned to magnesium and 7% assigned to placebo commented on GI changes at any point in the study. Specific GI comments, by intervention day, are provided in Table 5.

One person in the intervention group experienced side effects, which led the participant to discontinue blinded study treatment.

At the end of the study, when asked to which group they were assigned, among those assigned to the active treatment, 15% guessed magnesium supplements, 14.3% guessed placebo, and 35.7% reported not knowing (15 participants did not respond). Of those assigned to the placebo, 4.3% guessed magnesium supplements, 26.1% guessed placebo, and 69.6% reported not knowing (7 participants did not respond).

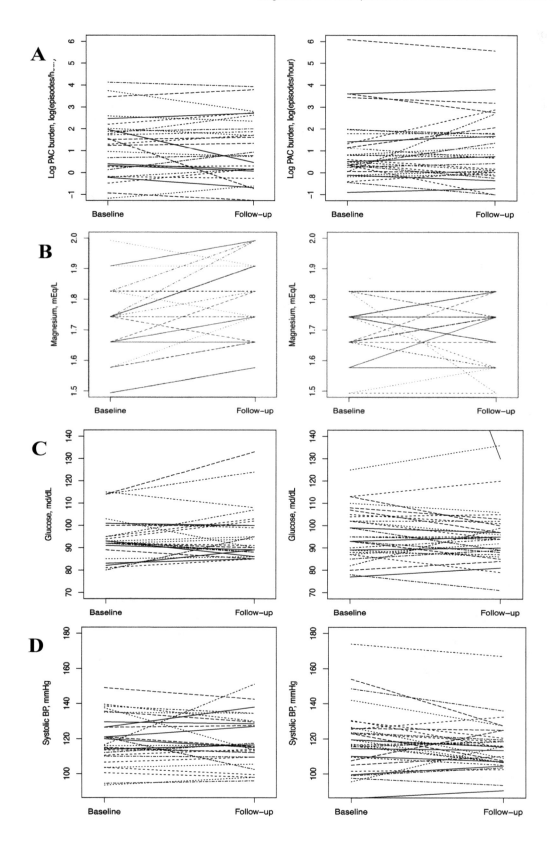

Figure 2. Spaghetti plots for change in (**A**) log PAC burden, (**B**) change in serum magnesium, (**C**) serum glucose *, and (**D**) SBP (systolic blood pressure). * One participant had a baseline glucose concentration of 307 mg/dL. The baseline value for this participant is outside the frame. PAC, premature atrial contractions; and BP, blood pressure.

Table 5. Gastrointestinal (GI)-related responses to the open-ended question, "Since starting the study, have you experienced anything out of the ordinary?" *.

Intervention Day #	Intervention	Comment
Day #21	Magnesium	Less solid stools
	Magnesium	Initially, I took the pill before bed with calcium and fish oil and a blood pressure med. It did not really make me sick, but I felt some bloating and cramping. I switched to taking it in the am, and that works better. That was the reason for missing.
	Magnesium	Diarrhea
	Magnesium	My stools have changed in consistency and color.
	Magnesium	I have had some diarrhea but that could be due to my innards. They have been unpredictable since my abdominal/colorectal surgeries.
	Magnesium	After 4 pills, I quit taking them due to intestinal issues. I was in the bathroom the third and fourth day and very crampy all day. I emailed and was told I could quit taking them.
	Magnesium	The first two days, I experienced brief bouts of diarrhea about 90 min after taking the pills. No problems since.
	Magnesium	Some diarrhea and gas
	Placebo	Sudden onset of nausea lasting about 30 s about an hour after taking the pill.
	Placebo	Increase in diarrhea but could be from the increase in nuts in my diet.
Day #42	Magnesium	Slightly often stools
	Magnesium	Diarrhea
	Magnesium	Slight nausea, slight pain in stomach, increased flatulence
	Magnesium	Upset Stomach
	Magnesium	The initial 4 pills made me sick. Also, I am currently stressed as my (spouse) is scheduled for (major) surgery next week.
	Magnesium	A little diarrhea an hour or so after taking the pill, but this only happened on the first two days.
	Magnesium	Had gastrointestional issues when taking the pill.
	Magnesium	Loose stools, some diarrhea, and cramps after taking pill in the morning.
	Placebo	Diarrhea, but could be due to increased nut intake,
Day #80	Magnesium	Some difficulty with digestion
	Magnesium	My fingernails have gotten must stronger, and my bowels were loose and somewhat sluggish.
	Magnesium	I have been a lot 'looser' since taking the pills.
	Magnesium	Upset stomach
	Magnesium	Small bouts of diarrhea the first two days of taking the pills; nothing since.

#, number .* Some details were modified slightly to reduce the likelihood of identifying a participant. Minor spelling and punctuation changes were made to improve clarity.

4. Discussion

In this pilot trial of 59 relatively healthy adults aged 55 and older, supplementation with 400 mg of magnesium daily over 12 weeks was safe and well tolerated and led to a change of 0.07 mEq/L in serum magnesium, which is substantial enough in magnitude that in a larger sample size it may translate to health outcomes. The intervention was not associated with change in PACs, but estimates of association had wide confidence intervals, and the study was not powered to identify important differences. Likewise, there was no association between supplemental magnesium and changes in glucose, systolic blood pressure, or diastolic blood pressure.

The mechanisms through which magnesium supplementation could reduce the risk of supraventricular arrhythmias and AF are not fully understood. However, magnesium is known to play a direct role in cardiac contractility [21]. Small studies in healthy individuals and in patients with cardiac disease have found that intravenous magnesium administration prolongs sinoatrial, intra-atrial, and atrioventricular node conduction and the atrial refractory period, which in turn may contribute to prevent the onset of AF [22–24]. Also, randomization to 148 mg of oral magnesium (and 296 mg of potassium) intake (vs. the placebo) had antiarrhythmic effects among 232 patients with frequent ventricular arrhythmias [25].

Blood pressure and diabetes are also established risk factors for AF [26,27], through which magnesium may lower AF risk. In the present pilot trial, changes in blood pressure and serum glucose did not differ significantly for those given the magnesium supplementation and those given the placebo. This is in contrast with the existing literature; however, our study was small, and confidence intervals around the treatment differences were wide. Meta-analyses of randomized controlled trials have consistently demonstrated that magnesium supplementation lowers blood pressure in a dose-dependent manner [28–30]. In the most recent meta-analysis, a median dose of 368 mg/d for a median duration of 3 months significantly reduced systolic blood pressure (BP) by 2.0 mm Hg (95% CI: 0.4, 3.6) and diastolic BP by 1.8 mm Hg (95% CI: 0.7, 2.8) [30]. Based partly on this evidence, in November 2016, a petition was filed with the Food and Drug Administration (FDA) for a qualified health claim for magnesium and reduced risk of high blood pressure (FDA-2016-Q-3770). A comparable meta-analysis of RCTs, including a total of 370 patients with type 2 diabetes, found that magnesium supplementation (median dosage 360 mg/day) reduced concentrations of fasting blood glucose (-10.1 mg/dL, 95% CI -19.8, -0.2) over a median intervention duration of 13 weeks [31]. These meta-analyses suggest that magnesium is causally related to hypertension and abnormal glucose homeostasis. However, their interpretation is complicated by the fact that the individual studies included in the meta-analyses were highly heterogeneous in terms of magnesium formulation and dosage and participant characteristics.

In terms of serum magnesium, the intervention of 400 mg of magnesium oxide daily was associated with a serum increase of 0.07 mEq/L. This finding is concordant with results from a meta-analysis of the effect of magnesium supplementation dosage on serum magnesium response. In the meta-analysis the median dose was 360 mg of magnesium/day, the intervention length was 12 weeks, and the response was 0.08 mEq/L [32]. In the meta-analysis there was evidence of an inverse relationship between the baseline magnesium concentration and responsiveness to the supplementation. A similar phenomenon was not observed in the present trial; however, in our sample, the baseline magnesium concentrations were quite high, and power was exceedingly low for subgroup comparisons.

The results from this study provide additional evidence about compliance with magnesium supplementation at the dosage of 400 mg of magnesium daily, as well as safety and tolerability. Among the participants randomized to magnesium, only 1 out of 29 participants (3.5%) ceased the intervention due to side effects. The compliance in this study was good, at 75% in the intervention group and 83% in the placebo group, according to pill counts. The low drop-out rate and high compliance provides support for the tolerability of this dosage. However, the fact that 50% in the intervention group commented on GI changes at some point in the follow-up should not be dismissed. Unfortunately, given the way side effects were assessed, it is not possible to quantify the severity of the GI complaints. Notably, several individuals only commented about GI changes in the first few days after taking the study treatment.

The primary limitation of this study is the small size, which led to an imbalance of some key potential confounding factors, such as sex. Among those randomized to magnesium, 86.2% were female, whereas among those randomized to the placebo, 60.0% were female. This is important, because AF risk is known to be greater among men [3]. However, the findings were similar in post-hoc sensitivity analyses where we adjusted for sex. An additional consideration is that the baseline serum concentrations of the trial participants were quite high; it is unclear how serum magnesium would have changed in a context of low baseline magnesium concentrations or how that may translate to change in other physiologic outcomes. Lastly, we assessed tolerability with a simple open-ended question, not a checklist of specific signs and symptoms graded for severity according to a standard toxicity table.

5. Conclusions

In sum, this small pilot double-blinded randomized controlled trial of supplementation with 400 mg of magnesium daily provides evidence to support the safety and tolerability of this intervention and for adherence to the ZioPatch heart rhythm monitoring device. Despite our study population being largely magnesium replete, a change in serum magnesium was observed. Magnesium supplementation was not associated with change in PACs, glucose, or blood pressure; however, this small pilot study was short-term and not powered to identify small-to-moderate clinically relevant differences. The results of this pilot study will guide the design of a larger trial to evaluate the effect of supplemental magnesium on arrhythmias.

Author Contributions: P.L.L. and A.A. conceived of the study. P.L.L., A.A., M.J., K.D.R., and J.D.N. designed the study. P.L.L., A.A., L.Y.C., and M.J. collected the data. A.E. conducted the data analysis. All authors were involved in the drafting and critical review of the manuscript.

Acknowledgments: We thank the study participants, for taking part in this study.

1. Go, A.S.; Hylek, E.M.; Phillips, K.A.; Chang, Y.C.; Henault, L.E.; Selby, J.V.; Singer, D.E. Prevalence of diagnosed atrial fibrillation in adults. National implications for rhythm management and stroke prevention: The Anticoagulation and Risk Factors in Atrial Fibrillation (ATRIA) study. *JAMA* **2001**, *285*, 2370–2375. [CrossRef] [PubMed]
2. Miyasaka, Y.; Barnes, M.E.; Gersh, B.J.; Cha, S.S.; Bailey, K.R.; Abhayaratna, W.P.; Seward, J.B.; Tsang, T.S.M. Secular trends in incidence of atrial fibrillation in Olmsted County, Minnesota, 1980 to 2000, and implications on the projections for future prevalence. *Circulation* **2006**, *114*, 119–125. [CrossRef] [PubMed]
3. Benjamin, E.J.; Virani, S.S.; Callaway, C.W.; Chang, A.R.; Cheng, S.; Chiuve, S.E.; Cushman, M.; Delling, F.N.; Deo, R.; de Ferranti, S.D.; et al. Heart Disease and Stroke Statistics—2018 Update: A Report From the American Heart Association. *Circulation* **2018**. [CrossRef] [PubMed]
4. January, C.T.; Wann, L.S.; Alpert, J.S.; Calkins, H.; Cigarroa, J.E.; Cleveland, J.C.; Conti, J.B.; Ellinor, P.T.; Ezekowitz, M.D.; Field, M.E.; et al. 2014 AHA/ACC/HRS guideline for the management of patients with atrial fibrillation: A report of the American College of Cardiology/American Heart Association Task Force on Practice Guidelines and the Heart Rhythm Society. *Circulation* **2014**, *130*, e199–e267. [CrossRef] [PubMed]
5. Benjamin, E.J.; Chen, P.-S.; Bild, D.E.; Mascette, A.M.; Albert, C.M.; Alonso, A.; Calkins, H.; Connolly, S.J.; Curtis, A.B.; Darbar, D.; et al. Prevention of atrial fibrillation: Report from an NHLBI workshop. *Circulation* **2009**, *119*, 606–618. [CrossRef] [PubMed]
6. Van Wagoner, D.R.; Piccini, J.P.; Albert, C.M.; Anderson, M.E.; Benjamin, E.J.; Brundel, B.; Califf, R.M.; Calkins, H.; Chen, P.-S.; Chiamvimonvat, N.; et al. Progress toward the prevention and treatment of atrial fibrillation: A summary of the Heart Rhythm Society Research Forum on the Treatment and Prevention of Atrial Fibrillation, Washington, DC, December 9–10, 2013. *Heart Rhythm* **2015**, *12*, e5–e29. [CrossRef] [PubMed]
7. Arsenault, K.A.; Yusuf, A.M.; Crystal, E.; Healey, J.S.; Morillo, C.A.; Nair, G.M.; Whitlock, R.P. Interventions for preventing post-operative atrial fibrillation in patients undergoing heart surgery. *Cochrane Database Syst. Rev.* **2013**, *1*, CD003611. [CrossRef] [PubMed]
8. Khan, A.M.; Lubitz, S.A.; Sullivan, L.M.; Sun, J.X.; Levy, D.; Vasan, R.S.; Magnani, J.W.; Ellinor, P.T.; Benjamin, E.J.; Wang, T.J. Low serum magnesium and the development of atrial fibrillation in the community: The Framingham Heart Study. *Circulation* **2013**, *127*, 33–38. [CrossRef] [PubMed]
9. Misialek, J.R.; Lopez, F.L.; Lutsey, P.L.; Huxley, R.R.; Peacock, J.M.; Chen, L.Y.; Soliman, E.Z.; Agarwal, S.K.; Alonso, A. Serum and dietary magnesium and incidence of atrial fibrillation in whites and in African Americans—Atherosclerosis Risk in Communities (ARIC) Study. *Circ. J.* **2013**, *77*, 323–329. [CrossRef] [PubMed]
10. Markovits, N.; Kurnik, D.; Halkin, H.; Margalit, R.; Bialik, M.; Lomnicky, Y.; Loebstein, R. Database evaluation of the association between serum magnesium levels and the risk of atrial fibrillation in the community. *Int. J. Cardiol.* **2016**, *205*, 142–146. [CrossRef] [PubMed]

11. Nielsen, F.H.; Milne, D.B.; Klevay, L.M.; Gallagher, S.; Johnson, L. Dietary magnesium deficiency induces heart rhythm changes, impairs glucose tolerance, and decreases serum cholesterol in post menopausal women. *J. Am. Coll. Nutr.* **2007**, *26*, 121–132. [CrossRef] [PubMed]

12. Wardlaw, G.M.; Byrd-Bredbenner, C.; Moe, G.; Berning, J.R.; Kelley, D.S. *Wardlaw's Perspectives in Nutrition*, 10th ed.; McGraw-Hill Education: New York, NY, USA, 2016.

13. Worwag, M.; Classen, H.G.; Schumacher, E. Prevalence of magnesium and zinc deficiencies in nursing home residents in Germany. *Magn. Res.* **1999**, *12*, 181–189.

14. Dietary Guidelines for Americans 2015–2020. Available online: https://health.gov/dietaryguidelines/2015/resources/2015-2020_Dietary_Guidelines.pdf (accessed on 2 October 2017).

15. Harris, P.A.; Taylor, R.; Thielke, R.; Payne, J.; Gonzalez, N.; Conde, J.G. Research Electronic Data Capture (REDCap)—A metadata-driven methodology and workflow process for providing translational research informatics support. *J. Biomed. Inform.* **2009**, *42*, 377–381. [CrossRef] [PubMed]

16. Dewland, T.A.; Vittinghoff, E.; Mandyam, M.C.; Heckbert, S.R.; Siscovick, D.S.; Stein, P.K.; Psaty, B.M.; Sotoodehnia, N.; Gottdiener, J.S.; Marcus, G.M. Atrial Ectopy as a Predictor of Incident Atrial Fibrillation A Cohort Study. *Ann. Intern. Med.* **2013**, *159*, 721–728. [CrossRef] [PubMed]

17. Chong, B.H.; Pong, V.; Lam, K.F.; Liu, S.; Zuo, M.L.; Lau, Y.F.; Lau, C.P.; Tse, H.F.; Siu, C.W. Frequent premature atrial complexes predict new occurrence of atrial fibrillation and adverse cardiovascular events. *Europace* **2012**, *14*, 942–947. [CrossRef] [PubMed]

18. Conen, D.; Adam, M.; Roche, F.; Barthelemy, J.C.; Felber Dietrich, D.; Imboden, M.; Kunzli, N.; von Eckardstein, A.; Regenass, S.; Hornemann, T.; et al. Premature atrial contractions in the general population: Frequency and risk factors. *Circulation* **2012**, *126*, 2302–2308. [CrossRef] [PubMed]

19. Turakhia, M.P.; Hoang, D.D.; Zimetbaum, P.; Miller, J.D.; Froelicher, V.F.; Kumar, U.N.; Xu, X.; Yang, F.; Heidenreich, P.A. Diagnostic utility of a novel leadless arrhythmia monitoring device. *Am. J. Cardiol.* **2013**, *112*, 520–524. [CrossRef] [PubMed]

20. R Development Core Team. *R: A Language and Environment for Statistical Computing*; R Foundation for Statistical Computing: Vienna, Austria, 2015.

21. Byrd-Bredbenner, C.; Moe, G.; Beshgetoor, D.; Berning, J. *Wardlaw's Perspectives in Nutrition*, 9th ed.; McGraw-Hill: New York, NY, USA, 2013; 259p.

22. Christiansen, E.H.; Frost, L.; Andreasen, F.; Mortensen, P.; Thomsen, P.E.; Pedersen, A.K. Dose-related cardiac electrophysiological effects of intravenous magnesium. A double-blind placebo-controlled dose-response study in patients with paroxysmal supraventricular tachycardia. *Europace* **2000**, *2*, 320–326. [CrossRef] [PubMed]

23. Rasmussen, H.S.; Thomsen, P.E. The electrophysiological effects of intravenous magnesium on human sinus node, atrioventricular node, atrium, and ventricle. *Clin. Cardiol.* **1989**, *12*, 85–90. [CrossRef] [PubMed]

24. Kulick, D.L.; Hong, R.; Ryzen, E.; Rude, R.K.; Rubin, J.N.; Elkayam, U.; Rahimtoola, S.H.; Bhandari, A.K. Electrophysiologic effects of intravenous magnesium in patients with normal conduction systems and no clinical evidence of significant cardiac disease. *Am. Heart J.* **1988**, *115*, 367–373. [CrossRef]

25. Zehender, M.; Meinertz, T.; Faber, T.; Caspary, A.; Jeron, A.; Bremm, K.; Just, H. Antiarrhythmic Effects of Increasing the Daily Intake of Magnesium and Potassium in Patients With Frequent Ventricular Arrhythmias fn1fn1This study was supported by Trommsdorff GmbH and Company, Alsdorf, Germany and Hexal AG, Holzkirchen, Germany. *J. Am. Coll. Cardiol.* **1997**, *29*, 1028–1034. [CrossRef]

26. Huxley, R.R.; Filion, K.B.; Konety, S.; Alonso, A. Meta-analysis of cohort and case-control studies of type 2 diabetes mellitus and risk of atrial fibrillation. *Am. J. Cardiol.* **2011**, *108*, 56–62. [CrossRef] [PubMed]

27. Roetker, N.S.; Chen, L.Y.; Heckbert, S.R.; Nazarian, S.; Soliman, E.Z.; Bluemke, D.A.; Lima, J.A.; Alonso, A. Relation of systolic, diastolic, and pulse pressure and aortic distensibility with atrial fibrillation (from the Multi-Ethnic Study of Atherosclerosis). *Am. J. Cardiol.* **2014**, *114*, 587–592. [CrossRef] [PubMed]

28. Jee, S.H.; Miller, E.R., 3rd; Guallar, E.; Singh, V.K.; Appel, L.J.; Klag, M.J. The effect of magnesium supplementation on blood pressure: A meta-analysis of randomized clinical trials. *Am. J. Hypertens.* **2002**, *15*, 691–696. [CrossRef]

29. Kass, L.; Weekes, J.; Carpenter, L. Effect of magnesium supplementation on blood pressure: A meta-analysis. *Eur. J. Clin. Nutr.* **2012**, *66*, 411–418. [CrossRef] [PubMed]

30. Zhang, X.; Li, Y.; Del Gobbo, L.C.; Rosanoff, A.; Wang, J.; Zhang, W.; Song, Y. Effects of Magnesium Supplementation on Blood Pressure: A Meta-Analysis of Randomized Double-Blind Placebo-Controlled

Trials. *Hypertension* **2016**, *68*, 324–333. [CrossRef] [PubMed]

31. Song, Y.; He, K.; Levitan, E.B.; Manson, J.E.; Liu, S. Effects of oral magnesium supplementation on glycaemic control in type 2 diabetes: A meta-analysis of randomized double-blind controlled trials. *Diabet. Med.* **2006**, *23*, 1050–1056. [CrossRef] [PubMed]

32. Zhang, X.; Del Gobbo, L.C.; Hruby, A.; Rosanoff, A.; He, K.; Dai, Q.; Costello, R.B.; Zhang, W.; Song, Y. The circulating concentration and 24-h urine excretion of magnesium dose- and time-dependently respond to oral magnesium supplementation in a meta-analysis of randomized controlled trials. *J. Nutr.* **2016**, *146*, 595–602. [CrossRef] [PubMed]

11

The Role of Magnesium in Neurological Disorders

Anna E. Kirkland [1], Gabrielle L. Sarlo [1] and Kathleen F. Holton [2,3,*]

[1] Department of Psychology, Behavior, Cognition and Neuroscience Program, American University, Washington, DC 20016, USA; ak0698a@american.edu (A.E.K.); gs0703a@american.edu (G.L.S.)
[2] Department of Health Studies, American University, Washington, DC 20016, USA
[3] Center for Behavioral Neuroscience, American University, Washington, DC 20016, USA
[*] Correspondence: holton@american.edu

Abstract: Magnesium is well known for its diverse actions within the human body. From a neurological standpoint, magnesium plays an essential role in nerve transmission and neuromuscular conduction. It also functions in a protective role against excessive excitation that can lead to neuronal cell death (excitotoxicity), and has been implicated in multiple neurological disorders. Due to these important functions within the nervous system, magnesium is a mineral of intense interest for the potential prevention and treatment of neurological disorders. Current literature is reviewed for migraine, chronic pain, epilepsy, Alzheimer's, Parkinson's, and stroke, as well as the commonly comorbid conditions of anxiety and depression. Previous reviews and meta-analyses are used to set the scene for magnesium research across neurological conditions, while current research is reviewed in greater detail to update the literature and demonstrate the progress (or lack thereof) in the field. There is strong data to suggest a role for magnesium in migraine and depression, and emerging data to suggest a protective effect of magnesium for chronic pain, anxiety, and stroke. More research is needed on magnesium as an adjunct treatment in epilepsy, and to further clarify its role in Alzheimer's and Parkinson's. Overall, the mechanistic attributes of magnesium in neurological diseases connote the macromineral as a potential target for neurological disease prevention and treatment.

Keywords: magnesium; excitotoxicity; glutamate; migraine; chronic pain; epilepsy; Alzheimer's; Parkinson's; stroke

1. Introduction

Magnesium is a very important macromineral in the diet with a multitude of roles in the human body, including serving as a cofactor in more than 300 enzymatic reactions. Magnesium is essential for regulation of muscle contraction (including that of the heart), blood pressure, insulin metabolism, and is required for the synthesis of DNA, RNA, and proteins [1]. In the nervous system, magnesium is important for optimal nerve transmission and neuromuscular coordination, as well as serving to protect against excitotoxicity (excessive excitation leading to cell death) [1,2].

One of the main neurological functions of magnesium is due to magnesium's interaction with the *N*-methyl-D-aspartate (NMDA) receptor. Magnesium serves as a blockade to the calcium channel in the NMDA receptor (Figure 1), and must be removed for glutamatergic excitatory signaling to occur [3]. Low magnesium levels may theoretically potentiate glutamatergic neurotransmission, leading to a supportive environment for excitotoxicity, which can lead to oxidative stress and neuronal cell death [4]. Abnormal glutamatergic neurotransmission has been implicated in many neurological and psychiatric disorders [5] including: migraine, chronic pain, epilepsy, Alzheimer's, Parkinson's, and stroke, in addition to depression and anxiety, which are commonly comorbid with these neurological disorders. Molecular studies [6] and animal studies [7] have shown neuronal protection from pre-treatment with magnesium, making this mineral of intense interest for its potential neuroprotective role in humans.

Thus, magnesium could be an important dietary factor in the prevention and/or treatment of the above conditions.

Figure 1. Glutamatergic *N*-methyl-D-aspartate receptor with magnesium block of calcium channel. Reprinted from [8] with permission from Elsevier.

It has been estimated that approximately half of the US population is consuming inadequate amounts of magnesium [9]. Due to the wide-ranging functions of magnesium, inadequate intake could predispose individuals to multiple health issues, including those related to neurological conditions. This review aims to summarize the recent human literature on what is known about magnesium and the following neurological disorders: migraine, chronic pain, epilepsy, Alzheimer's, Parkinson's, and stroke, as well as anxiety and depression. Recommendations will also be made for future research directions.

2. Materials and Methods

A search was completed using PubMed, MEDLINE, PsychINFO, and Wiley-Blackwell Cochrane Library. Abstracts were pulled for all available literature and were then reviewed by all three authors and a consensus decision was made about which papers met inclusion criteria. Studies of adult human populations from any year were included if they were written in English. Papers were reviewed for every article that met the review criteria, including magnesium levels (e.g., blood serum, cerebrospinal fluid, etc.) or magnesium treatment in human populations with migraine, chronic pain, anxiety, depression, epilepsy, Alzheimer's disease, Parkinson's disease, and stroke. Search strings included the neurological or commonly comorbid disorder AND "magnesium", "intravenous magnesium", "oral magnesium", or "magnesium treatment". Reviews and meta-analyses were used to gain an understanding of where the current literature stands in magnesium research across neurological disorders. The most recent reviews and meta-analyses are discussed in order to reduce duplication and provide a wide scope of the literature previously reviewed. New studies are described in detail to provide an update on the literature. If there was not a review or meta-analysis, like in the case of

Parkinson's disease, available research was compiled and reviewed. Figure 2 summarizes the search strategy and demonstrates the disparity in the number of magnesium research studies ranging from the most studied (i.e., migraine) to the least studied (i.e., Parkinson's disease).

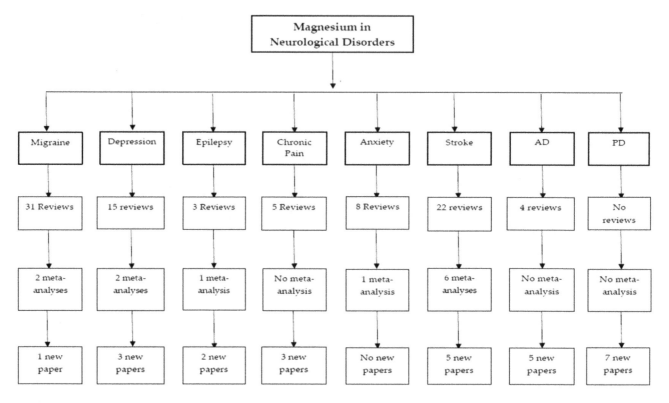

Figure 2. Flow chart of magnesium in neurological disorders literature. New papers refer to published research not included in previously-published reviews and meta-analyses. AD = Alzheimer's Disease; PD = Parkinson's Disease.

3. Results

3.1. Migraine

Migraine is the most common neurological disorder in the United Sates with a prevalence rate of 16.2% [10]. It is classified by recurrent moderate to severe headaches with or without aura, often lasting between 4 and 27 h with many associated symptoms, including nausea, vomiting, and sensitivity to various environmental stimuli [11,12]. Although the exact mechanisms are not yet fully understood, alterations in the excitability of the central nervous system, spontaneous neuronal depolarization, and abnormal mitochondria functioning have been connected to migraines. Since glutamate is the most abundant excitatory neurotransmitter, it is often linked to etiological, prevention, and treatment discussions concerning migraines [13]. Magnesium has been a proposed treatment option for migraines due to its blockade of the glutamatergic N-methyl-D-aspartate (NMDA) receptor, a receptor known to be an active contributor to pain transmission and cortical spreading depression [14]. Magnesium is also known to be a key metabolic factor in mitochondrial functioning and lowers membrane permeability reducing the possibility of spontaneous neuronal depression due to hyperexcitability [15]. Past research has shown that significantly lower levels of magnesium have been reported in serum, saliva, and cerebrospinal fluid of individuals with migraines during, and between, migraine attacks [12,16–18], along with evidence suggesting lower brain concentrations of magnesium based on MR spectroscopy [18].

Oral and intravenous magnesium administration has been proposed as a treatment option for migraines since the late 1980s and the results have been analyzed by several meta-analyses and reviews over the past three decades. In 2014, Choi and Parmer completed a meta-analysis using odds ratio (OR) on 5 randomized controlled trials published between 2000 and 2005 [19–23] and did not find strong evidence for magnesium as an effective treatment. It was concluded that i.v. magnesium resulted in a 7% lower relief rate 30 min post administration than the control groups (OR = −0.07), 37% greater side effect response rate (OR = 0.37), and no significant difference between the use of i.v. magnesium, placebo, or other migraine medications tested. However, 1 study included in the meta-analysis showed differences between migraines with and without aura; i.v. magnesium was significantly more effective at migraine relief in individuals with aura than placebo at 60 min post administration ($p < 0.05$) [24]. A more recent meta-analysis by Chiu et al. in 2016, reviewed a larger sample of randomized clinical trials with 11 studies investigating the effects of intravenous magnesium on acute migraines [19–21,25–30] and 10 studies investigating the effects of oral magnesium on migraine prophylaxis [16,31–39]. Using odds ratios, it was concluded that i.v. magnesium treatment for acute migraines resulted in significant relief across 15–45 min (OR = 0.23), 120 min (OR = 0.20), and 24 h (OR = 0.27) post magnesium administration. Similarly, oral magnesium treatment resulted in significantly reduced frequency of migraine attacks (OR = 0.20) and intensity of the attacks (OR = 0.27). Overall, this meta-analysis presents evidence for the usefulness of magnesium in both i.v. or oral forms on the treatment of migraines [40]. It also expands on the previous meta-analysis since it included randomized clinical trials published in English and Chinese investigating i.v. magnesium or oral magnesium treatment. This broadened the scope, sample size, and external validity of their work.

One quasi-experimental study has been published since the most current review comparing 2 g of i.v. magnesium sulfate compared to 60 mg of caffeine citrate on individuals presenting with a migraine at two hospitals. While both groups displayed improved pain scores over 1 hour, the magnesium group had significantly greater improvement when compared to the group receiving caffeine ($p < 0.001$) [41].

The beneficial use of magnesium in the prevention of migraine and the quality of life improvement has a Grade C evidence classification, meaning it is possibly an effective treatment based on current data. This classification is based on finding a reduction in migraine days between 22–43% across five clinical trials reviewed from 1990–2016. It is suggested that 600 mg of magnesium daily may be a safe and cost effective component of migraine care [42]. While Grade C evidence is not ideal, evidence of the effectiveness for the prevention and treatment of migraines using oral or i.v. magnesium may very well become stronger over time with the publication of more intervention and prospective cohort studies. Overall, while recent evidence does point towards i.v. and oral magnesium as potentially effective treatment options, randomized controlled clinical trials with larger sample sizes and standardized experimental designs need to be conducted in order to have more confidence in the efficacy of magnesium treatment for migraines, and to better understand how magnesium compares to current pharmaceuticals used in the prevention and treatment of migraines.

3.2. Chronic Pain

Pain is a universal sensation that can be presented in several different forms, ranging from acute to chronic. Chronic pain is broadly defined as persistent pain lasting at least three months often spurred on by central pain amplification, although the exact mechanism of pain can vary (e.g., nociceptive, neuropathic, central, etc.) or is sometimes unidentified [43]. It is estimated that chronic regional pain may be present in 20–25% of the population and chronic widespread pain may be present in 10% of the population [44]. As discussed earlier, magnesium blocks the NMDA receptor channels limiting the influx of calcium. Therefore, moderate doses of magnesium may be able to reduce the risk of excitotoxicity [45]. It is proposed that the pain relieving effects of magnesium may be dependent on the blockade of NMDA receptors in the spinal cord [46]. Magnesium is thought to produce antinociceptive and analgesic effects in patients with chronic pain and has been studied as a treatment target for chronic pain in several forms [45].

Research exploring the analgesic use of magnesium in chronic pain disorders is limited by the type and severity of chronic pain evaluated. A review on the use of magnesium as an alternative treatment for chronic pain was recently published [47]. Chronic pain was defined as pain lasting more than three months in any body part, including chronic complex regional pain syndrome, chronic low back pain, fibromyalgia, neuropathy, or pain of vascular origin. Two double-blind randomized clinical trials on complex regional pain syndrome (CRPS) [48,49] and 1 double-blind randomized clinical trial on chronic low back pain [50] were reviewed. The studies used intravenous, intradermal, and oral magnesium administration compared to placebo. The 2 CRPS randomized clinical trials had conflicting results; Fischer et al. reported no differences in CRPS pain between patients who received i.v. magnesium and those who received a placebo using several outcome measures [48]. However, van de Plas reported significant differences between intramuscular magnesium administration and a placebo on the numeric rating scale (NRS) pain assessment scores, but not on the McGill Pain Questionnaire [49]. Both studies reported more adverse effects in the groups receiving magnesium than placebo. Yousef and Al-deeb investigated the use of i.v. magnesium followed by oral magnesium compared to a placebo on chronic lower back pain over six months using NRS pain assessment scores. Beginning at two weeks, and continuing throughout the six months of follow up, the group receiving magnesium treatment had significantly improved scores from baseline measurements. Furthermore, the magnesium group had significantly lower pain scores than the placebo group at six months [50]. Based on the review of these studies, magnesium may be a viable treatment option for some types of chronic pain. A protocol was published in 2015 describing a clinical trial that is currently investigating the effects of oral magnesium administration in patients with peripheral arterial occlusive disease [51]. This trial will add much needed evidence on the potential validity of using oral magnesium as a treatment for chronic pain.

Fibromyalgia was initially considered a rheumatic disorder, but is now known to be a neurological condition, with intense widespread pain and tenderness coupled with other unpleasant symptoms, such as severe fatigue, cognitive dysfunction, memory loss, headache, and sleep problems [52,53]. As with other chronic widespread pain conditions, it is thought that pain neurotransmission occurs through glutamate's action on the NMDA receptor [54]; thus, magnesium is likely to play a protective role. It has also been proposed that fibromyalgia may be a result of insufficient levels of substances necessary for ATP synthesis, such as oxygen, magnesium, ADP, and inorganic phosphate. Magnesium is a key component within this process as it is needed for both aerobic and anaerobic glycolysis. It also aids in maintaining low cytosolic calcium in order to limit the inhibition of ATP synthesis within the mitochondria, ultimately reducing the chances of cell death caused by mitochondrial calcification [55]. Due to the overlap in symptomatology and the mechanistic actions of magnesium, researchers have studied magnesium levels in individuals with fibromyalgia, resulting in conflicting findings between modes of magnesium detection. Erythrocyte [56–59] and intracellular muscle magnesium levels [60] are decreased in fibromyalgia patients while there has been evidence that plasma and serum levels remain in normal ranges [57–59,61]. However, other studies have shown significantly decreased magnesium serum levels in fibromyalgia patients, as compared to controls [53,62,63]. Based on these findings, a recent study examined the effects of 300 mg magnesium citrate and 10 mg of amitriptyline, alone and in combination, in 60 women with fibromyalgia and 20 age- and sex-matched controls over eight weeks. Both erythrocyte and serum magnesium levels were significantly lower in the fibromyalgia group. Furthermore, the group receiving the combination of magnesium and amitriptyline reported significantly decreased pain across various pain and tenderness index scores, while magnesium alone resulted in an improvement in the number of tender points and the intensity of fibromyalgia pain [53]. Another study reported improved scores on the Fibromyalgia Impact Questionnaire-Revised (FIQR) after 8 weeks of transdermal magnesium chloride solution use [64].

It is too early to conclude whether or not magnesium is a viable treatment option for general or specific forms of chronic pain. However, the preliminary data concerning varying levels of systemic magnesium and supplementation of magnesium orally, transdermally, and intravenously for fibromyalgia and other forms of chronic pain, suggest the potential for magnesium to be an important player in the treatment and prevention of chronic pain.

3.3. Anxiety and Depression

Anxiety and depression are both common comorbid conditions with neurological illness [65] especially with chronic pain conditions [66], including migraine [67]. Anxiety and depression are also similarly mediated by altered glutamatergic neurotransmission, which may account for this comorbidity [68,69]. Since magnesium has the ability to modulate glutamatergic neurotransmission through its action at the N-methyl-D-asparate (NMDA) receptor [70], it may be possible for hypomagnesaemia to contribute to both the neurological symptoms, as well as the psychiatric symptoms.

With a lifetime prevalence rate of 15% in the general population, anxiety is considered the most pervasive psychiatric affective disorder [71]. Magnesium is involved in several physiological processes in the psychoneuroendrocrine system and modulates the hypothalamic pituitary adrenal (HPA) axis, along with blocking the calcium influx of NMDA glutamatergic receptors, all of which help prevent feelings of stress and anxiety [72]. While the data on serum and cerebrospinal fluid levels of magnesium are limited, these concentrations have been shown to be modified by exposing individuals to various types of stress, resulting in a reduction in serum magnesium due to excretion by the kidneys [73], and increasing serum levels when magnesium is administered resulting in anxiolytic-like effects [74]. Dietary intake of magnesium was also found to have a slight inverse relationship with subjective anxiety scores in a large community-based sample [75]. However, one study found no difference between the serum magnesium concentrations in patients with Generalized Anxiety Disorders when compared to controls [76].

In 2017, Boyle and Dye published a review on the available studies investigating the effects of magnesium, alone or in combination, on the experience of subjective anxiety or stress (i.e., mild anxiety, premenstrual syndrome, postpartum status, and hypertension) in adult populations [72]. Eight studies were reviewed which focused on the treatment of mild anxiety with magnesium alone [77], magnesium in combination with vitamin B_6 [78–81], magnesium with fermented cow's drink with protein hydrolysate [82], or magnesium in combination with Hawthorn extract and California poppy [83]. Modest evidence of the beneficial use of various forms of magnesium for treatment of mild to moderate anxiety was found. However, limitations were present including the occurrence of significant placebo effects and the inability to know the exact effects of magnesium when studying multiple combined compounds. Of the 7 studies which were reviewed for anxiety associated with PMS, 5 investigated the effects of oral or i.v. magnesium administration alone [84–87] and 2 investigated the effects of magnesium in combination with vitamin B_6 [88,89]. Despite methodological and sample selection issues presented by Boyle and Dye, the authors concluded that there is a potential positive effect of magnesium alone, and even more so in combination with vitamin B_6 on PMS. One study was reviewed for the effects of 64.4 mg of oral magnesium on anxiety related to postpartum depression with no significant effects reported [90]. Overall, the summarized findings allow for marginal support of magnesium as a treatment for mild anxiety and anxiety with PMS, with several of the studies reviewed reporting positive outcomes when administering magnesium as the sole or adjunct treatment.

An earlier review by Lakhan and Vieira in 2010 had a similar conclusion: magnesium administration may have a positive impact on the treatment of multiple anxiety disorders. The authors also note that many studies and clinical trials conducted do not look at the effects of magnesium alone, a comment that holds true today [91]. To our knowledge, no new magnesium studies examining the effects of magnesium on anxiety disorders have been published since the 2017 review. There is currently a strong need for methodologically sound clinical trials exploring this treatment option, as it could improve the lives of those with anxiety disorders while eliminating the negative side effects from current medications to treat anxiety.

Depression is a psychiatric disorder that affects hundreds of millions of people around the world, with major depressive disorder (MDD) accounting for 40% of the neuropsychiatric disorders in the United States [92]. Depression is linked to poor quality of life with severe impairments and, as mentioned earlier, often presents with other comorbid disorders. While there are some beneficial biomedical and clinical therapies for depression, dietary magnesium intake could be an important adjunct treatment [93,94].

Restoring the balance of magnesium within patients with depression has been proposed to have anti-depressive effects by protecting brain structures associated with depression by reducing the cascade of cell death caused by excitotoxicity [95–97]. Magnesium may also impact depressive symptoms by interacting with the HPA system, as discussed with anxiety disorders [97,98]. As seen in several other neurological disorders, lower magnesium levels have been associated with depression. One recent study reported a negative correlation between dietary intake of magnesium and depression [93]. Studies have also observed lower cerebrospinal fluid (CSF) and serum magnesium levels in individuals diagnosed with depression as compared to controls [94] along with moderately lower levels of erythrocyte magnesium levels in patients with major depression [99]. Moreover, plasma levels of magnesium were observed to be significantly lower among those with depression, as compared to healthy controls, while also being correlated with treatment response success [100] and the severity of depressive symptoms [101,102]. However, another study reported no differences in CSF, blood, and serum magnesium levels between groups [103]. This latter finding could have been due to inaccurate assessment technique, since 99% of magnesium within the human body is located intracellularly [103].

There is neurobiological evidence to support magnesium supplementation as a treatment for depression, however, the results from the limited number of randomized controlled trials (RCTs) is not clear cut. In 2016, Rechenberg reviewed RCTs examining the use of magnesium in depressed populations. However, only three studies, with limited insight into the potential use of magnesium as a treatment, are discussed due to the lack of literature on the subject [94]. Bhudi and colleagues compared the use of magnesium to a placebo over three months as a neuroprotective agent for patients undergoing cardiac surgery. Depressive symptoms were reported at baseline and three months postsurgery as one of the outcomes measured. While depressive symptoms decreased, no significant differences were noted between the magnesium and placebo groups [104]. An RCT was conducted in 2007 to study the utility of oral magnesium as a treatment for newly-depressed elderly individuals with type 2 diabetes. After establishing the presence of hypomagnesemia, individuals were randomized to either the magnesium or imipramine treatment group for twelve weeks of treatment administration. At follow-up, there was no significant difference between the magnesium treatment group or the imipramine treatment group, with similar improvements in both arms of the clinical trial. Thus, magnesium performed as well as imipramine, an anti-depressant drug [101]. Lastly, Walker et al. showed no significant differences in reported depressive symptoms when administering 200 mg of magnesium or placebo daily, for two menstrual cycles, in a double-blind placebo-controlled crossover study, among individuals who typically report monthly depressive symptoms with PMS [85].

A meta-analysis of 11 studies was recently published examining the relationship between dietary magnesium intake and the risk of depression. Using pooled measurements of relative risk (RR) and a dose-response analysis, the authors concluded that over half of the reviewed studies supported significant effects of dietary magnesium intake in relation to a decreased risk of depression (pooled RR = 0.81) with a distinct nonlinear relationship ($p = 0.0038$) between the two factors. Furthermore, the largest risk reduction was observed with 320 mg/day of magnesium [93]. This meta-analysis adds more evidence to the theory that magnesium supplementation, either through dietary intake or other routes of administration, should be continued to be researched as a potential target for the treatment of depression.

Three newly-published studies were found since the review by Rechenberg [94] and the meta-analysis by Li et al. [93]. One clinical trial studied the use of intravenous magnesium combined with dextrose in adults with treatment-resistant depression as compared to dextrose alone in a crossover study. The authors observed significant differences in serum magnesium levels measured at two time points: baseline compared to day 8 (the last day of administration) and day 2 compared to day 8. However, depression rating scale results were not as substantial as the only difference seen was a reduction on the Patient Health Questionnaire-9 from baseline to day 7 [105]. This study was limited by its short duration of treatment. Tarleton and colleagues performed an open-label randomized trial with 126 adults comparing 248 mg of magnesium to a placebo over six weeks, resulting in the significant improvement of depression scores within the magnesium group. In fact, improvement was noted within the first two weeks of treatment [106]. Lastly, a study of 60 patients with depression and lab-confirmed hypomagnesaemia were randomized to receive either 250 mg of magnesium or a placebo for eight weeks. Using the Beck Depression Inventory-II as an outcome measure, magnesium levels and Beck scores significantly improved in the magnesium group, as compared to the placebo group [107]. It is important to note that the amount of magnesium supplemented in these latter studies was less than the recommended dietary allowance (RDA) for adults of 310–420 mg/day.

Unfortunately, the current research implementing magnesium as a treatment option for depression has not shown consistently significant results, although this does not mean it is not an effective treatment option [103,108]. There is a need for more well-designed randomized clinical trials and prospective studies of longer duration with adequately powered sample sizes to fully understand the effects of magnesium on depression.

3.4. Epilepsy

Epilepsy is a disease classified by seizure occurrence that is believed to affect 50 million people worldwide [109–111]. The widespread and debilitating effects of this disorder have resulted in the investigation of treatments that fall outside the classic treatment with anti-epileptic drugs (AEDs), especially when research suggests that new AEDs are no better at significantly reducing seizures or improving prognosis than older AEDs [112–114]. The search for alternative treatment possibilities has directed some attention towards magnesium. Magnesium is an essential element involved in many bodily processes and, as mentioned earlier, has been found to be deficient in the modern Western diet [114–116]. Moreover, seizure activity has been strongly linked to excessive glutamatergic neurotransmission, thus, magnesium could potentially modulate the excitotoxicity connected to epilepsy [117]. Extracellular magnesium has been reported to reduce spontaneous spikes in seizure activity via the NMDA receptor, while also decreasing the hyperexcitability of the neuronal surface [114,118,119]. In fact, it is well known that hypomagnesaemia, itself, can cause seizure activity with more severe deficiency [120].

Two recent reviews [114,121] have examined the literature on magnesium and epilepsy. Both reviews stress the lack of large-scale, randomized controlled trials that are essential to gaining insight into the potential role of magnesium as a treatment for epilepsy, in general, as well as more specifically, refractory epilepsy. Refractory epilepsy is of particular interest due to its lack of response to AEDs, usually resulting in the seizures and other symptoms going untreated.

In humans, magnesium deficiency has been found to result in seizures, as well as lower levels of magnesium being observed in epileptic patients when compared to healthy controls [114,121–128]. A recent meta-analysis that included 60 studies (40 on epilepsy and 25 on febrile seizures) found that magnesium levels were not significantly different in patients with epilepsy versus controls, or in patients with febrile seizures versus controls. Yet, that same study found that hair magnesium concentrations were significantly lower in both non-treated and treated epilepsy patients versus controls [129]. Another study reported lower magnesium levels in more severe cases of epilepsy and status epilepticus as compared to moderate and mild cases [124]. The relationship between disease severity and magnesium concentration is not an area that has been explored at length and could result in valuable information if more work focused on this potential association.

In regards to magnesium as a treatment, magnesium supplementation has been found to be beneficial for hypomagnesaemia, a known risk factor for seizures in both infants and adults [130,131]. Other conditions associated with symptomatic seizures, such as pre-eclampsia and eclampsia, have demonstrated an improvement as a result of magnesium supplementation, as well [132–134]. Additionally, studies that have examined subjects with a *TRPM6* gene mutation [135–137], juvenile onset Alpers syndrome [138], and a case of refractory status epilepticus in a subject with a normal MRI, have also reported therapeutic benefit from the administration of magnesium supplementation [114,121,139].

Despite the supporting evidence from these research studies, only one randomized controlled trial has been conducted on magnesium treatment for epilepsy, which focused on infantile spasms. The study found that intravenous administration of adrenocorticotropic hormone (ACTH) with magnesium supplementation for a three week period resulted in a significant reduction in seizures compared to receiving ACTH on its own. At eight weeks post administration, the group that received the magnesium supplementation had a 79% seizure-free rate compared to only a 53% seizure-free rate of the ACTH only group [140]. While this study offers promising results, there have been no other randomized controlled studies completed since the last review in 2015. A recent study investigated the interictal total serum magnesium concentrations along with serum ionized magnesium concentrations in 104 drug-resistant epileptic individuals. Data was collected at baseline and 14 years later, with results demonstrating that 60.6% (OR = 29.19) of the sample had low interictal ionized magnesium and total serum magnesium ratio [141].

More randomized controlled trials are needed to better understand the potential of magnesium as a treatment option for epilepsy. Such trials, with more accurate measuring of magnesium levels, would provide greater and more specific insight into the potential role of magnesium as a treatment (or adjunct treatment) for various types of epilepsy.

3.5. Parkinson's Disease

Parkinson's disease (PD) is a neurological disorder with symptoms such as loss of balance, muscle tension, slowed body movements, resting limb tremors, and cognitive impairment [142] caused by a selective loss of dopamine in the basal ganglia. Other factors that impact PD include mitochondrial dysfunction, oxidative stress, and protein dysfunction [143]. It has been suggested that excitotoxicity caused by excessive glutamatergic neurotransmission may mediate the dopaminergic cell loss seen in Parkinson's disease, making modulators of excitotoxicity an area of growing research interest [144]. Human research that investigates the potential role of magnesium in PD is scarce [145]. To our knowledge, no in-depth review articles focusing on magnesium and PD in humans exist. The most recently-published study was a multicenter hospital-based case-control study in Japan that examined dietary intake of metals in patients who were found to be within six years of onset for PD. The results of the study found that higher magnesium concentrations were associated with a reduced risk of PD [146].

Research examining magnesium levels in PD patients have yielded mixed results. Older research from the 1960s reported no differences in serum magnesium levels in PD patients compared to controls [147]; however, this research was likely limited by the types of magnesium testing available at that time. A more recent study found similar results, with no significant differences noted in hair magnesium levels between those with and without PD. Furthermore, no association between magnesium levels and disease duration or severity was observed [142]. In contrast, a study examining cerebrospinal fluid (CSF), blood, serum, urine, and hair magnesium levels of 18 controls and 91 PD patients found that CSF magnesium levels were inversely associated with disease duration and severity. The same study also concluded that PD patients with less than a year of the disease had higher magnesium levels than PD patients with more than eight years of the disease [148]. Finally, older studies comparing magnesium levels in brain areas of PD patients versus controls found that PD patients had lower magnesium levels in the cortex, white matter, basal ganglia, caudate nucleus, and brain stem as compared to controls [149,150]. It is essential to note that these studies utilized different methods to measure magnesium concentrations, which could be a factor in the contradictory results. Future research examining the role of magnesium in PD should include measurements of magnesium concentrations in the cerebral spinal fluid (CSF) (as a measure of magnesium in the central nervous system), rather than solely in the periphery. This measurement technique may be of use in other neurological disorders as well.

In short, human research of magnesium concentrations in PD is severely lacking, despite growing evidence implicating magnesium in animal studies. There is a need for more studies in PD patients focusing on magnesium concentrations in order to get a better consensus on the relationship between magnesium and PD. These few studies have provided a small window of insight into the possible role of magnesium as a treatment for PD; however, many more studies are needed before any conclusions can be drawn.

3.6. Alzheimer's Disease

Alzheimer's disease (AD) is a degenerative neurological disorder that is characterized by synaptic loss and cognitive impairments that include deterioration in learning and memory [1]. AD presents with accumulations of beta-amyloid and tau tangles, along with inflammation and atrophy [151]. Excitotoxicity, neuroinflammation, and mitochondrial dysfunction have all been implicated in Alzheimer's disease [152], thus, hypomagnesaemia could further impair neuronal function. Factors related to lower magnesium availability, such as malnutrition and poor nutrient intake, are also present in AD patients [153,154], making magnesium deficiency more likely. Research suggests that ionized magnesium [155], cerebral spinal fluid (CSF) magnesium, hair magnesium, plasma magnesium, and red blood cell magnesium concentrations are significantly reduced in AD patients compared to healthy and medical controls [154]. Additionally, postmortem brain examinations of AD brains have found decreased magnesium levels compared to healthy controls [154,156,157]. Magnesium depletion has been found in the hippocampus in patients with AD, providing more evidence that magnesium may be a target of treatment [156].

A systematic review analyzed 13 cross-sectional studies that included AD patients and healthy controls and/or medical controls [154]. The results demonstrated that AD patients had significantly lower magnesium concentrations in CSF [158,159] and in hair samples [160,161], but no such differences were found in serum [161–164], plasma [158,165,166], or ionized/ blood cell magnesium levels [165] compared to controls. Compared to medical controls, AD patients had reduced plasma [167] and ionized blood cell magnesium concentrations [168], but no differences in serum [155,169], or CSF concentrations [168]. Meanwhile, other research has found no differences between hair and serum magnesium levels in patients with AD compared to controls [170]. Hence, current research has found contradictory results on magnesium concentration levels and, thus, requires further investigation and standardized ways to measure magnesium levels. One specific study worth noting reported that ionized magnesium levels were significantly associated with cognitive function, but not with physical function, when comparing AD patients to age-matched controls [155]. Similar to Parkinson's disease, future AD research should include a greater focus on CNS magnesium concentrations from CSF measurements, as well as using magnetic resonance spectroscopy. The above findings suggest that AD patients may be commonly deficient in magnesium.

While previous reviews have demonstrated a link between magnesium deficiency and AD in humans, there is a distinct lack of research that looks at magnesium as a treatment for AD in humans. Research to date has focused mainly on dementia, as opposed to AD specifically, and has had mixed findings. One study observed low magnesium levels in patients with mild cognitive impairment and AD patients as compared to controls [171]. Yet, another study found that both low and high magnesium concentration levels were associated with a greater risk of all-cause dementia [172]. This is the only study that provides evidence for both high and low magnesium levels being related to the risk of dementia development. As the study insists, the replication of findings from large population-based research is essential for a better understanding of these findings. For dementia, focusing on magnesium treatment through diet has been shown to improve memory [173]. The PATH through Life Project found that higher magnesium intake was related to a reduced risk of developing mild cognitive impairment and mild cognitive disorders [173]. Similarly, one study in Japan found that the greater the magnesium intake, the lower the rates of all-cause dementia and vascular dementia. However, the same relationship was absent for AD patients [174]. It is important to remember that dementia has multiple causes, including that stemming from vascular origin. Magnesium is unique for its ability to affect vascular function in addition to neuronal function [1]. Thus, magnesium may be affecting cognitive function in multiple distinct ways. Future clinical trial research is needed in this area to add to the literature in examining whether magnesium should be an adjunct treatment option in AD and/or in other types of dementia.

3.7. Stroke

Stroke is a cerebrovascular accident that presents itself with symptoms such as slurred speech, paralysis/numbness, and difficulty walking. Stroke can be broken down into two types, ischemic (where blood flow is impeded, usually by a clot) and hemorrhagic (where a blood vessel ruptures, causing impaired blood flow in the brain) [175]. The induced hypoxia causes excitotoxicity and resultant cell death [176]. Magnesium's dual role in its ability to affect vascular function [177], as well as its ability to protect against excitotoxicity mediated by NMDA receptors [176], has made it an element of interest within the stroke research community. Studies examining risk of stroke and magnesium levels have yielded mixed results. Research has found no relationship between serum ionized magnesium levels and stroke risk, when based on ischemic stroke cases over a 16 years follow-up [178]. Similarly, another study reported that plasma magnesium levels were not associated with the risk of ischemic stroke in women, yet those with low ionized magnesium levels (<0.82 mmol/L) had a 57% higher risk of ischemic stroke, after controlling for potential confounds [179]. Yet, more recent studies have found that higher serum magnesium concentrations at the time of hospital admission were independently related to lower hematoma volume and lower intracerebral hemorrhage scores in patients with acute spontaneous intracerebral hemorrhage [180]. In a more general study of adults in the United States, very low serum magnesium concentrations were significantly related to increased risk of stroke mortality [181]. While magnesium levels and stroke risk have resulted in contradictory results, there is a clear suggestion of magnesium being protective against stroke.

Most of the research conducted on the association between risk of stroke and magnesium can be found in American, European, and Asian prospective cohort studies [182,183]. A recent publication on stroke reviewed multiple meta-analyses and reported a dose-dependent protective effect of magnesium against stroke [182]. Most of the meta-analyses reviewed found that each 100 mg/day increment of dietary magnesium intake provided between 2% and 13% protection against total stroke [183–186]. A recently updated meta-analysis by Fang et al. included 40 prospective cohort studies and found 22% protection against the risk of stroke when comparing people with the highest to the lowest categories of dietary magnesium intake [183]. These meta-analyses are noted in the review paper as exhibiting high homogeneity, low publication bias, and were careful to adjust for potential confounds [182]. Hence, these studies are highly reliable and support the notion of an inverse-dose dependent relationship between dietary magnesium intake and risk for total stroke. These meta-analyses suggest that increased magnesium intake, as well as higher levels of serum magnesium, appear to be beneficial in reducing total stroke risk.

It is important to note that there are many types of stroke, and that not all stroke subtypes have demonstrated a universal relationship with magnesium. For example, one meta-analysis [184] included 7 prospective studies and found that magnesium intake levels were inversely related to the risk of ischemic stroke [178,187–189]; however, this inverse relationship was absent for intracerebral hemorrhage or subarachnoid hemorrhage [184,187,188]. A later study investigating whether magnesium could reduce the risk of delayed cerebral ischemia in patients with aneurysmal subarachnoid hemorrhage, also found that magnesium was not beneficial and did not reduce the risk [190]. Such evidence suggests the possibility that different types of stroke have different relationships to magnesium, an important distinction to be made for understanding magnesium's role in the risk of stroke development.

Investigations on magnesium levels in stroke patients have suggested an association between low magnesium levels and poor outcomes post-stroke. A recent study confirms this notion, providing evidence that low serum magnesium levels at the time of hospital admission were independently related to in-hospital mortality of patients with acute ischemic stroke [191]. An earlier study reported that decreased CSF magnesium levels were observed in ischemic stroke patients compared to controls, and that a positive association existed between low CSF magnesium levels and mortality after 7 days [192]. In addition to ischemic stroke, an observational cohort study involving patients presenting with intracerebral hemorrhage found that three month post-observation, poor functional outcomes were associated with low magnesium levels at the time of hospital admission, even after adjusting for age and measures of disease severity. Furthermore, initial and final hematoma volumes, as well as hematoma growth, were all independently and inversely correlated with low admission serum magnesium levels [193]. It is important to address the major issue when studying hypomagnesemia in stroke patients, which is that the levels are measured post diagnosis, so a causal relationship cannot be assumed and consequently there is the possibility that the lower magnesium levels are a result of stroke and not a cause of stroke [182].

Despite what appears to be a protective effect of magnesium levels on stroke, magnesium as a treatment for stroke has yielded less clear results. A trial investigating acute stroke has found that intravenous magnesium administration within 12 h of stroke onset does not improve death or disability outcomes [194]. Similarly, a meta-analysis also reported no beneficial effect of magnesium on delayed cerebral ischemia when started early after an aneurysmal subarachnoid hemorrhage based on 5 trials [195–200].

Some studies have found magnesium sulfate to be beneficial for managing post-stroke outcomes [201,202]. A meta-analysis by Chen and Carter [203] investigated 8 controlled clinical trials, 4 of which provided evidence that magnesium sulfate reduces the risk of poor outcomes 3–6 months after aneurysmal subarachnoid hemorrhage when compared to controls [198,199,201,204]. The other studies reported that magnesium sulfate was not beneficial for treating aneurysmal subarachnoid hemorrhage [199,205,206]. The overall findings of the meta-analysis suggested that magnesium sulfate may be able to decrease the risk of poor functional outcome in subarachnoid hemorrhage.

In terms of overall stroke, Panahi et al. reviewed studies that demonstrate how magnesium sulfate has been found to improve scores on different measurement indices [196,201,207], neuroprotective properties [208,209], hospital stay length [207,210], and recovery outcomes [206,207]. An additional compound that has been studied as a potential treatment for stroke is an enriched salt that is made up of a combination of magnesium and potassium. In a double-blind randomized controlled trial study, the compound was found to improve neurologic deficits following a stroke when administered for a six month period [211].

In summary, there is research to suggest the use of magnesium to improve outcomes post-stroke. More research is needed to understand the potential protective role of maintaining adequate magnesium levels in the prevention of stroke occurrence.

4. Conclusions

In conclusion, the amount of quality data on the association of magnesium with various neurological disorders differs greatly. There is strong data for the role of magnesium in migraine and depression. There is also good potential for magnesium to be having an effect in chronic pain conditions, as well as commonly comorbid psychiatric disorders, such as anxiety and depression. Much more research is needed in regards to magnesium's effects on epilepsy, including clinical trials evaluating the use of magnesium as an adjunct treatment. Neurological disorders, like Parkinson's and Alzheimer's, would benefit greatly from additional research that include measures of CNS magnesium levels (via CSF measurements and MRS). Finally, there is some research to suggest a positive effect of magnesium for improving post-stroke outcomes, and as an important dietary strategy for potentially preventing stroke, though more prospective studies are needed in this regard.

Author Contributions: Conceptualization: K.F.H.; methodology: K.F.H., A.E.K. and G.L.S.: validation: K.F.H., A.E.K. and G.L.S.; Investigation: A.E.K. and G.L.S.; writing—original draft preparation: A.E.K., G.L.S. and K.F.H.; writing—review and editing: A.E.K., G.L.S. and K.F.H.; visualization: A.E.K., G.L.S. and K.F.H.; and supervision: K.F.H.

References

1. Grober, U.; Schmidt, J.; Kisters, K. Magnesium in prevention and therapy. *Nutrients* **2015**, *7*, 8199–8226. [CrossRef] [PubMed]

2. Vink, R.; Nechifor, M. *Magnesium in the Central Nervous System*; University of Adelaide Press: Adelaide, Australia, 2011; p. 342.

3. Stroebel, D.; Casado, M.; Paoletti, P. Triheteromeric nmda receptors: From structure to synaptic physiology. *Curr. Opin. Physiol.* **2018**, *2*, 1–12. [CrossRef] [PubMed]

4. Castilho, R.F.; Ward, M.W.; Nicholls, D.G. Oxidative stress, mitochondrial function, and acute glutamate excitotoxicity in cultured cerebellar granule cells. *J. Neurochem.* **1999**, *72*, 1394–1401. [CrossRef] [PubMed]

5. Olloquequi, J.; Cornejo-Cordova, E.; Verdaguer, E.; Soriano, F.X.; Binvignat, O.; Auladell, C.; Camins, A. Excitotoxicity in the pathogenesis of neurological and psychiatric disorders: Therapeutic implications. *J. Psychopharmacol.* **2018**, *32*, 265–275. [CrossRef] [PubMed]

6. Clerc, P.; Young, C.A.; Bordt, E.A.; Grigore, A.M.; Fiskum, G.; Polster, B.M. Magnesium sulfate protects against the bioenergetic consequences of chronic glutamate receptor stimulation. *PLoS ONE* **2013**, *8*, e79982. [CrossRef] [PubMed]

7. Lambuk, L.; Jafri, A.J.; Arfuzir, N.N.; Iezhitsa, I.; Agarwal, R.; Rozali, K.N.; Agarwal, P.; Bakar, N.S.; Kutty, M.K.; Yusof, A.P.; et al. Neuroprotective effect of magnesium acetyltaurate against NMDA-induced excitotoxicity in rat retina. *Neurotox. Res.* **2017**, *31*, 31–45. [CrossRef] [PubMed]

8. Kalia, L.V.; Kalia, S.K.; Salter, M.W. NMDA receptors in clinical neurology: Excitatory times ahead. *Lancet Neurol.* **2008**, *7*, 742–755. [CrossRef]

9. Rosanoff, A.; Weaver, C.M.; Rude, R.K. Suboptimal magnesium status in the United States: Are the health consequences underestimated? *Nutr. Rev.* **2012**, *70*, 153–164. [CrossRef] [PubMed]

10. Silberstein, S.; Loder, E.; Diamond, S.; Reed, M.L.; Bigal, M.E.; Lipton, R.B.; Group, A.A. Probable migraine in the United States: Results of the American migraine prevalence and prevention (AMPP) study. *Cephalalgia* **2007**, *27*, 220–229. [CrossRef] [PubMed]

11. Michael, J.; Aminoff, D.A.G.P.; David, A.; Greenburg, D.; Roger, P.; Simon, R. *Clinical Neurology*; McGraw-Hill: New York, NY, USA, 2009.

12. Nattagh-Eshtivani, E.; Sani, M.A.; Dahri, M.; Ghalichi, F.; Ghavami, A.; Arjang, P.; Tarighat-Esfanjani, A. The role of nutrients in the pathogenesis and treatment of migraine headaches. *Biomed. Pharmacother.* **2018**, *102*, 317–325. [CrossRef] [PubMed]

13. Goadsby, P.J.; Holland, P.R.; Martins-Oliveira, M.; Hoffmann, J.; Schankin, C.; Akerman, S. Pathophysiology of migraine: A disorder of sensory processing. *Physiol. Rev.* **2017**, *97*, 553–622. [CrossRef] [PubMed]

14. Hoffmann, J.; Charles, A. Glutamate and its receptors as therapeutic targets for migraine. *Neurotherapeutics* **2018**, 1–10. [CrossRef] [PubMed]

15. Welch, K.; Ramadan, N.M. Mitochondria, magnesium and migraine. *J. Neurol. Sci.* **1995**, *134*, 9–14. [CrossRef]

16. Peikert, A.; Wilimzig, C.; Köhne-Volland, R. Prophylaxis of migraine with oral magnesium: Results from a prospective, multi-center, placebo-controlled and double-blind randomized study. *Cephalalgia* **1996**, *16*, 257–263. [CrossRef] [PubMed]

17. Sarchielli, P.; Coata, G.; Firenze, C.; Morucci, P.; Abbritti, G.; Gallai, V. Serum and salivary magnesium levels in migraine and tension-type headache. Results in a group of adult patients. *Cephalalgia* **1992**, *12*, 21–27. [CrossRef] [PubMed]

18. Ramadan, N.; Halvorson, H.; Vande-Linde, A.; Levine, S.R.; Helpern, J.; Welch, K. Low brain magnesium in migraine. *Headache J. Head Face Pain* **1989**, *29*, 590–593. [CrossRef]

19. Bigal, M.; Bordini, C.; Tepper, S.; Speciali, J. Intravenous magnesium sulphate in the acute treatment of migraine without aura and migraine with aura. A randomized, double-blind, placebo-controlled study. *Cephalalgia* **2002**, *22*, 345–353. [CrossRef] [PubMed]

20. Cete, Y.; Dora, B.; Ertan, C.; Ozdemir, C.; Oktay, C. A randomized prospective placebo-controlled study of

intravenous magnesium sulphate vs. metoclopramide in the management of acute migraine attacks in the emergency department. *Cephalalgia* **2005**, *25*, 199–204. [CrossRef] [PubMed]

21. Corbo, J.; Esses, D.; Bijur, P.E.; Iannaccone, R.; Gallagher, E.J. Randomized clinical trial of intravenous magnesium sulfate as an adjunctive medication for emergency department treatment of migraine headache. *Ann. Emerg. Med.* **2001**, *38*, 621–627. [CrossRef] [PubMed]

22. Frank, L.R.; Olson, C.M.; Shuler, K.B.; Gharib, S.F. Intravenous magnesium for acute benign headache in the emergency department: A randomized double-blind placebo-controlled trial. *Can. J. Emerg. Med.* **2004**, *6*, 327–332. [CrossRef]

23. Ginder, S.; Oatman, B.; Pollack, M. A prospective study of i.v. magnesium and i.v. prochlorperazine in the treatment of headaches. *J. Emerg. Med.* **2000**, *18*, 311–315. [CrossRef]

24. Choi, H.; Parmar, N. The use of intravenous magnesium sulphate for acute migraine: Meta-analysis of randomized controlled trials. *Eur. J. Emerg. Med.* **2014**, *21*, 2–9. [CrossRef] [PubMed]

25. Demirkaya, Ş.; Vural, O.; Dora, B.; Topçuoğlu, M.A. Efficacy of intravenous magnesium sulfate in the treatment of acute migraine attacks. *Headache J. Head Face Pain* **2001**, *41*, 171–177. [CrossRef]

26. Shahrami, A.; Assarzadegan, F.; Hatamabadi, H.R.; Asgarzadeh, M.; Sarehbandi, B.; Asgarzadeh, S. Comparison of therapeutic effects of magnesium sulfate vs. Dexamethasone/metoclopramide on alleviating acute migraine headache. *J. Emerg. Med.* **2015**, *48*, 69–76. [CrossRef] [PubMed]

27. Liu, R. Clinical effects of ozagrel combined with magnesium for treating migraine. *China Med. Eng.* **2013**, *21*, 93.

28. Tang, L.; Zhou, Y. Clinical effects of ozagrel combined with magnesium for treating migraine. *J. Prac. Med.* **2011**, *27*, 2531.

29. Wang, Y. Clinical study of intravenous magnesium for treating migraine. *J. Qiqihar Med. Coll.* **2013**, *31*, 89.

30. Xu, L.; XU, Y. Observation of the effect of intravenous magnesium combined with lidocaine for treating migraine. *Med. Inf.* **2010**, *23*, 2103.

31. Maizels, M.; Blumenfeld, A.; Burchette, R. A combination of riboflavin, magnesium, and feverfew for migraine prophylaxis: A randomized trial. *Headache J. Head Face Pain* **2004**, *44*, 885–890. [CrossRef] [PubMed]

32. Observation of Clinical Effects of Magnesium Valproate Combined with Venlafaxine Hcl in 54 Individuals with Migraine. Available online: https://wenku.baidu.com/view/280201f404a1b0717fd5ddfc.html (accessed on 5 June 2018).

33. Köseoglu, E.; Talaslıoglu, A.; Gönül, A.S.; Kula, M. The effects of magnesium prophylaxis in migraine without aura. *Magnes. Res.* **2008**, *21*, 101–108. [PubMed]

34. Esfanjani, A.T.; Mahdavi, R.; Mameghani, M.E.; Talebi, M.; Nikniaz, Z.; Safaiyan, A. The effects of magnesium, L-carnitine, and concurrent cagnesium–L-carnitine supplementation in migraine prophylaxis. *Biol. Trace Elem. Res.* **2012**, *150*, 42–48. [CrossRef] [PubMed]

35. Wang, S.; Shan, H. Effects of magnesium sulphate, ergotamine, and flunarizine hydrochloride on treating migraine. *Prev. Med.* **2001**, *12*, 366–367.

36. Yang, X.; Yang, J.; Yuan, R.; Xu, X.; Zhang, L. Randomized double blind controlled trial of magnesium valproate in migraine prophylaxis. *China Hosp. Pharm.* **2005**, *25*, 649–651.

37. Bian, X.; Zhu, Y.; Xia, J.; Ai, H.; Guo, Q.; Lu, L.; Zhang, Q. Clinical observation on potassium magnesium asparate oral soluation combined with flinarizine capsule for migraine prophylaxis. *J. Commun. Med.* **2013**, *11*, 6–7.

38. Lan, Q.; Yang, C. Clinical observation of magnesium propylvalerate on treating migraine. *Youjiang Med. Coll. Natl.* **1998**, *21*, 639–640.

39. Tang, X.; Lin, W.; Zheng, X.; Liu, C. Observation of effects of nimodipine and magnesium sulfate combination for treating migraine. *Qiqihar Med. Coll.* **1998**, *19*, 5–6.

40. Chiu, H.Y.; Yeh, T.H.; Huang, Y.C.; Chen, P.Y. Effects of intravenous and oral magnesium on reducing migraine: A meta-analysis of randomized controlled trials. *Pain Phys.* **2016**, *19*, E97–E112.

41. Baratloo, A.; Mirbaha, S.; Delavar Kasmaei, H.; Payandemehr, P.; Elmaraezy, A.; Negida, A. Intravenous caffeine citrate vs. magnesium sulfate for reducing pain in patients with acute migraine headache; a prospective quasi-experimental study. *Korean J. Pain* **2017**, *30*, 176–182. [CrossRef] [PubMed]

42. Von Luckner, A.; Riederer, F. Magnesium in migraine prophylaxis—Is there an evidence-based rationale? A systematic review. *Headache J. Head Face Pain* **2018**, *58*, 199–209. [CrossRef] [PubMed]

43. Crofford, L.J. Chronic pain: Where the body meets the brain. *Trans. Am. Clin. Climatol. Assoc.* **2015**, *126*, 167. [PubMed]

44. McBeth, J.; Jones, K. Epidemiology of chronic musculoskeletal pain. *Best Prac. Res. Clin. Rheumatol.* **2007**, *21*, 403–425. [CrossRef] [PubMed]

45. Fisher, K.; Coderre, T.J.; Hagen, N.A. Targeting the *N*-methyl-D-aspartate receptor for chronic pain management: Preclinical animal studies, recent clinical experience and future research directions. *J. Pain Symptom Manag.* **2000**, *20*, 358–373. [CrossRef]

46. Srebro, D.; Vuckovic, S.; Milovanovic, A.; Kosutic, J.; Savic Vujovic, K.; Prostran, M. Magnesium in pain research: State of the art. *Curr. Med. Chem.* **2017**, *24*, 424–434.

47. Banerjee, S.; Jones, S. *Magnesium as an Alternative or Adjunct to Opioids for Migraine and Chronic Pain: A Review of the Clinical Effectiveness and Guidelines*; Canadian Agency for Drugs and Technologies in Health: Ottawa, ON, Canada, 2017.

48. Fischer, S.G.; Collins, S.; Boogaard, S.; Loer, S.A.; Zuurmond, W.W.; Perez, R.S. Intravenous magnesium for chronic complex regional pain syndrome type 1 (CRPS-1). *Pain Med.* **2013**, *14*, 1388–1399. [CrossRef] [PubMed]

49. Van der Plas, A.A.; Schilder, J.C.; Marinus, J.; van Hilten, J.J. An explanatory study evaluating the muscle relaxant effects of intramuscular magnesium sulphate for dystonia in complex regional pain syndrome. *J. Pain* **2013**, *14*, 1341–1348. [CrossRef] [PubMed]

50. Yousef, A.; Al-deeb, A. A double-blinded randomised controlled study of the value of sequential intravenous and oral magnesium therapy in patients with chronic low back pain with a neuropathic component. *Anaesthesia* **2013**, *68*, 260–266. [CrossRef] [PubMed]

51. Venturini, M.A.; Zappa, S.; Minelli, C.; Bonardelli, S.; Lamberti, L.; Bisighini, L.; Zangrandi, M.; Turin, M.; Rizzo, F.; Rizzolo, A. Magnesium-oral supplementation to reduce pain in patients with severe peripheral arterial occlusive disease: The mag-paper randomised clinical trial protocol. *BMJ Open* **2015**, *5*, e009137. [CrossRef] [PubMed]

52. Wolfe, F.; Smythe, H.A.; Yunus, M.B.; Bennett, R.M.; Bombardier, C.; Goldenberg, D.L.; Tugwell, P.; Campbell, S.M.; Abeles, M.; Clark, P. The american college of rheumatology 1990 criteria for the classification of fibromyalgia. *Arthr. Rheumatol.* **1990**, *33*, 160–172. [CrossRef]

53. Bagis, S.; Karabiber, M.; As, I.; Tamer, L.; Erdogan, C.; Atalay, A. Is magnesium citrate treatment effective on pain, clinical parameters and functional status in patients with fibromyalgia? *Rheumatol. Int.* **2013**, *33*, 167–172. [CrossRef] [PubMed]

54. Littlejohn, G.; Guymer, E. Modulation of NMDA receptor activity in fibromyalgia. *Biomedicines* **2017**, *5*, 15. [CrossRef] [PubMed]

55. Abraham, G.E.; Flechas, J.D. Management of fibromyalgia: Rationale for the use of magnesium and malic acid. *J. Nutr. Med.* **1992**, *3*, 49–59. [CrossRef]

56. Magaldi, M.; Moltoni, L.; Biasi, G.; Marcolongo, R. Role of intracellular calcium ions in the physiopathology of fibromyalgia syndrome. *Boll. Della Soc. Ital. Biol. Sper.* **2000**, *76*, 1–4.

57. Eisinger, J.; Plantamura, A.; Ayavou, T. Glycolysis abnormalities in fibromyalgia. *J. Am. Coll. Nutr.* **1994**, *13*, 144–148. [CrossRef] [PubMed]

58. Eisinger, J.; Zakarian, H.; Pouly, E.; Plantamura, A.; Ayavou, T. Protein peroxidation, magnesium deficiency and fibromyalgia. *Magnes. Res.* **1996**, *9*, 313–316. [PubMed]

59. Romano, T.J.; Stiller, J.W. Magnesium deficiency in fibromyalgia syndrome. *J. Nutr. Med.* **1994**, *4*, 165–167. [CrossRef]

60. Clauw, D.; Ward, K.; Katz, P.; Rajan, S. Muscle intracellular magnesium levels correlate with pain tolerance in fibromyalgia (FM). *Arthr. Rheum.* **1994**, *37*, R29.

61. Sakarya, S.T.; Akyol, Y.; Bedir, A.; Canturk, F. The relationship between serum antioxidant vitamins, magnesium levels, and clinical parameters in patients with primary fibromyalgia syndrome. *Clin. Rheumatol.* **2011**, *30*, 1039–1043. [CrossRef] [PubMed]

62. Sendur, O.F.; Tastaban, E.; Turan, Y.; Ulman, C. The relationship between serum trace element levels and clinical parameters in patients with fibromyalgia. *Rheumatol. Int.* **2008**, *28*, 1117. [CrossRef] [PubMed]

63. Kasim, A.A. Calcium, magnesium and phosphorous levels in serum of Iraqi women with fibromyalgia. *Iraqi J. Pharm. Sci.* **2017**, *20*, 34–37.

64. Engen, D.J.; McAllister, S.J.; Whipple, M.O.; Cha, S.S.; Dion, L.J.; Vincent, A.; Bauer, B.A.; Wahner-Roedler, D.L. Effects of transdermal magnesium chloride on quality of life for patients with

fibromyalgia: A feasibility study. *J. Integr. Med.* **2015**, *13*, 306–313. [CrossRef]

65. Calleo, J.; Amspoker, A.B.; Marsh, L.; Kunik, M.E. Mental health diagnoses and health care utilization in persons with dementia, Parkinson's disease, and stroke. *J. Neuropsychiatry Clin. Neurosci.* **2015**, *27*, e117–e121. [CrossRef] [PubMed]

66. Tsatali, M.; Papaliagkas, V.; Damigos, D.; Mavreas, V.; Gouva, M.; Tsolaki, M. Depression and anxiety levels increase chronic musculoskeletal pain in patients with alzheimer's disease. *Curr. Alzheimer Res.* **2014**, *11*, 574–579. [CrossRef] [PubMed]

67. Oh, K.; Cho, S.J.; Chung, Y.K.; Kim, J.M.; Chu, M.K. Combination of anxiety and depression is associated with an increased headache frequency in migraineurs: A population-based study. *BMC Neurol.* **2014**, *14*, 238. [CrossRef] [PubMed]

68. Riaza Bermudo-Soriano, C.; Perez-Rodriguez, M.M.; Vaquero-Lorenzo, C.; Baca-Garcia, E. New perspectives in glutamate and anxiety. *Pharmacol. Biochem. Behav.* **2012**, *100*, 752–774. [CrossRef] [PubMed]

69. Niciu, M.J.; Ionescu, D.F.; Richards, E.M.; Zarate, C.A., Jr. Glutamate and its receptors in the pathophysiology and treatment of major depressive disorder. *J. Neural Transm.* **2014**, *121*, 907–924. [CrossRef] [PubMed]

70. Pochwat, B.; Szewczyk, B.; Sowa-Kucma, M.; Siwek, A.; Doboszewska, U.; Piekoszewski, W.; Gruca, P.; Papp, M.; Nowak, G. Antidepressant-like activity of magnesium in the chronic mild stress model in rats: Alterations in the nmda receptor subunits. *Int. J. Neuropsychopharmacol.* **2014**, *17*, 393–405. [CrossRef] [PubMed]

71. Kessler, R.C.; Aguilar-Gaxiola, S.; Alonso, J.; Chatterji, S.; Lee, S.; Ormel, J.; Üstün, T.B.; Wang, P.S. The global burden of mental disorders: An update from the who world mental health (WMH) surveys. *Epidemiol. Psychiatr. Sci.* **2009**, *18*, 23–33. [CrossRef]

72. Boyle, N.B.; Lawton, C.; Dye, L. The effects of magnesium supplementation on subjective anxiety and stress-a systematic review. *Nutrients* **2017**, *9*, 429. [CrossRef] [PubMed]

73. Mocci, F.; Canalis, P.; Tomasi, P.; Casu, F.; Pettinato, S. The effect of noise on serum and urinary magnesium and catecholamines in humans. *Occup. Med.* **2001**, *51*, 56–61. [CrossRef]

74. Poleszak, E.; Szewczyk, B.; Kędzierska, E.; Wlaź, P.; Pilc, A.; Nowak, G. Antidepressant-and anxiolytic-like activity of magnesium in mice. *Pharmacol. Biochem. Behav.* **2004**, *78*, 7–12. [CrossRef] [PubMed]

75. Jacka, F.N.; Overland, S.; Stewart, R.; Tell, G.S.; Bjelland, I.; Mykletun, A. Association between magnesium intake and depression and anxiety in community-dwelling adults: The hordaland health study. *Aust. N. Z. J. Psychiatry* **2009**, *43*, 45–52. [CrossRef] [PubMed]

76. Islam, M.R.; Ahmed, M.U.; Mitu, S.A.; Islam, M.S.; Rahman, G.M.; Qusar, M.S.; Hasnat, A. Comparative analysis of serum zinc, copper, manganese, iron, calcium, and magnesium level and complexity of interelement relations in generalized anxiety disorder patients. *Biol. Trace Elem. Res.* **2013**, *154*, 21–27. [CrossRef] [PubMed]

77. Gendle, M.H.; O'Hara, K.P. Oral magnesium supplementation and test anxiety in university undergraduates. *J. Artic. Support Null Hypothesis* **2015**, *11*, 21–30.

78. Bourgeois, M. Rôle du magne-b6 dans les manifestations anxueuses en pratique medicale courante psychiatr. *Pract. Med* **1987**, *39*, 18–22.

79. Scharbach, H. Anxiété et magné-b6. *La Vie Médicale* **1988**, *69*, 867–869.

80. Caillard, V. *Sanofi Internal Report Mab6-26*; Paris, France. Unpublished work, 1992.

81. Caillard, V. *Sanofi Internal Report Mab6-32*; Paris, France. Unpublished work, 1996.

82. Cazaubiel, J.; Desor, D. Evaluation of the anti-stress effects of a fermented milk containing milk protein hydrolysate on healthy human subjects sensitive to the stress of everyday life. Proprietary data cited in scientific opinion of the panel on dietetic products, nutrition and allergies, No. 1924/20061. *Eur. Food Saf. Auth. J. Unpubl. Work* **2008**, *905*, 1–10.

83. Hanus, M.; Lafon, J.; Mathieu, M. Double-blind, randomised, placebo-controlled study to evaluate the efficacy and safety of a fixed combination containing two plant extracts (*Crataegus oxyacantha* and *Eschscholtzia californica*) and magnesium in mild-to-moderate anxiety disorders. *Curr. Med. Res. Opin.* **2004**, *20*, 63–71. [CrossRef] [PubMed]

84. Facchinetti, F.; Borella, P.; Sances, G.; Fioroni, L.; Nappi, R.E.; Genazzani, A.R. Oral magnesium successfully relieves premenstrual mood changes. *Obstetr. Gynecol.* **1991**, *78*, 177–181.

85. Walker, A.F.; De Souza, M.C.; Vickers, M.F.; Abeyasekera, S.; Collins, M.L.; Trinca, L.A. Magnesium supplementation alleviates premenstrual symptoms of fluid retention. *J. Women Health* **1998**, *7*, 1157–1165. [CrossRef]

86. Walker, A.F.; Marakis, G.; Christie, S.; Byng, M. Mg citrate found more bioavailable than other mg preparations in a randomised, double-blind study. *Magnes. Res.* **2003**, *16*, 183–191. [PubMed]

87. Khine, K.; Rosenstein, D.L.; Elin, R.J.; Niemela, J.E.; Schmidt, P.J.; Rubinow, D.R. Magnesium (MG) retention and mood effects after intravenous mg infusion in premenstrual dysphoric disorder. *Biol. Psychiatry* **2006**, *59*, 327–333. [CrossRef] [PubMed]

88. De Souza, M.C.; Walker, A.F.; Robinson, P.A.; Bolland, K. A synergistic effect of a daily supplement for 1 month of 200 mg magnesium plus 50 mg vitamin b6 for the relief of anxiety-related premenstrual symptoms: A randomized, double-blind, crossover study. *J. Women Health Gend. Based Med.* **2000**, *9*, 131–139. [CrossRef] [PubMed]

89. Fathizadeh, N.; Ebrahimi, E.; Valiani, M.; Tavakoli, N.; Yar, M.H. Evaluating the effect of magnesium and magnesium plus vitamin B_6 supplement on the severity of premenstrual syndrome. *Iran. J. Nurs. Midwifery Res.* **2010**, *15*, 401. [PubMed]

90. Fard, F.E.; Mirghafourvand, M.; Mohammad-Alizadeh Charandabi, S.; Farshbaf-Khalili, A.; Javadzadeh, Y.; Asgharian, H. Effects of zinc and magnesium supplements on postpartum depression and anxiety: A randomized controlled clinical trial. *Women Health* **2017**, *57*, 1115–1128. [CrossRef] [PubMed]

91. Lakhan, S.E.; Vieira, K.F. Nutritional and herbal supplements for anxiety and anxiety-related disorders: Systematic review. *Nutr. J.* **2010**, *9*, 42. [CrossRef] [PubMed]

92. Eby, G.A.; Eby, K.L. Magnesium for treatment-resistant depression: A review and hypothesis. *Med. Hypotheses* **2010**, *74*, 649–660. [CrossRef] [PubMed]

93. Li, B.; Lv, J.; Wang, W.; Zhang, D. Dietary magnesium and calcium intake and risk of depression in the general population: A meta-analysis. *Aust. N. Z. J. Psychiatry* **2017**, *51*, 219–229. [CrossRef] [PubMed]

94. Rechenberg, K. Nutritional interventions in clinical depression. *Clin. Psychol. Sci.* **2016**, *4*, 144–162. [CrossRef]

95. Paul, I.A. Antidepressant activity and calcium signaling cascades. *Hum. Psychopharmacol. Clin. Exp.* **2001**, *16*, 71–80. [CrossRef] [PubMed]

96. Hollister, L.E.; Trevino, E.S.G. Calcium channel blockers in psychiatric disorders: A review of the literature. *Can. J. Psychiatry* **1999**, *44*, 658–664. [CrossRef] [PubMed]

97. Eby, G.A.; Eby, K.L. Rapid recovery from major depression using magnesium treatment. *Med. Hypotheses* **2006**, *67*, 362–370. [CrossRef] [PubMed]

98. Murck, H. Magnesium and affective disorders. *Nutr. Neurosci.* **2002**, *5*, 375–389. [CrossRef] [PubMed]

99. Nechifor, M. Magnesium in major depression. *Magnes. Res.* **2009**, *22*, 163–166.

100. Camardese, G.; De Risio, L.; Pizi, G.; Mattioli, B.; Buccelletti, F.; Serrani, R.; Leone, B.; Sgambato, A.; Bria, P.; Janiri, L. Plasma magnesium levels and treatment outcome in depressed patients. *Nutr. Neurosci.* **2012**, *15*, 78–84. [CrossRef] [PubMed]

101. Barragan-Rodriguez, L.; Rodriguez-Moran, M.; Guerrero-Romero, F. Depressive symptoms and hypomagnesemia in older diabetic subjects. *Arch. Med. Res.* **2007**, *38*, 752–756. [CrossRef] [PubMed]

102. Hasey, G.M.; D'Alessandro, E.; Cooke, R.G.; Warsh, J.J. The interface between thyroid activity, magnesium, and depression: A pilot study. *Biol. Psychiatry* **1993**, *33*, 133–135. [CrossRef]

103. Derom, M.-L.; Sayón-Orea, C.; Martínez-Ortega, J.M.; Martínez-González, M.A. Magnesium and depression: A systematic review. *Nutr. Neurosci.* **2013**, *16*, 191–206. [CrossRef] [PubMed]

104. Bhudia, S.K.; Cosgrove, D.M.; Naugle, R.I.; Rajeswaran, J.; Lam, B.K.; Walton, E.; Petrich, J.; Palumbo, R.C.; Gillinov, A.M.; Apperson-Hansen, C.; et al. Magnesium as a neuroprotectant in cardiac surgery: A randomized clinical trial. *J. Thorac. Cardiovasc. Surg.* **2006**, *131*, 853–861. [CrossRef] [PubMed]

105. Mehdi, S.; Atlas, S.E.; Qadir, S.; Musselman, D.; Goldberg, S.; Woolger, J.M.; Corredor, R.; Abbas, M.H.; Arosemena, L.; Caccamo, S. Double-blind, randomized crossover study of intravenous infusion of magnesium sulfate versus 5% dextrose on depressive symptoms in adults with treatment-resistant depression. *Psychiatry Clin. Neurosci.* **2017**, *71*, 204–211. [CrossRef] [PubMed]

106. Tarleton, E.K.; Littenberg, B.; MacLean, C.D.; Kennedy, A.G.; Daley, C. Role of magnesium supplementation in the treatment of depression: A randomized clinical trial. *PLoS ONE* **2017**, *12*, e0180067. [CrossRef] [PubMed]

107. Rajizadeh, A.; Mozaffari-Khosravi, H.; Yassini-Ardakani, M.; Dehghani, A. Effect of magnesium supplementation on depression status in depressed patients with magnesium deficiency: A randomized, double-blind, placebo-controlled trial. *Nutrition* **2017**, *35*, 56–60. [CrossRef] [PubMed]

108. Wang, J.; Um, P.; Dickerman, B.; Liu, J. Zinc, magnesium, selenium and depression: A review of the evidence, potential mechanisms and implications. *Nutrients* **2018**, *10*, 584. [CrossRef] [PubMed]

109. Ivanova, J.I.; Birnbaum, H.G.; Kidolezi, Y.; Qiu, Y.; Mallett, D.; Caleo, S. Economic burden of epilepsy among the privately insured in the US. *Pharmacoeconomics* **2010**, *28*, 675–685. [CrossRef] [PubMed]
110. Organization, W.H. *Atlas: Country Resources for Neurological Disorders 2004: Results of a Collaborative Study of the World Health Organization and the World Federation of Neurology*; World Health Organization: Geneva, Switzerland, 2004.
111. Metcalfe, A.; Jette, N. Medical and employment-related costs of epilepsy in the USA. *Expert Rev. Pharmacoecon. Outcomes Res.* **2010**, *10*, 645–647. [CrossRef] [PubMed]
112. Kwan, P.; Brodie, M.J. Early identification of refractory epilepsy. *N. Engl. J. Med.* **2000**, *342*, 314–319. [CrossRef] [PubMed]
113. Pati, S.; Alexopoulos, A.V. Pharmacoresistant epilepsy: From pathogenesis to current and emerging therapies. *Cleve Clin. J. Med.* **2010**, *77*, 457–567. [CrossRef] [PubMed]
114. Yuen, A.W.; Sander, J.W. Can magnesium supplementation reduce seizures in people with epilepsy? A hypothesis. *Epilepsy Res.* **2012**, *100*, 152–156. [CrossRef] [PubMed]
115. Alaimo, K.; McDowell, M.A.; Briefel, R.; Bischof, A.; Caughman, C.; Loria, C.; Johnson, C. Dietary intake of vitamins, minerals, and fiber of persons ages 2 months and over in the united states: Third national health and nutrition examination survey, phase 1, 1988–1991. *Adv. Data* **1994**, *258*, 1–28.
116. Ismail, Y.; Ismail, A.A.; Ismail, A.A. The underestimated problem of using serum magnesium measurements to exclude magnesium deficiency in adults; a health warning is needed for "normal" results. *Clin. Chem. Lab. Med.* **2010**, *48*, 323–327. [CrossRef] [PubMed]
117. Barker-Haliski, M.; White, H.S. Glutamatergic mechanisms associated with seizures and epilepsy. *Cold Spring Harb. Perspect. Med.* **2015**, *5*, a022863. [CrossRef] [PubMed]
118. Coan, E.; Collingridge, G. Magnesium ions block an N-methyl-D-aspartate receptor-mediated component of synaptic transmission in rat hippocampus. *Neurosci. Lett.* **1985**, *53*, 21–26. [CrossRef]
119. Isaev, D.; Ivanchick, G.; Khmyz, V.; Isaeva, E.; Savrasova, A.; Krishtal, O.; Holmes, G.L.; Maximyuk, O. Surface charge impact in low-magnesium model of seizure in rat hippocampus. *J. Neurophysiol.* **2011**, *107*, 417–423. [CrossRef] [PubMed]
120. Chen, B.B.; Prasad, C.; Kobrzynski, M.; Campbell, C.; Filler, G. Seizures related to hypomagnesemia: A case series and review of the literature. *Child Neurol. Open* **2016**, *3*, 2329048X16674834. [CrossRef] [PubMed]
121. Osborn, K.E.; Shytle, R.D.; Frontera, A.T.; Soble, J.R.; Schoenberg, M.R. Addressing potential role of magnesium dyshomeostasis to improve treatment efficacy for epilepsy: A reexamination of the literature. *J. Clin. Pharmacol.* **2016**, *56*, 260–265. [CrossRef] [PubMed]
122. Oladipo, O.; Ajala, M.; Okubadejo, N.; Danesi, M.; Afonja, O. Plasma magnesium in adult nigerian patients with epilepsy. *Niger. Postgrad. Med. J.* **2003**, *10*, 234–237. [PubMed]
123. Sinert, R.; Zehtabchi, S.; Desai, S.; Peacock, P.; Altura, B.; Altura, B. Serum ionized magnesium and calcium levels in adult patients with seizures. *Scand. J. Clin. Lab. Investig.* **2007**, *67*, 317–326. [CrossRef] [PubMed]
124. Gupta, S.K.; Manhas, A.S.; Gupta, V.K.; Bhatt, R. Serum magnesium levels in idiopathic epilepsy. *J. Assoc. Phys. India* **1994**, *42*, 456–457.
125. Sood, A.; Handa, R.; Malhotra, R.; Gupta, B. Serum, CSF, RBC & urinary levels of magnesium & calcium in idiopathic generalised tonic clonic seizures. *Indian J. Med. Res.* **1993**, *98*, 152–154. [PubMed]
126. Prebble, J. Primary infantile hypomagnesaemia: Report of two cases. *J. Paediatr. Child Health* **1995**, *31*, 54–56. [CrossRef] [PubMed]
127. Unachak, K.; Louthrenoo, O.; Katanyuwong, K. Primary hypomagnesemia in thai infants: A case report with 7 years follow-up and review of literature. *J. Med. Assoc. Thai.* **2002**, *85*, 1226–1231.
128. Visudhiphan, P.; Visudtibhan, A.; Chiemchanya, S.; Khongkhatithum, C. Neonatal seizures and familial hypomagnesemia with secondary hypocalcemia. *Pediatr. Neurol.* **2005**, *33*, 202–205. [CrossRef] [PubMed]
129. Saghazadeh, A.; Mahmoudi, M.; Meysamie, A.; Gharedaghi, M.; Zamponi, G.W.; Rezaei, N. Possible role of trace elements in epilepsy and febrile seizures: A meta-analysis. *Nutr. Rev.* **2015**, *73*, 760–779. [CrossRef] [PubMed]
130. Fagan, C.; Phelan, D. Severe convulsant hypomagnesaemia and short bowel syndrome. *Anaesth. Intens. Care* **2001**, *29*, 281.
131. Weisleder, P.; Tobin, J.A.; Kerrigan, J.F.; Bodensteiner, J.B. Hypomagnesemic seizures: Case report and presumed pathophysiology. *J. Child Neurol.* **2002**, *17*, 59–61. [CrossRef] [PubMed]

132. Chien, P.F.; Khan, K.S.; Arnott, N. Magnesium sulphate in the treatment of eclampsia and pre-eclampsia: An overview of the evidence from randomised trials. *BJOG Int. J. Obstet. Gynaecol.* **1996**, *103*, 1085–1091. [CrossRef]

133. Duley, L.; Gülmezoglu, A.M.; Henderson-Smart, D.J.; Chou, D. Magnesium sulphate and other anticonvulsants for women with pre-eclampsia. *Cochrane Libr.* **2010**, *11*, 100. [CrossRef] [PubMed]

134. Duley, L.; Henderson-Smart, D.J.; Walker, G.J.; Chou, D. Magnesium sulphate versus diazepam for eclampsia. *Cochrane Libr.* **2010**, *12*, 127–186. [CrossRef] [PubMed]

135. Kamate, M.; Singh, N.; Patil, S. Familial hypomagnesemia with secondary hypocalcemia mimicking neurodegenerative disorder. *Indian Pediatr.* **2015**, *52*, 521–522. [CrossRef] [PubMed]

136. Katayama, K.; Povalko, N.; Yatsuga, S.; Nishioka, J.; Kakuma, T.; Matsuishi, T.; Koga, Y. New trpm6 mutation and management of hypomagnesaemia with secondary hypocalcaemia. *Brain Dev.* **2015**, *37*, 292–298. [CrossRef] [PubMed]

137. Schlingmann, K.P.; Sassen, M.C.; Weber, S.; Pechmann, U.; Kusch, K.; Pelken, L.; Lotan, D.; Syrrou, M.; Prebble, J.J.; Cole, D.E. Novel TRPM6 mutations in 21 families with primary hypomagnesemia and secondary hypocalcemia. *J. Am. Soc. Nephrol.* **2005**, *16*, 3061–3069. [CrossRef] [PubMed]

138. Visser, N.A.; Braun, K.P.; Leijten, F.S.; van Nieuwenhuizen, O.; Wokke, J.H.; van den Bergh, W.M. Magnesium treatment for patients with refractory status epilepticus due to POLG1-mutations. *J. Neurol.* **2011**, *258*, 218–222. [CrossRef] [PubMed]

139. Pandey, M.; Gupta, A.; Baduni, N.; Vijfdar, H.; Sinha, S.; Jain, A. Refractory status epilepticus-magnesium as rescue therapy. *Anaesth. Intens. Care* **2010**, *38*, 962.

140. Zou, L.P.; Wang, X.; Dong, C.H.; Chen, C.H.; Zhao, W.; Zhao, R.Y. Three-week combination treatment with acth + magnesium sulfate versus acth monotherapy for infantile spasms: A 24-week, randomized, open-label, follow-up study in China. *Clin. Ther.* **2010**, *32*, 692–700. [CrossRef] [PubMed]

141. Gorica, D.; Slavica, D.D.; Vladan, D.; Nebojsa, Z.; Curcic, D.; Rankovic, A.; Branimir, R.; Vladimir, J. Interictal ionized magnesium/total serum magnesium ratio in serbian population with drug resistant epilepsy-whether is severe epilepsy in fact brain injury? *Neuropsychiatry* **2017**, *7*, 629–636. [CrossRef]

142. Forte, G.; Alimonti, A.; Violante, N.; Di Gregorio, M.; Senofonte, O.; Petrucci, F.; Sancesario, G.; Bocca, B. Calcium, copper, iron, magnesium, silicon and zinc content of hair in parkinson's disease. *J. Trace Elem. Med. Biol.* **2005**, *19*, 195–201. [CrossRef] [PubMed]

143. De Lau, L.M.; Breteler, M.M. Epidemiology of Parkinson's disease. *Lancet Neurol.* **2006**, *5*, 525–535. [CrossRef]

144. Ambrosi, G.; Cerri, S.; Blandini, F. A further update on the role of excitotoxicity in the pathogenesis of parkinson's disease. *J. Neural Transm.* **2014**, *121*, 849–859. [CrossRef] [PubMed]

145. Kurup, R.K.; Kurup, P.A. Hypothalamic digoxin-mediated model for Parkinson's disease. *Int. J. Neurosci.* **2003**, *113*, 515–536. [CrossRef] [PubMed]

146. Miyake, Y.; Tanaka, K.; Fukushima, W.; Sasaki, S.; Kiyohara, C.; Tsuboi, Y.; Yamada, T.; Oeda, T.; Miki, T.; Kawamura, N.; et al. Dietary intake of metals and risk of Parkinson's disease: A case-control study in Japan. *J. Neurol. Sci.* **2011**, *306*, 98–102. [CrossRef] [PubMed]

147. Schwab, R.S.; Poryali, A.; Ames, A. Normal serum magnesium levels in Parkinson's disease. *Neurology* **1964**, *14*, 855–856. [CrossRef] [PubMed]

148. Bocca, B.; Alimonti, A.; Senofonte, O.; Pino, A.; Violante, N.; Petrucci, F.; Sancesario, G.; Forte, G. Metal changes in csf and peripheral compartments of Parkinsonian patients. *J. Neurol. Sci.* **2006**, *248*, 23–30. [CrossRef] [PubMed]

149. Yasui, M.; Kihira, T.; Ota, K. Calcium, magnesium and aluminum concentrations in Parkinson's disease. *Neurotoxicology* **1992**, *13*, 593–600. [PubMed]

150. Uitti, R.J.; Rajput, A.H.; Rozdilsky, B.; Bickis, M.; Wollin, T.; Yuen, W.K. Regional metal concentrations in Parkinson's disease, other chronic neurological diseases, and control brains. *Can. J. Neurol. Sci.* **1989**, *16*, 310–314. [CrossRef] [PubMed]

151. Alzheimer's Association. 2018 alzheimer's disease facts and figures. *Alzheimer Dement.* **2018**, *14*, 367–429.

152. Zadori, D.; Veres, G.; Szalardy, L.; Klivenyi, P.; Vecsei, L. Alzheimer's disease: Recent concepts on the relation of mitochondrial disturbances, excitotoxicity, neuroinflammation, and kynurenines. *J. Alzheimers Dis.* **2018**, *62*, 523–547. [CrossRef] [PubMed]

153. Shatenstein, B.; Kergoat, M.-J.; Reid, I. Poor nutrient intakes during 1-year follow-up with

community-dwelling older adults with early-stage Alzheimer dementia compared to cognitively intact matched controls. *J. Am. Diet. Assoc.* **2007**, *107*, 2091–2099. [CrossRef] [PubMed]

154. Veronese, N.; Zurlo, A.; Solmi, M.; Luchini, C.; Trevisan, C.; Bano, G.; Manzato, E.; Sergi, G.; Rylander, R. Magnesium status in Alzheimer's disease: A systematic review. *Am. J. Alzheimers Dis. Other Demen.* **2016**, *31*, 208–213. [CrossRef] [PubMed]

155. Barbagallo, M.; Belvedere, M.; Di Bella, G.; Dominguez, L.J. Altered ionized magnesium levels in mild-to-moderate Alzheimer's disease. *Magnes. Res.* **2011**, *24*, 115–121.

156. Andrasi, E.; Igaz, S.; Molnár, Z.; Mako, S. Disturbances of magnesium concentrations in various brain areas in alzheimer's disease. *Magnes. Res.* **2000**, *13*, 189–196. [PubMed]

157. Glick, J.L. Dementias: The role of magnesium deficiency and an hypothesis concerning the pathogenesis of alzheimer's disease. *Med. Hypotheses* **1990**, *31*, 211–225. [CrossRef]

158. Basun, H.; Forssell, L.; Wetterberg, L.; Winblad, B. Metals and trace elements in plasma and cerebrospinal fluid in normal aging and Alzheimer's disease. *J. Neural Transm. Parkinson Dis. Dement. Sect.* **1991**, *3*, 231–258.

159. Boström, F.; Hansson, O.; Gerhardsson, L.; Lundh, T.; Minthon, L.; Stomrud, E.; Zetterberg, H.; Londos, E. Csf mg and Ca as diagnostic markers for dementia with lewy bodies. *Neurobiol. Aging* **2009**, *30*, 1265–1271. [CrossRef] [PubMed]

160. Kobayashi, S.; Fujiwara, S.; Arimoto, S.; Koide, H.; Fukuda, J.; Shimode, K.; Yamaguchi, S.; Okada, K.; Tsunematsu, T. Hair aluminium in normal aged and senile dementia of alzheimer type. *Progress Clin. Biol. Res.* **1989**, *317*, 1095–1109. [CrossRef]

161. Shore, D.; Henkin, R.I.; Nelson, N.R.; Agarwal, R.P.; Wyatt, R.J. Hair and serum copper, zinc, calcium, and magnesium concentrations in alzheimer-type dementia. *J. Am. Geriatr. Soc.* **1984**, *32*, 892–895. [CrossRef] [PubMed]

162. Gustaw-Rothenberg, K.; Lerner, A.; Bonda, D.J.; Lee, H.-G.; Zhu, X.; Perry, G.; Smith, M.A. Biomarkers in Alzheimer's disease: Past, present and future. *Biomark. Med.* **2010**, *4*, 15–26. [CrossRef] [PubMed]

163. Singh, N.K.; Banerjee, B.; Bala, K.; Basu, M.; Chhillar, N. Polymorphism in cytochrome P450 2D6, glutathione S-transferases Pi 1 genes, and organochlorine pesticides in Alzheimer disease: A case–control study in north indian population. *J. Geriatr. Psychiatry Neurol.* **2014**, *27*, 119–127. [CrossRef] [PubMed]

164. Vural, H.; Demirin, H.; Kara, Y.; Eren, I.; Delibas, N. Alterations of plasma magnesium, copper, zinc, iron and selenium concentrations and some related erythrocyte antioxidant enzyme activities in patients with Alzheimer's disease. *J. Trace Elem. Med. Biol.* **2010**, *24*, 169–173. [CrossRef] [PubMed]

165. Borella, P.; Giardino, A.; Neri, M.; Andermarker, E. Magnesium and potassium status in elderly subjects with and without dementia of the Alzheimer type. *Magnes. Res.* **1990**, *3*, 283–289. [PubMed]

166. Brackenridge, C.; McDonald, C. The concentrations of magnesium and potassium in erythrocytes and plasma of geriatric patients with psychiatric disorders. *Med. J. Aust.* **1969**, *2*, 390. [PubMed]

167. Lemke, M.R. Plasma magnesium decrease and altered calcium/magnesium ratio in severe dementia of the Alzheimer type. *Biol. Psychiatry* **1995**, *37*, 341–343. [CrossRef]

168. Hozumi, I.; Hasegawa, T.; Honda, A.; Ozawa, K.; Hayashi, Y.; Hashimoto, K.; Yamada, M.; Koumura, A.; Sakurai, T.; Kimura, A. Patterns of levels of biological metals in CSF differ among neurodegenerative diseases. *J. Neurol. Sci.* **2011**, *303*, 95–99. [CrossRef] [PubMed]

169. Çilliler, A.E.; Öztürk, Ş.; Özbakır, Ş. Serum magnesium level and clinical deterioration in alzheimer's disease. *Gerontology* **2007**, *53*, 419–422. [CrossRef] [PubMed]

170. Koc, E.R.; Ilhan, A.; Ayturk, Z.; Acar, B.; Gurler, M.; Altuntas, A., Karapirli, M.; Bodur, A.S. A comparison of hair and serum trace elements in patients with Alzheimer disease and healthy participants. *Turk. J. Med. Sci.* **2015**, *45*, 1034–1039. [CrossRef] [PubMed]

171. Balmus, I.M.; Strungaru, S.A.; Ciobica, A.; Nicoara, M.N.; Dobrin, R.; Plavan, G.; Stefanescu, C. Preliminary data on the interaction between some biometals and oxidative stress status in mild cognitive impairment and Alzheimer's disease patients. *Oxid. Med. Cell. Longev.* **2017**, *2017*, 1–7. [CrossRef] [PubMed]

172. Kieboom, B.C.T.; Licher, S.; Wolters, F.J.; Ikram, M.K.; Hoorn, E.J.; Zietse, R.; Stricker, B.H.; Ikram, M.A. Serum magnesium is associated with the risk of dementia. *Neurology* **2017**, *89*, 1716–1722. [CrossRef] [PubMed]

173. Cherbuin, N.; Kumar, R.; Sachdev, P.; Anstey, K.J. Dietary mineral intake and risk of mild cognitive impairment: The path through life project. *Front. Aging Neurosci.* **2014**, *6*, 4. [CrossRef] [PubMed]

174. Ozawa, M.; Ninomiya, T.; Ohara, T.; Hirakawa, Y.; Doi, Y.; Hata, J.; Uchida, K.; Shirota, T.; Kitazono, T.;

Kiyohara, Y. Self-reported dietary intake of potassium, calcium, and magnesium and risk of dementia in the Japanese: The hisayama study. *J. Am. Geriatr. Soc.* **2012**, *60*, 1515–1520. [CrossRef] [PubMed]

175. Majid, A. Neuroprotection in stroke: Past, present, and future. *ISRN Neurol.* **2014**, *2014*, 515716. [CrossRef] [PubMed]

176. Lai, T.W.; Zhang, S.; Wang, Y.T. Excitotoxicity and stroke: Identifying novel targets for neuroprotection. *Prog. Neurobiol.* **2014**, *115*, 157–188. [CrossRef] [PubMed]

177. Laurant, P.; Touyz, R.M. Physiological and pathophysiological role of magnesium in the cardiovascular system: Implications in hypertension. *J. Hypertens.* **2000**, *18*, 1177–1191. [CrossRef] [PubMed]

178. Ohira, T.; Peacock, J.M.; Iso, H.; Chambless, L.E.; Rosamond, W.D.; Folsom, A.R. Serum and dietary magnesium and risk of ischemic stroke: The atherosclerosis risk in communities study. *Am. J. Epidemiol.* **2009**, *169*, 1437–1444. [CrossRef] [PubMed]

179. Adebamowo, S.N.; Jimenez, M.C.; Chiuve, S.E.; Spiegelman, D.; Willett, W.C.; Rexrode, K.M. Plasma magnesium and risk of ischemic stroke among women. *Stroke* **2014**, *45*, 2881–2886. [CrossRef] [PubMed]

180. Goyal, N.; Tsivgoulis, G.; Malhotra, K.; Houck, A.L.; Khorchid, Y.M.; Pandhi, A.; Inoa, V.; Alsherbini, K.; Alexandrov, A.V.; Arthur, A.S.; et al. Serum magnesium levels and outcomes in patients with acute spontaneous intracerebral hemorrhage. *J. Am. Heart Assoc.* **2018**, *7*, e008698. [CrossRef] [PubMed]

181. Zhang, X.; Xia, J.; Del Gobbo, L.C.; Hruby, A.; Dai, Q.; Song, Y. Serum magnesium concentrations and all-cause, cardiovascular, and cancer mortality among U.S. Adults: Results from the NHANES I epidemiologic follow-up study. *Clin. Nutr.* **2017**, 30304–30307. [CrossRef] [PubMed]

182. Rosique-Esteban, N.; Guasch-Ferré, M.; Hernández-Alonso, P.; Salas-Salvadó, J. Dietary magnesium and cardiovascular disease: A review with emphasis in epidemiological studies. *Nutrients* **2018**, *10*, 168. [CrossRef] [PubMed]

183. Fang, X.; Wang, K.; Han, D.; He, X.; Wei, J.; Zhao, L.; Imam, M.U.; Ping, Z.; Li, Y.; Xu, Y.; et al. Dietary magnesium intake and the risk of cardiovascular disease, type 2 diabetes, and all-cause mortality: A dose–response meta-analysis of prospective cohort studies. *BMC Med.* **2016**, *14*, 210. [CrossRef] [PubMed]

184. Larsson, S.C.; Orsini, N.; Wolk, A. Dietary magnesium intake and risk of stroke: A meta-analysis of prospective studies. *Am. J. Clin. Nutr.* **2011**, *95*, 362–366. [CrossRef] [PubMed]

185. Nie, Z.-L.; Wang, Z.-M.; Zhou, B.; Tang, Z.-P.; Wang, S.-K. Magnesium intake and incidence of stroke: Meta-analysis of cohort studies. *Nutr. Metab. Cardiovasc. Dis.* **2013**, *23*, 169–176. [CrossRef] [PubMed]

186. Adebamowo, S.N.; Spiegelman, D.; Flint, A.J.; Willett, W.C.; Rexrode, K.M. Intakes of magnesium, potassium, and calcium and the risk of stroke among men. *Int. J. Stroke* **2015**, *10*, 1093–1100. [CrossRef] [PubMed]

187. Iso, H.; Stampfer, M.J.; Manson, J.E.; Rexrode, K.; Hennekens, C.H.; Colditz, G.A.; Speizer, F.E.; Willett, W.C. Prospective study of calcium, potassium, and magnesium intake and risk of stroke in women. *Stroke* **1999**, *30*, 1772–1779. [CrossRef] [PubMed]

188. Larsson, S.C.; Virtanen, M.J.; Mars, M.; Männistö, S.; Pietinen, P.; Albanes, D.; Virtamo, J. Magnesium, calcium, potassium, and sodium intakes and risk of stroke in male smokers. *Arch. Int. Med.* **2008**, *168*, 459–465. [CrossRef] [PubMed]

189. Weng, L.-C.; Yeh, W.-T.; Bai, C.-H.; Chen, H.-J.; Chuang, S.-Y.; Chang, H.-Y.; Lin, B.-F.; Chen, K.-J.; Pan, W.-H. Is ischemic stroke risk related to folate status or other nutrients correlated with folate intake? *Stroke* **2008**, *39*, 3152–3158. [CrossRef] [PubMed]

190. Leijenaar, J.F.; Dorhout Mees, S.M.; Algra, A.; van den Bergh, W.M.; Rinkel, G.J.; Group, M.-I.S. Effect of magnesium treatment and glucose levels on delayed cerebral ischemia in patients with subarachnoid hemorrhage: A substudy of the magnesium in aneurysmal subarachnoid haemorrhage trial (MASH-II). *Int. J. Stroke* **2015**, *10* (Suppl. A100), 108–112. [CrossRef] [PubMed]

191. You, S.; Zhong, C.; Du, H.; Zhang, Y.; Zheng, D.; Wang, X.; Qiu, C.; Zhao, H.; Cao, Y.; Liu, C.F. Admission low magnesium level is associated with in-hospital mortality in acute ischemic stroke patients. *Cerebrovasc. Dis.* **2017**, *44*, 35–42. [CrossRef] [PubMed]

192. Bayir, A.; Kara, H.; Ak, A.; Cander, B.; Kara, F. Magnesium sulfate in emergency department patients with hypertension. *Biol. Trace Elem. Res.* **2009**, *128*, 38–44. [CrossRef] [PubMed]

193. Liotta, E.M.; Prabhakaran, S.; Sangha, R.S.; Bush, R.A.; Long, A.E.; Trevick, S.A.; Potts, M.B.; Jahromi, B.S.; Kim, M.; Manno, E.M.; et al. Magnesium, hemostasis, and outcomes in patients with intracerebral hemorrhage. *Neurology* **2017**, *89*, 813–819. [CrossRef] [PubMed]

194. Mozaffarian, D.; Benjamin, E.J.; Go, A.S.; Arnett, D.K.; Blaha, M.J.; Cushman, M.; Das, S.R.; de Ferranti, S.; Despres, J.P.; Fullerton, H.J.; et al. Heart disease and stroke statistics-2016 update: A report from the American heart association. *Circulation* **2016**, *133*, e38–e360. [CrossRef] [PubMed]

195. Mees, S.M.D.; Algra, A.; Vandertop, W.P.; van Kooten, F.; Kuijsten, H.A.; Boiten, J.; van Oostenbrugge, R.J.; Salman, R.A.-S.; Lavados, P.M.; Rinkel, G.J. Magnesium for aneurysmal subarachnoid haemorrhage (MASH-2): A randomised placebo-controlled trial. *Lancet* **2012**, *380*, 44–49. [CrossRef]

196. Saver, J.L.; Starkman, S.; Eckstein, M.; Stratton, S.J.; Pratt, F.D.; Hamilton, S.; Conwit, R.; Liebeskind, D.S.; Sung, G.; Kramer, I. Prehospital use of magnesium sulfate as neuroprotection in acute stroke. *N. Engl. J. Med.* **2015**, *372*, 528–536. [CrossRef] [PubMed]

197. Bradford, C.M.; Finfer, S.; O'Connor, A.; Yarad, E.; Firth, R.; McCallister, R.; Harrington, T.; Steinfort, B.; Faulder, K.; Assaad, N. A randomised controlled trial of induced hypermagnesaemia following aneurysmal subarachnoid haemorrhage. *Crit. Care Resusc.* **2013**, *15*, 119. [PubMed]

198. Van den Bergh, W.M.; van der Schaaf, I.; van Gijn, J. The spectrum of presentations of venous infarction caused by deep cerebral vein thrombosis. *Neurology* **2005**, *65*, 192–196. [CrossRef] [PubMed]

199. Wong, G.K.C.; Poon, W.S.; Chan, M.T.; Boet, R.; Gin, T.; Ng, S.C.; Zee, B.C. Intravenous magnesium sulphate for aneurysmal subarachnoid hemorrhage (IMASH): A randomized, double-blinded, placebo-controlled, multicenter phase III trial. *Stroke* **2010**, *41*, 921–926. [CrossRef] [PubMed]

200. Dorhout Mees, S.M.; Algra, A.; Wong, G.K.; Poon, W.S.; Bradford, C.M.; Saver, J.L.; Starkman, S.; Rinkel, G.J.; van den Bergh, W.M.; et al. Early magnesium treatment after aneurysmal subarachnoid hemorrhage: Individual patient data meta-analysis. *Stroke* **2015**, *46*, 3190–3193. [CrossRef] [PubMed]

201. Veyna, R.S.; Seyfried, D.; Burke, D.G.; Zimmerman, C.; Mlynarek, M.; Nichols, V.; Marrocco, A.; Thomas, A.J.; Mitsias, P.D.; Malik, G.M. Magnesium sulfate therapy after aneurysmal subarachnoid hemorrhage. *J. Neurosurg.* **2002**, *96*, 510–514. [CrossRef] [PubMed]

202. Van Norden, A.; Van Den Bergh, W.; Rinkel, G. Dose evaluation for long-term magnesium treatment in aneurysmal subarachnoid haemorrhage. *J. Clin. Pharm. Ther.* **2005**, *30*, 439–442. [CrossRef] [PubMed]

203. Chen, M.-D.; Rimmer, J.H. Effects of exercise on quality of life in stroke survivors: A meta-analysis. *Stroke* **2011**, *42*, 832–837. [CrossRef] [PubMed]

204. Chia, R.; Hughes, R.; Morgan, M.K. Magnesium: A useful adjunct in the prevention of cerebral vasospasm following aneurysmal subarachnoid haemorrhage. *J. Clin. Neurosci.* **2002**, *9*, 279–281. [CrossRef] [PubMed]

205. Akdemir, H.; Kulakszoğlu, E.O.; Tucer, B.; Menkü, A.; Postalc, L.; Günald, Ö. Magnesium sulfate therapy for cerebral vasospasm after aneurysmal subarachnoid hemorrhage. *Neurosurg. Q.* **2009**, *19*, 35–39. [CrossRef]

206. Panahi, Y.; Mojtahedzadeh, M.; Najafi, A.; Ghaini, M.R.; Abdollahi, M.; Sharifzadeh, M.; Ahmadi, A.; Rajaee, S.M.; Sahebkar, A. The role of magnesium sulfate in the intensive care unit. *EXCLI J.* **2017**, *16*, 464. [PubMed]

207. Lampl, Y.; Gilad, R.; Geva, D.; Eshel, Y.; Sadeh, M. Intravenous administration of magnesium sulfate in acute stroke: A randomized double-blind study. *Clin. Neuropharmacol.* **2001**, *24*, 11–15. [CrossRef] [PubMed]

208. Hassan, A.E.; Chaudhry, S.A.; Grigoryan, M.; Tekle, W.G.; Qureshi, A.I. National trends in utilization and outcomes of endovascular treatment of acute ischemic stroke patients in the mechanical thrombectomy era. *Stroke* **2012**, *43*, 3012–3017. [CrossRef] [PubMed]

209. Singh, N.N.; Pan, Y.; Muengtaweeponsa, S.; Geller, T.J.; Cruz-Flores, S. Cannabis-related stroke: Case series and review of literature. *J. Stroke Cerebrovasc. Dis.* **2012**, *21*, 555–560. [CrossRef] [PubMed]

210. Afshari, D.; Moradian, N.; Rezaei, M. Evaluation of the intravenous magnesium sulfate effect in clinical improvement of patients with acute ischemic stroke. *Clin. Neurol. Neurosurg.* **2013**, *115*, 400–404. [CrossRef] [PubMed]

211. Pan, W.H.; Lai, Y.H.; Yeh, W.T.; Chen, J.R.; Jeng, J.S.; Bai, C.H.; Lin, R.T.; Lee, T.H.; Chang, K.C.; Lin, H.J.; et al. Intake of potassium- and magnesium-enriched salt improves functional outcome after stroke: A randomized, multicenter, double-blind controlled trial. *Am. J. Clin. Nutr.* **2017**, *106*, 1267–1273. [CrossRef] [PubMed]

12

Variations in Magnesium Concentration are Associated with Increased Mortality: Study in an Unselected Population of Hospitalized Patients

Justyna Malinowska [1], Milena Małecka [2] and Olga Ciepiela [2],*

[1] Students Scientific Group of Laboratory Medicine, Medical University of Warsaw, 02-097 Warsaw, Poland; malinowska_justyna@interia.pl

[2] Department of Laboratory Medicine, Medical University of Warsaw, 02-097 Warsaw, Poland; milena.malecka@wum.edu.pl

* Correspondence: olga.ciepiela@wum.edu.pl

Abstract: Dysmagnesemia is a serious disturbance of microelement homeostasis. The aim of this study was to analyze the distribution of serum magnesium concentrations in hospitalized patients according to gender, age, and result of hospitalization. The study was conducted from February 2018 to January 2019 at the Central Clinical Hospital in Warsaw. Laboratory test results from 20,438 patients were included in this retrospective analysis. When a lower reference value 0.65 mmol/L was applied, hypermagnesemia occurred in 196 patients (1%), hypomagnesemia in 1505 patients (7%), and normomagnesemia in 18,711 patients (92%). At a lower reference value of 0.75 mmol/L, hypomagnesemia was found in 25% and normomagnesemia in 74% of patients. At a lower reference value of 0.85 mmol/L, hypomagnesemia was found in 60% and normomagnesemia in 39% of patients. Either hypo- or hyper-magnesemia was associated with increased risk of in-hospital mortality. This risk is the highest in patients with hypermagnesemia (40.1% of deaths), but also increases inversely with magnesium concentration below 0.85 mmol/L. Serum magnesium concentration was not gender-dependent, and there was a slight positive correlation with age ($p < 0.0001$, r = 0.07). Large fluctuations in serum magnesium level were associated with increased mortality ($p = 0.0017$). The results indicate that dysmagnesemia is associated with severe diseases and generally severe conditions. To avoid misdiagnosis, an increase of a lower cut-off for serum magnesium concentration to at least 0.75 mmol/L is suggested.

Keywords: cut-off value; hypomagnesemia; hospitalization; mortality; serum magnesium

---

1. Introduction

Magnesium is one of the most important minerals for maintaining microelement homeostasis. It acts as a cofactor or activator for over 800 enzymes, is essential for neuromuscular conduction, and affects blood glucose level and blood pressure [1–3]. Its absorption and excretion are regulated by the kidneys, gut and bones [4]. Magnesium is absorbed primarily in the intestine in an amount of 30–50% of daily intake (~100 mg daily, at a daily recommended intake of 320–420 mg per day for women and men, respectively). There are two pathways in which Mg^{2+} is absorbed: one is a paracellular transport within the small intestine, and the other is a transcellular transport in the cecum and colon [1,4–6]. Total storage of magnesium is estimated for 2400 mg, among which 50–60% is stored in bones bound to the hydroxyapatite crystals, 25–30% is stored in muscles, and 20–25% in other soft tissues [5–7]. Daily, ~2400 mg of magnesium is filtered by the kidneys' glomeruli, and up to 99% of this microelement is reabsorbed. This results in daily excretion of magnesium by kidneys in an amount of approximately

100 mg [1,4,5,7]. Unabsorbed magnesium from daily intake is excreted with feces (approximately 270 mg per day) [6]. Mg^{2+} concentration is measured routinely in serum during medical laboratory testing, however it does not provide full information about magnesium homeostasis in the body, since serum concentration constitutes ca. 1% of the total amount of the body's magnesium [6]. Despite being the second most abundant ion in the cells, its free concentration remains low (up to 1.2 mM). Nevertheless, its role in the cells metabolism is inestimable: bound to polynucleotides, ribosomes, or adenosine triphosphate (ATP), it takes part in nucleotide binding, supports variable enzymatic reaction as a crucial activator or cofactor, allows protein synthesis, and controls cell proliferation [6]. Magnesium homeostasis is connected to calcium and phosphates. Imbalances of those element concentrations result in serious disorders, i.e., arrhythmia, convulsions, and respiratory distress. Renal regulation of its serum concentration occurs through glomerular filtration, tubular reabsorption, or secretion. Under physiological conditions, calcium, phosphates, and magnesium are metabolized by adjusting the amounts excreted in urine to the amount of supply [4].

Hypomagnesemia is reported to be a frequent condition. From the clinical laboratory point of view, hypomagnesemia is defined as decreased serum magnesium concentration below reference ranges. The discussion about reference values for magnesium is still ongoing, since several studies show discrepancies between clinical symptoms of Mg deficiency and the threshold in serum magnesium concentration applied to diagnose magnesium deficiency [8–10]. Despite the fact that serum magnesium concentration is routinely used to assess body magnesium status, it has to be underlined that Mg in serum may not correspond with total body magnesium content, since it reflects only 1% of total body stores [2,6,11,12]. Serum magnesium concentration depends, among others, on the daily intake [2,11]. In the NHANES (National Health and Nutrition Examination Survey) results, 45% of the American population was found to be dietary deficient [13], and other studies also point to populational inappropriate magnesium intake [14–16]. Magnesium deficiency is associated with enhanced oxidative stress, inflammation, impaired glucose transport, reduced pancreatic insulin secretion, increased insulin resistance, and impaired endothelial function [6,17–19]. It is a part of the pathophysiology of type 2 diabetes mellitus, ischemic heart disease, hypertension, dyslipidemia, metabolic syndrome, liver diseases, migraines, and depression [17,19–27].

Hypermagnesemia is a less common condition and usually remains undetected. It occurs mostly as a result of chronic kidney disease or the misuse of magnesium-containing supplements or medicines [5]. Despite being a rare condition, extreme hypermagnesemia has serious clinical manifestation and may lead to hypotension, complete heart block, coma, and death [6].

As mentioned above, the most commonly used method as an assessment of serum magnesium concentration is a total Mg concentration assessment, which does not provide full information about body magnesium status. Approximately 2% of clinical laboratories offer measurement of ionized magnesium, which represents 55–70% of total magnesium and is biologically active [5,11]. Twenty-four-hour excretion of magnesium in urine gives reliable information about Mg metabolism but should be very carefully used in patients with renal disorders. Insufficient glomerular filtration rate would falsify results of magnesium turnover [5,7,11]. The aforementioned method is particularly useful in assessment of magnesium retention during oral or parenteral loading tests. Decreased excretion of Mg with urine suggests increased magnesium embedding to the bones, which might suggest its depletion. On the other hand, excretion exceeding 60% of magnesium load with the highest probability excludes Mg deficiency [5]. Other methods, which are not routinely and commonly used, are assessment of red blood cell magnesium concentration, soft and hard tissue tests for magnesium content, or isotope studies [5,11].

The aim of this study was to assess the frequency of total serum magnesium imbalance among unselected subjects from inpatient departments using different lower reference values (0.65, 0.75, and 0.85 mmol/L) and its association with in-hospital mortality.

2. Materials and Methods

We performed a retrospective analysis of serum magnesium assessment among 20,438 patients hospitalized between February 2018 and January 2019 in the Central Clinical Hospital of the Medical University of Warsaw. Among all subjects included, there were 11,537 men (56%) and 8901 women (44%). Average mortality among included subjects was estimated for 3.6%, while overall mortality in the corresponding period of time among all hospitalized patients was 2.3%. Mean age was 60.96 ± 16.90 years, median 61 years (18–99 years). Magnesium concentration was tested upon admission. The frequency of magnesium measurement was dependent on patients' condition and clinical requirements. For the analysis, the first time-measurements and measurements repeated at least 10 times were included. Peripheral blood was taken by venipuncture into tubes with clotting accelerator and left for 30 min for clotting. Then, samples were centrifuged for 10 min at 1500× g and magnesium in serum was measured using a Cobas C702 analyzer (Roche). The principle of the method is based on the reaction of magnesium with xylidyl blue in alkaline solution, which produces a purple diazonium salt. Absorbance of the purple product is directly proportional to the magnesium concentration. The measuring range was 0.10–2.0 mmol/L (0.243–4.86 mg/dL), with high precision (coefficient of variation(CV) 0.7–1.3%).

All data were anonymized. The study included analysis of magnesium concentration, age, gender, and outcome of hospitalization (mortality or survival). As a retrospective analysis, this study was conducted according to rules of the Bioethical Committee of the Medical University of Warsaw.

Statistical analysis was performed using Microsoft Office Excel 2019, GraphPad Prism 6.0, and Statsoft Statistica. A nonparametric analysis was performed using the Mann–Whitney test (difference in magnesium concentration between 2 groups), one-way analysis of variance (ANOVA) (difference in magnesium concentration between age groups), the Fisher exact test (sex difference among different magnesium state groups), and the Kruskal–Wallis test (difference in magnesium concentration between 3 groups), where appropriate. The correlation between age and magnesium concentration was estimated with nonparametric Spearman correlation. Variations in magnesium concentration in patients who were tested at least 10 times were calculated as a delta (Δ) between the lowest and the highest serum magnesium concentration during one hospitalization. Normality of distribution of the results was assessed using Shapiro–Wilk and Kolmogorov–Smirnov tests. Results were considered statistically significant at $p < 0.05$.

3. Results

The mean serum magnesium concentration was 0.82 ± 0.13 mmol/L. According to different lower reference values of serum magnesium that are recommended in the literature [8,9,11,12], analyses were performed separately for cut-offs of 0.65, 0.75, and 0.85 mmol/L.

3.1. Reference Valuesof 0.65–1.2 mmol/L

Hypomagnesemia (Mg < 0.65 mmol/L) was found in 1505 subjects (7%), among which 840 were men (56%) and 665 were women (44%). Patients with hypomagnesemia had a mean Mg concentration of 0.57 ± 0.06 mmol/L.

Normomagnesemia (Mg 0.65–1.2 mmol/L) was found in 18,711 (92%) subjects, among which 10,580 (57%) were men and 8131 (43%) were women. Mean Mg concentration in the normomagnesemic group was 0.83 ± 0.1 mmol/L.

Hypermagnesemia (Mg >1.2 mmol/L) was found in 196 subjects (1%), among which 105 (54%) were men and 91 (46%) were women. Mean Mg concentration in this group was 1.36 ± 0.22 mmol/L. All three groups differed significantly in serum magnesium concentration, $p < 0.0001$ (the Kruskal–Wallis test) (Figure 1A).

THRESHOLD 0.65%

A

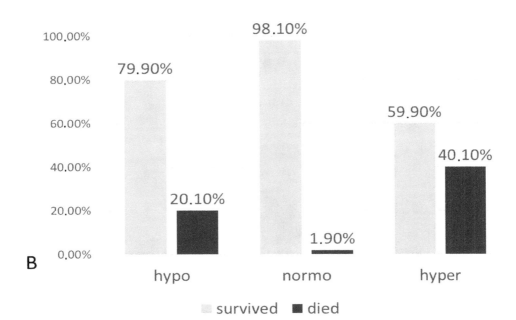

B

Figure 1. (**A**) Percentages of subjects assigned to hypo-, normo- and hyper-magnesemia groups at reference values of 0.65–1.2 mmol/L, and (**B**) in-hospital mortality ratio among separated groups. The difference between death ratio is statistically significant (Chi-square test), $p < 0.0001$.

The highest ratio of in-hospital mortality was found in the group of hypermagnesemic subjects (40.1%). In the group of hypomagnesemic patients, in-hospital mortality was significantly lower (20.1%) than in hypermagnesemic, but also significantly higher than in the normomagnesemic group (1.9%), $p < 0.0001$ (Chi-square test) (Figure 1B).

3.2. Reference Values 0.75–1.2 mmol/L

Hypomagnesemia (Mg < 0.75 mmol/L) was found in 5109 subjects (25%), among which 2878 were men (56%) and 2231 were women (44%). Patients with hypomagnesemia had a mean Mg concentration of 0.66 ± 0.07 mmol/L.

Normomagnesemia (Mg 0.75–1.2 mmol/L) was found in 15,183 (74%) subjects, among which 8553 (56%) were men and 6630 (44%) were women. Mean Mg concentration in the normomagnesemic group was 0.86 ± 0.08 mmol/L.

Hypermagnesemia (Mg >1.2 mmol/L) was found in 196 subjects (1%), among which 105 (54%) were men and 91 (46%) were women. Mean Mg concentration in this group was 1.36 ± 0.22 mmol/L. All three groups differed significantly in serum magnesium concentration, $p < 0.0001$ (Figure 2A).

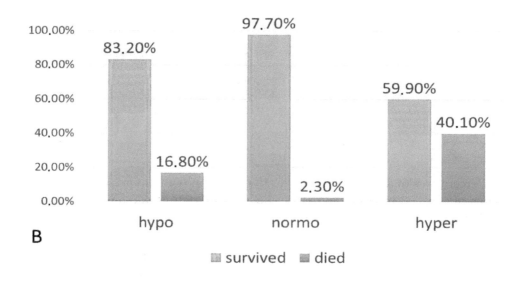

Figure 2. (**A**) Percentages of subjects assigned to hypo-, normo- and hyper-magnesemia groups at reference values of 0.75–1.2 mmol/L, and (**B**) in-hospital mortality ratio among separated groups. The difference between death ratio is statistically significant (Chi-square test), $p < 0.0001$.

In the group of hypomagnesemic patients, in-hospital mortality was significantly lower (16.8%) than in hypermagnesemic (40.1%), but also significantly higher than in the normomagnesemic group (2.3%), $p < 0.0001$ (Chi-square test) (Figure 2B).

3.3. Reference Values 0.85–1.2 mmol/L

Hypomagnesemia (Mg < 0.85 mmol/L) was found in 12,177 subjects (60%), among which 840 were men (56%) and 665 were women (44%). Patients with hypomagnesemia had a mean Mg concentration of 0.74 ± 0.08 mmol/L.

Normomagnesemia (Mg 0.85–1.2 mmol/L) was found in 8064 (39%) subjects, among which 4596 (57%) were men and 3468 (43%) were women. Mean Mg concentration in the normomagnesemic group was 0.92 ± 0.07 mmol/L.

Hypermagnesemia (Mg >1.2 mmol/L) was found in 196 subjects (1%), among which 105 (54%) were men and 91 (46%) were women. Mean Mg concentration in this group was 1.36 ± 0.22 mmol/L. All three groups differed significantly in serum magnesium concentration, $p < 0.0001$ (Figure 3A).

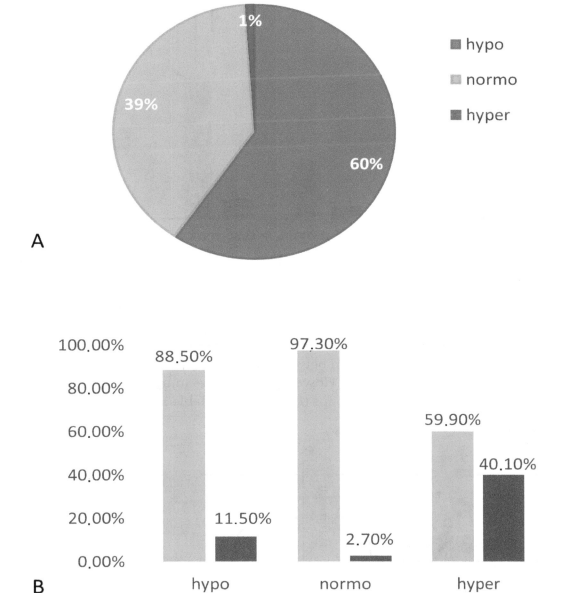

Figure 3. (**A**) Percentages of subjects assigned to hypo-, normo- and hyper-magnesemia groups at reference values of 0.85–1.2 mmol/L, and (**B**) in-hospital mortality ratio among separated groups. The difference between death ratio is statistically significant (Chi-square test), $p < 0.0001$.

In the group of hypomagnesemic patients, in-hospital mortality was significantly lower (11.5%) than in hypermagnesemic (40.1%), but also significantly higher than in the normomagnesemic group (2.7%), $p < 0.0001$ (Chi-square test) (Figure 3B).

There was a statistically significant difference in in-hospital mortality between hypomagnesemic groups, when using different lower reference values of serum magnesium (0.65 mmol/L, 0.75 mmol/L, and 0.85 mmol/L), with the highest ratio of mortality in the group with the lowest reference value applied (Figure 4).

Figure 4. Differences in in-hospital mortality ratio between hypomagnesemic groups in dependence on lower reference value applied. Analysis was performed using Chi-square test, $p < 0.0001$.

There was no difference in magnesium concentration between men and women, either in all enrolled subjects, or in hypo-, normo-, and hyper-magnesemia groups at all reference values applied, $p > 0.05$ (the Mann–Whitney test).

There was a slight positive correlation between magnesium concentration and age of studied subjects (r = 0.07, $p < 0.0001$) (Figure 5A). However, differences in magnesium concentration were found between different analyzed aged groups (Figure 5B and Table 1)

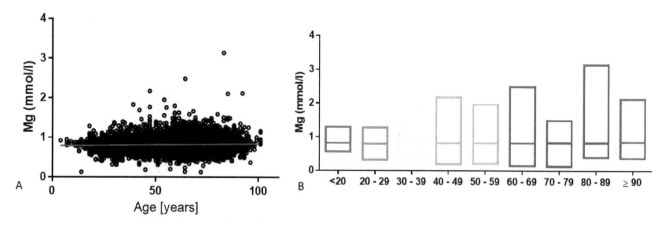

Figure 5. (**A**) Magnesium concentration showed a slight positive correlation with patient age (r = 0.07, $p < 0.0001$), assessed with nonparametric Spearman correlation. (**B**) Median and minimum/maximum values in different age groups.

Table 1. Statistical differences in median magnesium concentration among studied aged groups (Kruskal–Wallis test).

Compared Aged Groups	Median Mg Values	p-Value
<20 vs ≥90	0.82 vs 0.85	<0.01
20–29 vs 40–49	0.80 vs 0.82	<0.001
20–29 vs 50–59	0.80 vs 0.82	<0.0001
20–29 vs 60–69	0.80 vs 0.82	<0.0001
20–29 vs 70–79	0.80 vs 0.83	<0.0001
20–29 vs 80–89	0.80 vs 0.83	<0.0001
20–29 vs ≥90	0.80 vs 0.85	<0.0001
30–39 vs 50–59	0.81 vs 0.82	<0.01
30–39 vs 60–69	0.81 vs 0.82	<0.01
30–39 vs 70–79	0.81 vs 0.83	<0.0001
30–39 vs 80–89	0.81 vs 0.83	<0.0001
30–39 vs ≥90	0.81 vs 0.85	<0.0001
40–49 vs 80–89	0.82 vs 0.83	<0.001
40–49 vs ≥90	0.82 vs 0.85	<0.01
50–59 vs 80–89	0.82 vs 0.83	<0.01
50–59 vs ≥90	0.82 vs 0.85	<0.01
60–69 vs 80–89	0.82 vs 0.83	<0.001
60–69 vs ≥90	0.82 vs 0.85	<0.01
70–79 vs ≥90	0.83 vs 0.85	<0.05

In the study, we also analyzed variation in magnesium concentration in patients who were examined more than 10 times during one hospitalization. This group ($n = 52$) was divided into two subgroups, depending on the outcome of hospitalization: death ($n = 17$, 33%) or survival ($n = 35$, 67%). The variation in magnesium concentration was expressed as a difference between the lowest and highest serum magnesium concentration during one hospitalization (Δ). In the group of patients with in-hospital mortality, variations in serum magnesium concentration were higher than in the group of subjects who survived (0.64 ± 0.47 mmol/L vs 0.39 ± 0.2 mmol/L; $p = 0.0017$; Figure 6). We also found that the highest instability in magnesium concentration in the group of subjects with in-hospital mortality was associated with hematological malignancies (0.94 ± 0.79 mmol/L, $n = 5$), septic shock (0.6 ± 0.1 mmol/L, $n = 2$), and multi-organ failure (0.6 ± 0.16 mmol/L, $n = 4$). In the group of patients who survived, magnesium variations were as follows: hematological malignancies 0.44 ± 0.22 mmol/L ($n = 14$, $p = 0.03$), septic shock 0.69 ± 0.15 mmol/L ($n = 4$, $p = 0.53$), and multi-organ failure 0.40 ± 0.13 mmol/L ($n = 5$, $p = 0.19$).

Based on different lower reference values for magnesium concentration in serum, we analyzed how many patients from the group which was tested at least 10 times were hypo-, normo- or hyper-magnesemic upon hospital admission. When setting the reference value for 0.65 mmol/L, there were 44 normomagnesemic and 8 hypomagnesemic patients, among which there was only 1 patient with hypomagnesemia who died during hospitalization (16 were normomagnesemic upon admission). If the lower reference value is set to 0.75 mmol/L, among these 52 subjects, there were 17 hypomagnesemic and 35 normomagnesemic; moreover, 4 hypomagnesemic patients did not survive hospitalization (and 13 normomagnesemic). If we use 0.85 mmol/L as a lower reference value, among 52 patients who were tested at least 10 times, there were 32 hypomagnesemic and 20 normomagnesemic upon admission. Ten patients with hypomagnesemia and seven with normomagnesemia died. None of the patients who were tested at least 10 times had hypermagnesemia upon submission (Table 2).

Figure 6. Variation in magnesium concentration in group of patients who were examined at least 10 times and whose hospitalization resulted in (**A**) death or (**B**) survival. Figures A and B present variations in magnesium concentration of ten subjects from each group, in which these fluctuations were expressed the most. The value of magnesium variation was expressed as a difference between the lowest and the highest serum Mg concentration during hospitalization. (**C**) The difference between these two groups assessed with Mann–Whitney test (death, $n = 17$ and survival, $n = 35$) was statistically significant ($p = 0.0017$).

Table 2. Number of patients ($n = 52$) tested at least 10 times who died ($n = 17$) or survived hospitalization ($n = 35$) with regard to their magnesium status. Data are separately presented for different lower cut-off for reference magnesium concentration in serum.

	0.65–1.2 mmol/L		0.75–1.2 mmol/L		0.85–1.2 mmol/L	
	Dead (n)	**Survived (n)**	**Dead (n)**	**Survived (n)**	**Dead (n)**	**Survived (n)**
Hypomagnesemia	1	7	4	13	10	22
Normomagnesemia	16	28	13	22	7	13

4. Discussion

In the present study, disturbances in magnesium homeostasis were assessed with regard to different lower cut-offs for reference values of serum magnesium concentration: 0.65 mmol/L (applied in the authors' clinical laboratory), 0.75 mmol/L, and 0.85 mmol/L. At the lowest cut-off value, normomagnesemia was found in 92% of patients, hypomagnesemia was found in 7%, and hypermagnesemia in 1% of studied cases. An increase of the lower reference value for serum magnesium allowed to increase hypomagnesemia frequency to 25% and 60% respectively, and decrease normomagnesemia to 74% and 39%, respectively.

Laboratory relevant hypomagnesemia is recognized when total serum magnesium concentration is below the lower reference value. However, discussion concerning an adequate cut-off for normomagnesemia has been going on since the end of the 20th century. Wong et al. defined hypomagnesemia when total serum Mg concentration was below 0.6 mmol/L, and this value was obtained after assessment of serum magnesium in 341 individuals [10]. von Ehrlich [8] was considering two cut-off values: 0.70 and 0.75 mmol/L to diagnose hypomagnesemia, and found that approximately 9% of patients with a syndrome of magnesium deficiency would remain omitted in clinical practice if the lower cut-off value would be set for 0.7 mmol/L. Increasing the cut-off to 0.75 mmol/L allows to increase the ratio of appropriately diagnosed patients four times. Other studies suggest setting the lower reference value in a range of 0.65-0.95 mmol/L [12,28–33]. Nevertheless, it has to be underlined that magnesium deficiency should be assessed clinically, based on deficiency syndromes, not only based on reference values provided by local laboratories or test manufacturers. Costello et al. underline that clinical magnesium deficiency is accurately diagnosed at a cut-off value of 0.82 mmol/L, with proper urinary magnesium excretion (40–80 mg/day) [12]. Liebscher and Liebscher point out that the misdiagnosis ratio of magnesium disturbances could be decreased in a vast majority of patients (99%), if the cut-off value was 0.9 mmol/L. They based their conviction on clinical studies in patients with magnesium disorders, who expressed unspecific symptoms of Mg deficiency attributed to underlying disease [9,11].

Here, we found that the hypomagnesemia ratio strictly depends on the cut-off value of serum magnesium concentration. We found hypomagnesemia in 7%, 25%, and 60% of in-patients, using cut-off values of 0.65, 0.75, and 0.85 mmol/L in hospitalized patients. Wong et al., based on a cut-off value of 0.6 mmol/L, recognized hypomagnesemia in 11% of in-patients [10], which is similar to our data and the results of a study performed last year in Italy [29]. Our observation is in contrast to the recent study of Lorenzoni et al., who found that hypomagnesemia at a cut-off value of 0.65 mmol/L is recognized in over 58% of elderly in-patients [28]. We have obtained such a level of hypomagnesemia diagnosis at a cut-off value of 0.85 mmol/L. Our data obtained when a 0.75 mmol/L cut-off value was applied are also in line with Cheungpasitporn et al.'s results, who diagnosed hypomagnesemia (<0.7 mmol/L) in 20.2% of in-patients [31].

Literature data show that increased magnesium concentration in patients with severe conditions is associated with a high risk of mortality. Here, we also confirmed this observation. Similar to an aforementioned study performed in the Mayo Clinic, Rochester, USA [31], we assessed mortality ratio in patients regarding their serum magnesium status. Comparably, we obtained a high mortality rate in subjects of serum magnesium upon admission, with less than 0.75 mmol/L (16.8%) and 0.65 mmol/L (20.1%) [31], but in our study, significantly higher mortality was associated with hypermagnesemia upon admission (40.1%), a group that is much smaller (1%) than hypomagnesemia upon admission (7%, 25%, or 60% depending upon cutoff). Our results are in line with a study by Lorenzoni et al., who assessed a mortality rate in hypermagnesemic subjects of 45% [28]. A higher mortality rate in patients with hypermagnesemia has been also confirmed in other studies [33,34]. This phenomenon may be associated with the influence of magnesium excess on heart muscle function—arrhythmia associated with high magnesium levels may lead to death [34–36]. On the other hand, severe conditions may disturb electrolyte homeostasis and induce the release of magnesium from cells, which leads to hypermagnesemia. Moreover, it has been shown that, in general, hypermagnesemia bears a high risk of in-hospital mortality, as well as of 30-day and 12-month mortality [33]. We also observed that mortality in the group of enrolled subjects was higher than overall mortality among all hospitalized subjects in a corresponding period of time. It suggests that, firstly, patients in whom magnesium concentration is assessed upon admission are, in general, in worse condition than others, and secondly, that hypo- (regardless, defined as less than 0.65 or 0.85 mmol/L) and, what is more expressed, hyper-magnesemia, may characterize patients who are more susceptible to in-hospital mortality.

In our study, hypermagnesemia was less frequent than in other studies (1.78–12%) [5,29–31]. The differences may be associated with the selection of study group—we did not focus on patients hospitalized due to calcium–phosphate–magnesium disorders, rather we analyzed the general hospitalized population. Regardless of the reference value applied, disturbed magnesium homeostasis is an adverse prognostic factor in in-patient subjects, especially in intensive care units, thus constant and sufficient magnesium concentration might contribute to a decrease of in-hospital mortality [28,37].

Here, we did not observe significant changes in magnesium concentration with patient age—there was only a very slight correlation, which showed that magnesium concentration increases with age. A similar observation was reported by Cheungpasitporn et al. [31]. Interestingly, the mean age of patients with hypomagnesemia was 57.5 years, and with hypermagnesemia, 63 years. Similar observations were reported in other studies, where the mean age with hypomagnesemia was 60 years, and with hypermagnesemia, 65 years [31]. This phenomenon could be associated with inadequate Mg intake in elderly people or decreased kidney function, which appears with age [37]; however, we did not analyze estimated glomerular filtration rate (eGFR) in enrolled subjects and we cannot confirm this observation. Wakai et al. showed that the risk of hypermagnesemia in patients administering magnesium oxide increases in subjects who are ≥68 years old or have decreased eGFR (≤55.4 mL/min), or urea nitrogen of ≥22.4 mg/dL, and their daily administration of magnesium oxide exceeds 1650 mg [38].

Here, we showed that variations in magnesium concentration are associated with in-hospital mortality. This is in line with the observations of Rhee et al., who showed that fluctuations in magnesium concentration in dialyzed patients constitute a risk factor for increased mortality [39]. In our study, the highest variations in magnesium concentration were associated with hematological malignancies, septic shock, and multi-organ disfunction. Literature data show that both hypo- and hyper-magnesemia increase the risk of septic shock in patients who are recognized with systemic inflammatory response syndrome [40]. On the other hand, magnesium was not found as a marker that could help to predict organ failure in critically ill adult patients [41]. Here, we also found differences in magnesium concentration in a group of patients who suffered from different hematological malignancies with different hospitalization outcomes. Significantly higher values were found in subjects with in-hospital mortality. Variation in magnesium concentrations in patients suffering from acute leukemias have already been reported [42] and may be associated with either tumor lysis syndrome triggered by chemotherapy or improper parenteral nutrition. Regardless of etiology, variations in magnesium concentration in these patients may lead to increased mortality due to arrythmia and cardiotoxicity [43].

5. Conclusions

To conclude, it has been shown that disturbances in magnesium homeostasis accompany systemic diseases and severe conditions [39,40,43]. Either hypo- or hyper-magnesemia are associated with increased risk of mortality, and, for this reason, primarily, hypermagnesemia should be treated as a laboratory biomarker of critical value. Despite local laboratory reference values for serum magnesium concentration, its deficiency should always be diagnosed based on clinical symptoms. To avoid misdiagnosis, the increase of a lower cut-off value is suggested. High variation in magnesium levels during hospitalization may be associated with increased in-hospital mortality [40,42]; thus, magnesium levels should be routinely tested in hospitalized subjects.

Author Contributions: Conceptualization, O.C.; methodology, J.M. and O.C.; software, J.M. and M.M.; validation, J.M., M.M., and O.C.; formal analysis, J.M., M.M., and O.C. investigation J.M., M.M., and O.C.; resources, J.M. and O.C.; data curation, O.C.; writing—original draft preparation, J.M. and O.C. writing—review and editing, J.M., M.M., and O.C.; visualization, J.M., M.M., and O.C.; supervision, O.C.; project administration, O.C. All authors have read and agreed to the published version of the manuscript

References

1.   Grober, U.; Schmidt, J.; Kisters, K. Magnesium in Prevention and Therapy. *Nutrients* **2015**, *7*, 8199–8226. [CrossRef] [PubMed]
2.   Razzaque, M.S. Magnesium: Are We Consuming Enough? *Nutrients* **2018**, *10*, 1863. [CrossRef] [PubMed]
3.   Volpe, S.L. Magnesium in disease prevention and overall health. *Adv. Nutr.* **2013**, *4*, 378S–383S. [CrossRef]
4.   Blaine, J.; Chonchol, M.; Levi, M. Renal control of calcium, phosphate, and magnesium homeostasis. *Clin. J. Am. Soc. Nephrol.* **2015**, *10*, 1257–1272. [CrossRef] [PubMed]
5.   Jahnen-Dechent, W.; Ketteler, M. Magnesium basics. *Clin. Kidney J.* **2012**, *5* (Suppl. 1), i3–i14. [CrossRef] [PubMed]
6.   de Baaij, J.H.; Hoenderop, J.G.; Bindels, R.J. Magnesium in man: Implications for health and disease. *Physiol. Rev.* **2015**, *95*, 1–46. [CrossRef]

7.   Elin, R.J. Magnesium metabolism in health and disease. *Dis. Mon.* **1988**, *34*, 161–218. [CrossRef]
8.   Ehrlich, B. Magnesiummangelsyndrom in der internischen Praxis. *Magnes.-Bull.* **1997**, *19*, 29–30.
9.   Liebscher, D.H.; Liebscher, D.E. About the misdiagnosis of magnesium deficiency. *J. Am. Coll. Nutr.* **2004**, *23*, 730S–731S. [CrossRef]
10. Wong, E.T.; Rude, R.K.; Singer, F.R.; Shaw, S.T., Jr. A high prevalence of hypomagnesemia and hypermagnesemia in hospitalized patients. *Am. J. Clin. Pathol.* **1983**, *79*, 348–352. [CrossRef]
11. Elin, R.J. Assessment of magnesium status for diagnosis and therapy. *Magnes. Res.* **2010**, *23*, S194–S198. [PubMed]
12. Costello, R.B.; Elin, R.J.; Rosanoff, A.; Wallace, T.C.; Guerrero-Romero, F.; Hruby, A.; Lutsey, P.L.; Nielsen, F.H.; Rodriguez-Moran, M.; Song, Y.; et al. Perspective: The Case for an Evidence-Based Reference Interval for Serum Magnesium: The Time Has Come. *Adv. Nutr.* **2016**, *7*, 977–993. [CrossRef]
13. Moshfegh Alanna, G.J.; Jaspreet, A.; Donna, R.; Randy, L. *What We Eat in America, NHANES 2005–2006: Usual Nutrient Intakes from Food and Water Compared to 1997 Dietary Reference Intakes for Vitamin D. Calcium, Phosphorus, and Magnesium*; US Department of Agriculture, Agricultural Research Service: Washington, DC, USA, 2009.
14. Elwood, P.C.; Fehily, A.M.; Ising, H.; Poor, D.J.; Pickering, J.; Kamel, F. Dietary magnesium does not predict ischaemic heart disease in the Caerphilly cohort. *Eur. J. Clin. Nutr.* **1996**, *50*, 694–697.
15. Choi, M.K.; Weaver, C.M. Daily Intake of Magnesium and its Relation to Urinary Excretion in Korean Healthy Adults Consuming Self-Selected Diets. *Biol. Trace Elem. Res.* **2017**, *176*, 105–113. [CrossRef] [PubMed]
16. McKay, J.; Ho, S.; Jane, M.; Pal, S. Overweight & obese Australian adults and micronutrient deficiency. *BMC Nutr.* **2020**, *6*, 12.
17. Del Gobbo, L.C.; Song, Y.; Poirier, P.; Dewailly, E.; Elin, R.J.; Egeland, G.M. Low serum magnesium concentrations are associated with a high prevalence of premature ventricular complexes in obese adults with type 2 diabetes. *Cardiovasc. Diabetol.* **2012**, *11*, 23. [CrossRef] [PubMed]
18. Lecube, A.; Baena-Fustegueras, J.A.; Fort, J.M.; Pelegri, D.; Hernandez, C.; Simo, R. Diabetes is the main factor accounting for hypomagnesemia in obese subjects. *PLoS ONE* **2012**, *7*, e30599. [CrossRef] [PubMed]
19. Wu, J.; Xun, P.; Tang, Q.; Cai, W.; He, K. Circulating magnesium levels and incidence of coronary heart diseases, hypertension, and type 2 diabetes mellitus: A meta-analysis of prospective cohort studies. *Nutr. J.* **2017**, *16*, 60. [CrossRef] [PubMed]
20. Fang, X.; Han, H.; Li, M.; Liang, C.; Fan, Z.; Aaseth, J.; He, J.; Montgomery, S.; Cao, Y. Dose-Response Relationship between Dietary Magnesium Intake and Risk of Type 2 Diabetes Mellitus: A Systematic Review and Meta-Regression Analysis of Prospective Cohort Studies. *Nutrients* **2016**, *8*, 739. [CrossRef] [PubMed]
21. Peters, K.E.; Chubb, S.A.; Davis, W.A.; Davis, T.M. The relationship between hypomagnesemia, metformin therapy and cardiovascular disease complicating type 2 diabetes: The Fremantle Diabetes Study. *PLoS ONE* **2013**, *8*, e74355. [CrossRef]
22. Spiga, R.; Mannino, G.C.; Mancuso, E.; Averta, C.; Paone, C.; Rubino, M.; Sciacqua, A.; Succurro, E.; Perticone, F.; Andreozzi, F.; et al. Are Circulating Mg(2+) Levels Associated with Glucose Tolerance Profiles and Incident Type 2 Diabetes? *Nutrients* **2019**, *11*, 2460. [CrossRef] [PubMed]
23. Sarrafzadegan, N.; Khosravi-Boroujeni, H.; Lotfizadeh, M.; Pourmogaddas, A.; Salehi-Abargouei, A. Magnesium status and the metabolic syndrome: A systematic review and meta-analysis. *Nutrition* **2016**, *32*, 409–417. [CrossRef]
24. Tarleton, E.K.; Littenberg, B. Magnesium intake and depression in adults. *J. Am. Board Fam. Med.* **2015**, *28*, 249–256. [CrossRef] [PubMed]
25. Liu, M.; Yang, H.; Mao, Y. Magnesium and liver disease. *Ann. Transl. Med.* **2019**, *7*, 578. [CrossRef] [PubMed]
26. Dolati, S.; Rikhtegar, R.; Mehdizadeh, A.; Yousefi, M. The Role of Magnesium in Pathophysiology and Migraine Treatment. *Biol. Trace Elem. Res.* **2019**. [CrossRef] [PubMed]
27. Altura, B.M.; Altura, B.T. New perspectives on the role of magnesium in the pathophysiology of the cardiovascular system. I. Clinical aspects. *Magnesium* **1985**, *4*, 226–244.
28. Lorenzoni, G.; Swain, S.; Lanera, C.; Florin, M.; Baldi, I.; Iliceto, S.; Gregori, D. High- and low-inpatients' serum magnesium levels are associated with in-hospital mortality in elderly patients: A neglected marker? *Aging Clin. Exp. Res.* **2020**, *32*, 407–413. [CrossRef]
29. Catalano, A.; Bellone, F.; Chila, D.; Loddo, S.; Corica, F. Magnesium disorders: Myth or facts? *Eur. J. Intern. Med.* **2019**, *70*, e22–e24. [CrossRef]

30. Ayuk, J.; Gittoes, N.J. Contemporary view of the clinical relevance of magnesium homeostasis. *Ann. Clin Biochem.* **2014**, *51 Pt. 2*, 179–188. [CrossRef]

31. Cheungpasitporn, W.; Thongprayoon, C.; Qian, Q. Dysmagnesemia in Hospitalized Patients: Prevalence and Prognostic Importance. *Mayo Clin. Proc.* **2015**, *90*, 1001–1010. [CrossRef]

32. Assadi, F. Hypomagnesemia: An evidence-based approach to clinical cases. *Iran. J. Kidney Dis.* **2010**, *4*, 13–19. [PubMed]

33. Tazmini, K.; Nymo, S.H.; Louch, W.E.; Ranhoff, A.H.; Oie, E. Electrolyte imbalances in an unselected population in an emergency department: A retrospective cohort study. *PLoS ONE* **2019**, *14*, e0215673. [CrossRef] [PubMed]

34. Naksuk, N.; Hu, T.; Krittanawong, C.; Thongprayoon, C.; Sharma, S.; Park, J.Y.; Rosenbaum, A.N.; Gaba, P.; Killu, A.M.; Sugrue, A.M.; et al. Association of Serum Magnesium on Mortality in Patients Admitted to the Intensive Cardiac Care Unit. *Am. J. Med.* **2017**, *130*, 229.e5–229.e13. [CrossRef] [PubMed]

35. Haider, D.G.; Lindner, G.; Ahmad, S.S.; Sauter, T.; Wolzt, M.; Leichtle, A.B.; Fiedler, G.; Exadaktylos, A.K.; Fuhrmann, V. Hypermagnesemia is a strong independent risk factor for mortality in critically ill patients: Results from a cross-sectional study. *Eur. J. Intern. Med.* **2015**, *26*, 504–507. [CrossRef]

36. Cascella, M.; Vaqar, S. *Hypermagnesemia*; StatPearls: Treasure Island, FL, USA, 2020.

37. Van Laecke, S. Hypomagnesemia and hypermagnesemia. *Acta Clin. Belg.* **2019**, *74*, 41–47. [CrossRef]

38. Wakai, E.; Ikemura, K.; Sugimoto, H.; Iwamoto, T.; Okuda, M. Risk factors for the development of hypermagnesemia in patients prescribed magnesium oxide: A retrospective cohort study. *J. Pharm. Health Care Sci.* **2019**, *5*, 4. [CrossRef]

39. Rhee, C.M.; Chou, J.A.; Kalantar-Zadeh, K. Dialysis Prescription and Sudden Death. *Semin. Nephrol.* **2018**, *38*, 570–581. [CrossRef]

40. Thongprayoon, C.; Cheungpasitporn, W.; Erickson, S.B. Admission hypomagnesemia linked to septic shock in patients with systemic inflammatory response syndrome. *Ren. Fail.* **2015**, *37*, 1518–1521. [CrossRef]

41. Helliksson, F.; Wernerman, J.; Wiklund, L.; Rosell, J.; Karlsson, M. The combined use of three widely available biochemical markers as predictor of organ failure in critically ill patients. *Scand. J. Clin. Lab. Investig.* **2016**, *76*, 479–485. [CrossRef] [PubMed]

42. Afridi, H.I.; Kazi, T.G.; Talpur, F.N. Correlation of Calcium and Magnesium Levels in the Biological Samples of Different Types of Acute Leukemia Children. *Biol. Trace Elem. Res.* **2018**, *186*, 395–406. [CrossRef] [PubMed]

43. British Committee for Standards in Haematology; Milligan, D.W.; Grimwade, D.; Cullis, J.O.; Bond, L.; Swirsky, D.; Craddock, C.; Kell, J.; Homewood, J.; Campbell, K.; et al. Guidelines on the management of acute myeloid leukaemia in adults. *Br. J. Haematol.* **2006**, *135*, 450–474. [CrossRef] [PubMed]

13

Longitudinal Study of the Role of Epidermal Growth Factor on the Fractional Excretion of Magnesium in Children: Effect of Calcineurin Inhibitors

Kristien J. Ledeganck [1,*], Charlotte Anné [1], Amandine De Monie [1], Sarang Meybosch [1], Gert A. Verpooten [1], Marleen Vinckx [1], Koen Van Hoeck [1,2], Annelies Van Eyck [1], Benedicte Y. De Winter [1] and Dominique Trouet [1,2]

[1]   Laboratory of Experimental Medicine and Pediatrics, University of Antwerp, Universiteitsplein 1, T3.34, 2610 Antwerp, Belgium; charlotte.anne@student.uantwerpen.be (C.A.); amandine.demonie@student.uantwerpen.be (A.D.M.); sarang.meybosch@student.uantwerpen.be (S.M.); gert.verpooten@uantwerpen.be (G.A.V.); marleen.vinckx@uantwerpen.be (M.V.); Koen.vanhoeck@uza.be (K.V.H.); annelies.vaneyck@uantwerpen.be (A.V.E.); benedicte.dewinter@uantwerpen.be (B.Y.D.W); Dominique.trouet@uza.be (D.T.)
[2]   Department of Pediatric Nephrology, Antwerp University Hospital, Wilrijkstraat 10, 2650 Edegem, Belgium
*   Correspondence: kristien.ledeganck@uantwerp.be

Abstract: Background: It was shown in animal models and adults that the epidermal growth factor (EGF) is involved in the pathophysiology of calcineurin inhibitor (CNI) induced renal magnesium loss. In children, however, the exact mechanism remains unclear, which was set as the purpose of the present study. Methods: Children with nephrotic syndrome and renal transplant children treated with CNI ($n = 50$) and non-CNI treated children ($n = 46$) were included in this study. Urine and serum samples were collected at three time points to determine magnesium, creatinine, and EGF. The magnesium intake was calculated from a food frequency questionnaire. Results: Serum Mg^{2+} and urinary EGF/creatinine were significantly lower in the CNI treated children, with significantly more CNI-treated children developing hypomagnesaemia. In the latter patients, the fractional excretion of magnesium (FE Mg^{2+}) was significantly higher. Urinary EGF, age, renal function, and serum magnesium were independent predictors of the FE Mg^{2+}. Only 29% of the children reached the recommended daily intake of magnesium. The magnesium intake did not differ between hypomagnesemic and normomagnesemic patients and was not a predictor of the FE Mg^{2+}. Conclusions: In CNI-treated children who developed hypomagnesemia, the FE Mg^{2+} was increased. The urinary EGF concentration, age, and renal function are independent predictors of the FE Mg^{2+}.

Keywords: epidermal growth factor; magnesium; children; magnesium intake; fractional excretion; calcineurin inhibitor; kidney transplantation; nephrotic syndrome

1. Introduction

Magnesium (Mg^{2+}) is an intracellular cation with roles in multiple physiologic processes, such as parathyroid metabolism, cardiovascular tone, nerve conduction, and the proper function of adenosine triphosphate complexes [1]. Furthermore, it also plays an important role in bone metabolism [2]. In the growing child, it is, therefore, essential to maintain a positive Mg^{2+} balance so that the amount of Mg^{2+} needed for growth and metabolic needs is ensured [2]. This balance requires interaction between the gut, the kidney, and the bone. Mg^{2+} is absorbed from the food in the gut and stored in the bone, while Mg^{2+} excess is excreted by the kidneys in the feces [3].

The recommended Mg^{2+} intake in children depends on their age, with increasing needs during adolescence to meet pubertal growth needs. The recommended intake approximates 130–150 mg/day for ages 4–8 year [2], 240 mg/day for ages 9–13 year, and 340 mg/day for boys and 300 mg/day for girls aged 14–18 year [4]. Magnesium deficiency is rare in healthy subjects as Mg^{2+} is widely present in food sources, such as dairy, nuts, whole cereal grains, green vegetables, dark chocolate, and legumes [5–7]. However, in a Cypriot population, none of the children aged 6–19 year met the recommended Mg^{2+} intake, with the highest prevalence of insufficiency in the adolescents [8]. Additionally, in chronic kidney disease (CKD) patients, magnesium intake has been shown to be below the recommended level [9]. The main nutrition-related goals for CKD patients involve slowing of the kidney failure progression rate, maintaining good nutritional status, and minimizing CKD complications, such as metabolic disorders and proteinuria. The nutrition requirements differ among patients with various stages of kidney function and proper nutrition is, therefore, difficult to fulfil in CKD patients [10]. Hypomagnesemia is defined as a serum Mg^{2+} concentration below 0.7 mmoL/L [11]. Most cases of hypomagnesemia in clinical practice, however, are asymptomatic. The clinical manifestation may depend more on the total body Mg^{2+} deficit rather than on the actual serum Mg^{2+} levels. Personality changes, muscle weakness, tremor, and dysphagia may occur at concentrations of <1.45 mg/dL, while confusion and a decreased consciousness develop at concentrations of ≤ 1.00 mg/dL [12]. Hypomagnesemia has been reported in children with malignancy and in those being treated for malnutrition [1]. In hospitalized children at the pediatric intensive care unit, a 20% to 60% incidence of hypomagnesemia has been reported [1].

Calcineurin inhibitors (CNIs), especially cyclosporine-A (CsA) and tacrolimus (TAC), are widely used immunosuppressive agents. Since the 1970s, CNIs are commonly administered to kidney transplant recipients or after other solid organ transplantation to reduce the rejection rate and improve early graft survival, although long-term nephrotoxicity is a serious side effect [13]. CNIs are also used for the treatment of steroid-resistant or steroid-dependent idiopathic nephrotic syndrome [13].

Besides nephrotoxicity, CNIs also induce functional alterations and ion homeostasis disturbances, such as hypomagnesemia and renal magnesium wasting, hyponatremia, hyperkalemia, hyperchloremic metabolic acidosis, and hyperuricemia [14,15]. Two ion channels play an important role in the Mg^{2+} homeostasis, TRPM6 and TRPM7. TRPM6 has an expression pattern predominantly present in absorbing epithelia. In the kidney, TRPM6 is expressed in the distal convoluted tubule, known as the main site of active transcellular Mg^{2+} reabsorption along the nephron. TRPM7 is ubiquitously expressed and implicated in cellular Mg^{2+} homeostasis, cell death, and cell cycle regulation [16,17]. A decade ago, it was demonstrated that epidermal growth factor (EGF) plays a crucial role in the stimulation of the renal Mg^{2+} channel TRPM6 [18,19]. Our research group demonstrated in a rat model that a combined decrease in the expression of renal EGF and the Mg^{2+} channel TRPM6 is responsible for CsA-induced renal Mg^{2+} loss [20]. In a translational clinical setting in adults, an increased FE Mg^{2+} was observed in CsA-treated patients who developed hypomagnesemia associated with decreased urinary renal EGF levels [21].

Besides its role in magnesium homeostasis, EGF is involved in many biological responses, including cell proliferation, differentiation, and migration, as well as pathophysiological events, such as tissue repair including ulcer and wound healing, or tissue repair, after ischemia/reperfusion injury [22,23]. EGF is also involved in inflammation, showing protective effects in animal models of pancreatitis [24]. Moreover, the correlation between EGF and other growth factors, such as transforming growth factor β (TGF-β) and platelet derived growth factor, needs to be considered [25,26].

In the present study, we aimed to investigate if children who were treated with CNIs developed hypomagnesemia and/or renal Mg^{2+} loss, and if the urinary EGF expression level is related to the fractional excretion of Mg^{2+} (FE Mg^{2+}). Furthermore, we investigated whether Mg^{2+} intake was related to the serum Mg^{2+} level and the FE Mg^{2+} in patients treated with CNIs.

2. Materials and Methods

2.1. Study Design

We performed a longitudinal observational clinical trial. Patients were included between March 2016 and February 2018 at the Antwerp University Hospital. Ninety-six patients were recruited in this study and divided into 2 subgroups. Group 1: Patients treated with CNI ($n = 50$); subdivided into renal transplant patients treated with CNI ($n = 23$; group 1A) and patients with nephrotic syndrome treated with CNI ($n = 27$; group 1B). Group 2: Non-CNI treated patients ($n = 46$); subdivided into patients with CKD as a control group for group 1A ($n = 24$; group 2A) and patients with nephrotic syndrome not treated with CNI as a control group for group 1B ($n = 22$; group 2B). Exclusion criteria were an estimated glomerular filtration rate (eGFR) < 20 mL/min/1.73 m^2, use of cisplatin, diuretics or aminoglycosides, diabetes mellitus, and an active urinary tract infection.

At 3 time points, with an interval of at least 1 month, blood and urine samples were collected from each patient to determine creatinine, magnesium, and EGF (urine). In the nephrotic syndrome patients, samples were collected during a period of remission. At one time point during the study, a Food Frequency Questionnaire was performed to obtain the frequency and portion size information.

A healthy control group ($n = 103$ healthy children) was included to determine serum and urine EGF reference values in children. From these patients, age, gender, weight, and length were obtained. From 42 patients, at 1 time point, both urine and serum were sampled, from 31 patients, only urine was sampled, and from 30 patients, only serum was sampled.

The study was conducted in accordance with the *Declaration of Helsinki* and the principles of Good Clinical Practice. The study protocol was approved by the Ethics Committee of the Antwerp University Hospital (file number 9/44/231). All patients and their parents and/or legal guardians gave a written informed consent.

2.2. Magnesium Intake Questionnaire and Nubel®

A Food Frequency Questionnaire was performed to obtain standardized information on food intake, with special attention to the frequency and portion size information. This information was then entered into the dietary software program Nubel® food planner (Nubel v.z.w. Eurostation, Brussels, Belgium) to analyse the daily Mg^{2+} intake. Nubel® is a Belgian non-profit organization responsible for the management of the nutritional and scientific information of food products in Belgium [27]. In patients treated with magnesium supplements, the amount of magnesium substitution was added to the daily magnesium intake from the food to calculate the total magnesium intake. The magnesium intake was then calculated as a percentage of the reference daily intake (RDI; Nubel) and thus corrected for age.

2.3. Determination of Creatinine, Magnesium, and CsA Levels

Serum and urine creatinine and magnesium, and whole blood CsA levels were analyzed with the Dimension Vista system (Siemens Healthcare Diagnostics, Deerfield, MA, USA) using an ECREA, Mg, or CsA flex® reagent cartridge, respectively. FE Mg^{2+} was calculated using the following equation: $FE_{Mg} = 100 \times (U_{Mg} \times S_{Cr})/[(0.8 \times S_{Mg}) \times U_{Cr}]$, with U_{Mg} urinary excretion of Mg^{2+} (mg/dL), S_{Cr} serum creatinine (mg/dL), S_{Mg} serum Mg^{2+} (mg/dL), and U_{Cr} urinary excretion of creatinine (mg/dL). The serum Mg^{2+} concentration was multiplied by 0.8, since, in children, only 80% of the serum Mg^{2+} is freely filtered by the glomerulus, with the remaining part being protein-bound [28].

Creatinine clearance was calculated using the Bedside Swartz equation, which is the recommended equation to estimate the GFR in children [29].

Since it is known that estradiol might influence renal magnesium reabsorption [30], serum estradiol levels were measured in female children using the Elecsys Estradiol III Assay (Cobas®, Roche Diagnostics GmbH, Mannheim, Germany). TAC levels were measured with the Elecsys Tacrolimus Assay.

2.4. Determination of Urinary EGF

Urinary EGF was measured using an EGF human Elisa kit® (Invitrogen, Waltham, MA, USA), according to the manufacturer's guidelines. The detection limit of this assay was 3.9 pg/mL. A preliminary experiment ($n = 10$) was performed to test the intra- and inter-variability of the EGF human Elisa kit®, showing a mean intra-assay coefficient of variance of 9.82% and an inter-assay coefficient of variation of 9.81%.

2.5. Statistical Analysis

All data were analysed using SPSS (version 24.0). Statistical significance was predetermined as p-value < 0.05. Normality of cross-sectional data (such as magnesium intake) was tested by applying the Kolmogorov-Smirnov test. Parametric data are expressed as mean $\pm$ standard deviation (SD) and non-parametric data are expressed as median (minimum-maximum). The correlation of magnesium intake with other variables was tested with a Pearson or Spearman correlation test for parametric or skewed data, respectively. Generalized Estimating Equations (GEE) were used to analyse the data collected per visit since the groups had unequal sample sizes. Moreover, the number of visits per patient varied from 1 to 3. GEEs were used to calculate the estimated means of variables and to compare them between groups. Models were constructed to study the time-dependency of the variables and to determine the relationship between outcome variables, such as FE Mg^{2+} and urinary EGF excretion, and a number of other predictors.

3. Results

3.1. Population Demographics

Group Descriptions

From 89% of the patients, three consecutive samples were collected, while from 9% of the patients only two samples were collected, and from 2% of the patients only one sample was collected. In the entire study population, the median age was 12.0 year (2.3–20.3 year). Seventy-one percent of the patients were male, the mean weight was 43.0 $\pm$ 18.0 kg, the median length was 147.5 cm (88–190 cm), and the median BMI z-score was 0.16 (-2.24–2.82).

The demographic data per group are displayed in Table 1.

Table 1. Demographic data of the study groups.

Group	Renal Tx + CNI (n = 23)	CKD − CNI (n = 24)	NS + CNI (n = 27)	NS − CNI (n = 22)
Age (year)	13.4 (2.2–20.3)	11.1 (3.2–18.9)	12.5 (3.1–19.5)	12.3 (3.7–18.7)
Gender (M/F; %)	87/13	62/38	71/29	64/36
Length (cm)	151 (88–183)	145 (95–176)	149 (92–190)	149 (101–183)
Weight (kg)	43 $\pm$ 17	42 $\pm$ 16	46 $\pm$ 23	42 $\pm$ 15
BMI z-score	0.40 (-2.10–1.13)	0.24 (-2.24–2.05)	0.17 (-1.57–2.12)	-0.09 (-1.86–2.82)
Mg^{2+} intake (% of RDI)	89 (37–684)	86 (63–436)	87 (45–299)	86 (41–383)
Patients who exceeded the RDI for Mg^{2+} intake (%)	27.3	30.4	30.8	42.1
Mg^{2+} supplements (%)	13.0	8.0	13.8	25.0

Normally distributed variables are presented as mean $\pm$ SD; skewed data are presented as median (minimum-maximum). None of the presented variables significantly differed between the groups. Tx: Transplantation; CNI: Calcineurin inhibitor, CKD: Chronic kidney disease, NS: Nephrotic syndrome, RDI: Reference daily intake (corrected for age).

3.2. Kidney Function, Magnesium, EGF, and CNI Levels

In the entire study population, the median serum creatinine was 0.77 mg/dL (0.27–2.97 mg/dL), the creatinine clearance was 80 mL/min/1.73 m^2 (19–180 mL/min/1.73 m^2), serum Mg^{2+} was 0.80 mg/dL (0.42–1.22 mg/dL), and the FE Mg^{2+} was 4.70% (0.16–21.47%). From all the patients, 29.3% developed hypomagnesemia at least at 1 time point during the study. The mean urinary EGF was 10.51 ng/mL (1.14–182.70 ng/mL) and the mean serum EGF was 811.73 pg/mL (33.07–2014.33 pg/mL). A detailed overview per group is shown in Table 2.

In the female patients ($n = 28$), the median estrogen level was 34.86 pg/mL (2.5–268.3 pg/mL) and did not differ between groups. From these patients, 29.6% had serum estrogen levels below the detection limit.

Table 2. Urine and serum analyses; data are presented in 4 groups.

Group	Renal Tx + CNI ($n = 23$)	CKD − CNI ($n = 24$)	NS + CNI ($n = 28$)	NS − CNI ($n = 22$)
Serum Creatinine (mg/dL)	1.11 (0.08) §#	1.27 (0.14) #§	0.72 (0.07) #$*	0.54 (0.03) $*§
Creatinine clearance (mL/min/1.73 m^2)	59 (3) §#	62 (6) #§	98 (5) #$*	117 (4) $*§
Urinary protein/creatinine (mg/g)	347.4 (71.8) $	613.2 (115.0) *	848.0 (333.9)	544.9 (215.8)
Serum Mg^{2+} (mg/dL)	0.76 (0.02) #$	0.82 (0.02) *§	0.78 (0.02) #$	0.84 (0.01) *§
HypoMg (%)	39.1 $#	16.0 *§	44.8 $#	10.0 *§
FE Mg^{2+} (%)	7.82 (0.84) §#	7.76 (0.84)	3.95 (0.32) *$	3.57 (0.28) *$
CsA levels (ng/mL)	666 (45)	-	579 (38)	-
Tacrolimus levels (ng/mL)	8.62 (0.91)	-	7.71 (0.79)	-
Serum EGF (pg/mL)	776.6 (39.9)	742.1 (47.8) §	865.5 (40.7) $	817.2 (55.0)
Urine EGF (ng/mL)	7.0 (1.1) #§	11.5 (2.4) #§	35.4 (6.0) $*$	47.7 (6.6) *$
Urine EGF/creatinine (ng/mg)	0.11 (0.01) $#§	0.19 (0.03) #*§	0.33 (0.05) #$*	0.51 (0.07) $*§

The renal Tx patients treated with CNI, the CKD patients, the nephrotic syndrome patients treated with CNI, and the nephrotic syndrome patients not treated with CNI. Data were analysed with GEE and, therefore, presented as mean (SE). Tx: Transplantation, CNI: Calcineurin inhibitor, CKD: Chronic kidney disease, NS: Nephrotic syndrome, CsA: Cyclosporine, EGF: Epidermal growth factor, FE: Fractional excretion. # $p < 0.05$ vs NS-CNI; $ $p < 0.05$ vs CKD-CNI; * $p < 0.05$ vs Renal Tx + CNI; § $p < 0.05$ vs NS+CNI.

Patients with Hypomagnesemia versus Patients with Normomagnesemia (presented in Table 3)

Twenty-nine percent of the patients developed hypomagnesemia. Patients who developed hypomagnesemia showed a higher FE Mg^{2+} when treated with CNI. The FE Mg^{2+} was 10.4% (1.8%) in the renal Tx group and 5.9% (1.7%) in the CKD group ($p = 0.073$), and 4.9% (0.6%) in the nephrotic syndrome group treated with CNI compared to 3.5% (<0.1%) in the nephrotic syndrome group not treated with CNI ($p = 0.023$). There was no difference in magnesium intake between hypomagnesemic patients treated with CNI and both control groups ($p = 0.243$).

Table 3. Comparison of clinical and laboratory data between patients who developed hypomagnesemia and nomomagnesemic patients.

Group	Normomagnesemic Patients (n = 69)	Hypomagnesemic Patients (n = 28)	p-Value
Age (year)	11.79 (3.20–18.66)	13.91 (3.14–19.53)	0.492
Length (cm)	147 (94.5–190)	155.4 (92–77.5)	0.582
Weight (kg)	42.95 ± 18.39	43.61 ± 19.31	0.683
BMI z-score	0.14 (−2.24–2.82)	0.13 (−1.66–2.12)	0.418
Mg^{2+} intake (% of RDI)	87 (41–436)	88 (37–684)	0.692
Patients who exceeded the RDI for Mg^{2+} intake (%)	31.3	34.6	0.419
Serum Creatinine (mg/dL)	0.88 (0.06)	1.01 (0.11)	0.287
Creatinine clearance (mL/min/1.73 m^2)	86 (4)	75 (6)	0.122
Urinary protein/creatinine (mg/g)	625.2 (155.8)	561.7 (120.5)	0.747
Serum estradiol (pg/mL)	60.28 (15.83)	67.24 (37.75)	0.865
Serum Mg^{2+} (mg/dL)	0.83 (0.01)	0.70 (0.01)	<0.001
FE Mg^{2+} (%)	5.41 (0.43)	6.55 (0.72)	0.178
CsA levels (ng/mL)	566.13 (30.70)	685.75 (53.56)	0.053
Tacrolimus levels (ng/mL)	6.90 (0.64)	8.55 (0.99)	0.163
Serum EGF (pg/mL)	802.77 (27.93)	795.60 (40.08)	0.883
Urine EGF (ng/mL)	27.46 (3.50)	18.58 (4.52)	0.120
Urine EGF/creatinine (ng/mg)	0.31 (0.03)	0.22 (0.05)	0.120

Cross-sectional data were analysed with Mann-Whitney-U test and presented as the median (minimum-maximum) or Student's t-test (mean ± SD). Longitudinal data were analysed with GEE and, therefore, presented as the mean (SE). RDI: Reference daily intake, EGF: Epidermal growth factor, FE: Fractional excretion, CsA: cyclosporine.

3.3. Magnesium Intake

The median amount of magnesium intake was 87% (37–684%) of the reference daily intake (RDI, corrected for age). Only 29% of all patients exceeded the RDI. Although the median magnesium intake remained stable from 8 year on, the number of children that reached the RDI for magnesium intake was decreasing with age: 63.2% of the children < 8 year exceeded the RDI for magnesium intake (median amount was 119% (62–684%)), while this was only 17.9% of children between 8–12 year (77% (41–151%)), 33.3% between 12–16 year (80% (56–436%), and 21.1% of the >16 year old children and adolescents (86% (37–323%)).

Magnesium intake was significantly correlated with age (Figure 1A; $p < 0.001$; $r = -0.375$), weight ($p = 0.009$; $r = -0.272$), and length ($p = 0.002$; $r = -0.318$). The use of Mg^{2+} supplements was negatively correlated with magnesium intake ($p = 0.095$; $r = -0.177$). Magnesium intake did not correlate with other variables, such as the BMI z-score, sex, serum Mg levels (Figure 1B), renal function, serum or urinary EGF concentration, or the presence of hypomagnesemia.

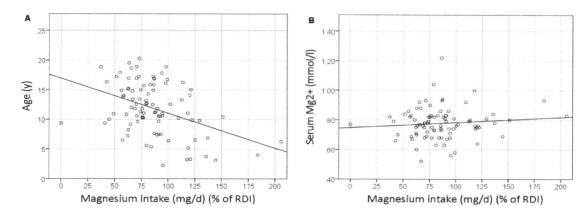

Figure 1. Correlation between the magnesium intake and age (**A**) and the serum magnesium level (**B**). RDI: Recommended daily intake.

3.4. The Healthy Control Group

The median age in the healthy control group was 13.2 year (3.3–17.9 year). Fifty-four percent of the healthy control children were male and length, weight, and BMI z-score was comparable to the study groups.

The serum creatinine was 0.54 mg/dL (0.32–1.09 mg/dL), the creatinine clearance was 108 mL/min/1.73 m^2 (66–143 mL/min/1.73 m^2), serum Mg^{2+} was 0.92 mg/dL (0.80–1.07 mg/dL), and the FE Mg^{2+} was 3.45% (0.81–5.82%). None of the patients developed hypomagnesemia.

The median urinary EGF was 67.4 ng/mL (17.9–218.8 ng/mL) and the median serum EGF was 807.7 pg/mL (141.6–2087.0 pg/mL). The urinary and serum EGF strongly correlated with age ($p < 0.001$; $r = -0.406$ for urinary EGF and $r = -0.447$ for serum EGF). Urinary EGF also correlated with creatinine clearance ($p = 0.011$; $r = 0.408$), but not with sex ($p = 0.514$; $r = -0.079$), FE Mg^{2+} ($p = 0.819$; $r = 0.038$), serum Mg^{2+} ($p = 0.478$; $r = 0.119$), or serum EGF ($p = 0.405$; $r = 0.135$). Serum EGF also correlated with the BMI z-score ($p = 0.001$; $r = 0.369$) but not with sex ($p = 0.054$; $r = 0.231$), creatinine clearance ($p = 0.520$; $r = 0.108$), serum Mg^{2+} ($p = 0.478$; $r = 0.119$), or FE Mg^{2+} ($p = 0.231$; $r = -0.199$).

3.5. Predictors of FE Mg^{2+}

In a univariate GEE analysis, the FE Mg^{2+} was predicted by the urinary EGF concentration, with $r = -0.57$ and $p < 0.001$ (depicted in Figure 2).

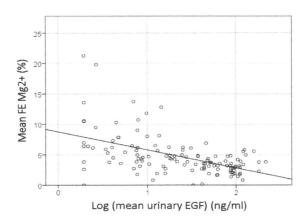

Figure 2. Correlation between the EGF and fractional excretion (FE) of magnesium. Logarithmic normalized data of the EGF are presented.

Urinary EGF, age, sex, renal function, serum magnesium concentration, the urinary protein/creatinine ratio, and Mg^{2+} intake were tested in a multivariate GEE model as predictors of FE Mg^{2+}. Except for sex ($p = 0.747$), urinary protein/creatinine ratio ($p = 0.192$), and Mg^{2+} intake ($p = 0.593$), the other factors appeared to be independent predictors of FE Mg^{2+} (data presented in Table 4).

Table 4. Log EGF as a predictor of FE Mg^{2+}.

	β	p-Value	95% CI	
			Lower	**Upper**
Log Urinary EGF (ng/mL)	−2.084	<0.001	−3.153	−1.015
eGFR (mL/min/1.73 m^2)	−0.049	<0.001	−0.067	−0.032
Serum Mg^{2+} (mg/dL)	−6.239	0.034	−12.014	−0.463
Age (year)	−0.239	0.001	−0.384	−0.094
Constant	20.078	<0.001		

In this population, the FE Mg^{2+} can be calculated using the following formula: FE Mg^{2+} = 20.078 − 2.084 × log Urinary EGF − 0.049 × eGFR − 0.239 × Age − 6.239 × serum Mg^{2+}. eGFR: estimated glomerular filtration rate, EGF: epidermal growth factor.

4. Discussion

This clinical study revealed several new insights into magnesium homeostasis in children: (1) Children treated with calcineurin inhibitors had lower serum magnesium levels and, more frequently, developed hypomagnesemia; (2) In children who developed hypomagnesemia, the FE Mg^{2+} was increased in patients treated with calcineurin inhibitors; (3) The urinary EGF concentration and the FE Mg^{2+} were inversely correlated in all research groups; (4) We defined a predictive model for the FE Mg^{2+} in children, including the urinary EGF concentration, age, renal function, and the serum magnesium concentration; (5) We found that only 29% of the children exceeded the RDI for magnesium intake, which further decreased with age; and (6) Magnesium intake was negatively correlated with the use of magnesium supplements.

In this study, we found that children treated with CNI showed significantly lower serum magnesium levels and that they were significantly more likely to develop hypomagnesemia. This is in line with previous findings in children [31–34] and adults [21]. In adults and animal models, it was shown that hypomagnesemia is caused by renal magnesium wasting [20,21,35]. CNI treatment lead to a decreased renal EGF production, resulting in a decreased magnesium channel TRPM6 expression in the distal convoluted tubule and, thus, a decreased renal magnesium reabsorption [20,35]. However, in children the pathogenesis of CNI induced hypomagnesemia is less clear as few studies have found a normal FE Mg^{2+} after CNI treatment, despite the development of hypomagnesemia [31,36]. In the present study, we demonstrated for the first time that the FE Mg^{2+} increased in children who developed hypomagnesemia when treated with CNI. This effect was independent from the magnesium intake as children who developed hypomagnesemia had an equal magnesium intake compared to normomagnesemic children. In addition to this finding, the urinary EGF concentration and the FE Mg^{2+} were inversely correlated, thus supporting the role of EGF in the renal magnesium reabsorption in children. In a multivariate model, EGF remained a significant predictor of the FE Mg^{2+}. Our results pinpoint to a similar mechanism of renal magnesium reabsorption in children as was demonstrated in adults and rats: Renal EGF stimulates the magnesium reabsorption via the TRPM6 channel in the distal convoluted tubule. To strengthen this hypothesis, a study should be conducted investigating EGF and TRPM6 in renal biopsies. However, as this would indicate an invasive procedure in children, ethical approval can never be obtained in a study context alone.

Additionally, from the multivariate model, age also appeared to be an independent predictor of the FE Mg^{2+} in children, with a positive correlation coefficient. In healthy children, it was shown that the FE Mg^{2+} did not correlate with age [37]. In the present study, only children with an underlying kidney disease were included. Several kidney diseases are accompanied by renal magnesium wasting in children, such as genetic disorders [38] or tubular dysfunction after acute tubular necrosis, or post-obstructive diuresis [39,40]. From our data, the FE Mg^{2+} increases with age in this population, which might indicate that the duration of the kidney disease is of importance in the development of renal magnesium wasting. As we did not go into detail on this finding, this would be an interesting topic for further research.

In children, the renal function also predicts the FE Mg^{2+}. A few other studies have already established a relation between the FE Mg^{2+} and the renal function. In children who recovered from ischemic acute tubular necrosis, it was shown that the FE Mg^{2+} declined, while the renal function improved [41]. This accords with the physiological principles as the FE Mg^{2+} is calculated from the serum creatinine (which is higher in patients with renal failure) and the urinary creatinine (which is lower in patients with renal failure). Therefore, an improvement of creatinine clearance would mathematically result in a decrease in the FE Mg^{2+}. To overcome this mathematical issue, biomarkers of kidney function other than creatinine should be determined, such as urine neutrophil gelatinase-associated lipocalin (NGAL), chromium-51 EDTA, or cystatin-C, which have been shown to be reliable markers of acute kidney injury as well as chronic kidney disease [42–44]. In the present study, the renal function of the children with CKD (the CKD group) was also determined with chromium-51 EDTA analysis (data not shown), which showed a significant relation with the FE Mg^{2+}. Also in pediatric patients after kidney transplantation, FE Mg^{2+} was negatively correlated with the renal function [45,46]. In adult patients, the renal function did not predict FE Mg^{2+} [21]. In that study, both the renal transplant group and the CKD control group were matched for renal function, which might explain why the relation was not found. In the present study, children with a decreased renal function (renal transplant group and CKD group), as well as children with a normal creatinine clearance (both nephrotic syndrome groups), were included.

The protein/creatinine ratio was increased in all groups in this study population, however, below the nephrotic range proteinuria. Normal protein/creatinine ratios up to 340 mg/g were reported in healthy children [47], while nephrotic range proteinuria is defined as protein/creatinine ratio >2 g/g creatinine [48]. The protein/creatinine ratio did not differ between patients with and without hypomagnesemia and was not independently related to the FE Mg^{2+}, suggesting that renal magnesium loss is not due to proteinuria.

Only 29% of the children reached the recommended amount of magnesium intake, which negatively correlated with age, with a higher magnesium intake more likely at a younger age. A few other European studies also found that older children had a higher prevalence of inadequate magnesium intake compared to younger children [8,49,50]. The average magnesium intake was the highest in the youngest children (<8 year), while the lowest intake was in the 8 to 12 year old children. From then on, the average magnesium intake increased with age which was also found in one other report [50]. In our study cohort, this was explained by the use of magnesium supplements, a treatment that is prescribed to patients with hypomagnesemia or patients susceptible to the development of hypomagnesemia. Our findings contrasted with a study of white and African-American girls, in which the magnesium intake decreased with age [51].

Our study has several strengths that led to new insights into the pathogenesis of CNI-induced magnesium loss in children. Despite the low incidence of nephrotic syndrome and renal transplantation in children, we were able to include sufficient numbers of patients. The longitudinal study design, with a low drop-out rate and age, gender, and renal function, matched the control groups and enabled us to draw sound conclusions. The most important limitation of the present study is that the CNI treated patients were included when they were already on treatment with CNI, sometimes for several years already. It would be of interest to include the patients at the moment CNIs are initiated and perform a long-term follow-up study over several years to study the time course influence of CNI on the renal EGF expression and renal magnesium loss. However, as CNI treatment is rare in children, with the low incidence of CNI-dependent nephrotic syndrome and kidney transplantation, the inclusion of sufficient children would take years.

5. Conclusions

In CNI-treated children who developed hypomagnesemia, the FE Mg^{2+} was increased. The urinary EGF concentration was an independent predictor of the FE Mg^2, as were age and renal function.

Author Contributions: Conceptualization, K.J.L., B.Y.D.W. and D.T.; Data curation, C.A., A.D.M., S.M. and M.V.; Formal analysis, K.J.L., C.A., S.M. and G.A.V.; Funding acquisition, D.T.; Investigation, K.J.L.; Methodology, K.J.L., A.V.E., B.Y.D.W. and D.T.; Project administration, K.J.L., A.D.M., M.V. and A.V.E.; Resources, K.V.H. and D.T.; Software, K.J.L.; Supervision, D.T.; Writing-original draft, K.J.L. and C.A.; Writing-review & editing, G.A.V., K.V.H., A.V.E., B.Y.D.W. and D.T.

Acknowledgments: We thank the nursing staff and all patients for making this observational study possible. We also like to thank Petra Aerts, Ilse Goolaerts, Angelika Jürgens and Lieve Vits for the technical assistance.

References

1. Narayanan, S.; Scalici, P. Serum magnesium levels in pediatric inpatients: A study in laboratory overuse. *Hosp. Pediatr.* **2015**, *5*, 9–17. [CrossRef] [PubMed]
2. Abrams, S.A.; Chen, Z.; Hawthorne, K.M. Magnesium metabolism in 4-year-old to 8-year-old children. *J. Bone Miner. Res.* **2014**, *29*, 118–122. [CrossRef] [PubMed]
3. Jahnen-Dechent, W.; Ketteler, M. Magnesium basics. *Clin. Kidney J.* **2012**, *5*, i3–i14. [CrossRef] [PubMed]
4. Weaver, C.M. Calcium and magnesium requirements of children and adolescents and peak bone mass. *Nutrition* **2000**, *16*, 514–516. [CrossRef]
5. Kris-Etherton, P.M.; Hu, F.B.; Ros, E.; Sabate, J. The role of tree nuts and peanuts in the prevention of coronary heart disease: Multiple potential mechanisms. *J. Nutr.* **2008**, *138*, 1746S–1751S. [CrossRef] [PubMed]
6. Heaney, R.P. Dairy and bone health. *J. Am. Coll. Nutr.* **2009**, *28* (Suppl. 1), 82S–90S. [CrossRef] [PubMed]
7. Hurrell, R.F. Influence of vegetable protein sources on trace element and mineral bioavailability. *J. Nutr.* **2003**, *133*, 2973S–2977S. [CrossRef] [PubMed]
8. Tornaritis, M.J.; Philippou, E.; Hadjigeorgiou, C.; Kourides, Y.A.; Panayi, A.; Savva, S.C. A study of the dietary intake of cypriot children and adolescents aged 6–18 years and the association of mother's educational status and children's weight status on adherence to nutritional recommendations. *BMC Public Health* **2014**, *14*, 13. [CrossRef] [PubMed]
9. Sanchez, C.; Aranda, P.; Perez de la Cruz, A.; Llopis, J. Magnesium and zinc status in patients with chronic renal failure: Influence of a nutritional intervention. *Magnes. Res.* **2009**, *22*, 72–80. [PubMed]
10. Gluba-Brzozka, A.; Franczyk, B.; Rysz, J. Vegetarian diet in chronic kidney disease-a friend or foe. *Nutrients* **2017**, *9*, 374. [CrossRef] [PubMed]
11. Lameris, A.L.; Monnens, L.A.; Bindels, R.J.; Hoenderop, J.G.J. Drug-induced alterations in mg2+ homoeostasis. *Clin. Sci.* **2012**, *123*, 1–14. [CrossRef] [PubMed]
12. Milbouw, S.; Verhaegen, J.; Verrijken, A.; Schepens, T.; De Winter, B.Y.; Van Gaal, L.F.; Ledeganck, K.J.; De Block, C.E.M. Predictors of insulin resistance in obesity and type 2 diabetes mellitus—The role of magnesium. *J. Metab. Syndr.* **2017**, *6*, 235. [CrossRef]
13. Liu, F.; Mao, J.H. Calcineurin inhibitors and nephrotoxicity in children. *World J. Pediatr.* **2018**, *14*, 121–126. [CrossRef] [PubMed]
14. Burdmann, E.A.; Andoh, T.F.; Lindsley, J.; Houghton, D.C.; Bennett, W.M. Effects of oral magnesium supplementation on acute experimental cyclosporin nephrotoxicity. *Nephrol. Dial. Transplant.* **1994**, *9*, 16–21. [PubMed]
15. Higgins, R.; Ramaiyan, K.; Dasgupta, T.; Kanji, H.; Fletcher, S.; Lam, F.; Kashi, H. Hyponatraemia and hyperkalaemia are more frequent in renal transplant recipients treated with tacrolimus than with cyclosporin. Further evidence for differences between cyclosporin and tacrolimus nephrotoxicities. *Nephrol. Dial. Transplant.* **2004**, *19*, 444–450. [CrossRef] [PubMed]
16. Hoenderop, J.G.J.; Bindels, R.J.M. Epithelial ca2+ and mg2+ channels in health and disease. *J. Am. Soc. Nephrol.* **2005**, *16*, 15–26. [CrossRef] [PubMed]
17. Schlingmann, K.P.; Waldegger, S.; Konrad, M.; Chubanov, V.; Gudermann, T. Trpm6 and trpm7—Gatekeepers of human magnesium metabolism. *Biochim. Biophys. Acta* **2007**, *1772*, 813–821. [CrossRef] [PubMed]
18. Thebault, S.P.; Alexander, R.T.; Tiel Groenestege, W.M.; Hoenderop, J.G.; Bindels, R.J. Egf increases trpm6 activity and surface expression. *J. Am. Soc. Nephrol.* **2009**, *20*, 78–85. [CrossRef] [PubMed]
19. Groenestege, W.M.; Thebault, S.; van der Wijst, J.; van den Berg, D.; Janssen, R.; Tejpar, S.; van den Heuvel, L.P.; van Cutsem, E.; Hoenderop, J.G.; Knoers, N.V.; et al. Impaired basolateral sorting of pro-egf causes isolated recessive renal hypomagnesemia. *J. Clin. Invest.* **2007**, *117*, 2260–2267. [CrossRef] [PubMed]
20. Ledeganck, K.J.; Boulet, G.A.; Horvath, C.A.; Vinckx, M.; Bogers, J.J.; Van den Bossche, R.; Verpooten, G.A.; De Winter, B.Y. Expression of renal distal tubule transporters trpm6 and ncc in a rat model of cyclosporine nephrotoxicity and effect of egf treatment. *Am. J. Physiol. Renal Physiol.* **2011**, *301*, F486–F493. [CrossRef] [PubMed]
21. Ledeganck, K.J.; De Winter, B.Y.; Van den Driessche, A.; Jurgens, A.; Bosmans, J.L.; Couttenye, M.M.; Verpooten, G.A. Magnesium loss in cyclosporine-treated patients is related to renal epidermal growth factor downregulation. *Nephrol. Dial. Transplant.* **2013**, *29*, 1097–1102. [CrossRef] [PubMed]

22. Zeng, F.; Harris, R.C. Epidermal growth factor, from gene organization to bedside. *Semin. Cell Dev. Biol.* **2014**, *28*, 2–11. [CrossRef] [PubMed]

23. Tomaszewska, R.; Dembinski, A.; Warzecha, Z.; Ceranowicz, P.; Konturek, S.J.; Stachura, J. The influence of epidermal growth factor on the course of ischemia-reperfusion induced pancreatitis in rats. *J. Physiol. Pharmacol.* **2002**, *53*, 183–198. [PubMed]

24. Warzecha, Z.; Dembinski, A.; Konturek, P.C.; Ceranowicz, P.; Konturek, S.J. Epidermal growth factor protects against pancreatic damage in cerulein-induced pancreatitis. *Digestion* **1999**, *60*, 314–323. [CrossRef] [PubMed]

25. Konturek, P.C.; Dembinski, A.; Warzecha, Z.; Ceranowicz, P.; Konturek, S.J.; Stachura, J.; Hahn, E.G. Expression of transforming growth factor-beta 1 and epidermal growth factor in caerulein-induced pancreatitis in rat. *J. Physiol. Pharmacol.* **1997**, *48*, 59–72. [PubMed]

26. Bennett, S.P.; Griffiths, G.D.; Schor, A.M.; Leese, G.P.; Schor, S.L. Growth factors in the treatment of diabetic foot ulcers. *Br. J. Surg.* **2003**, *90*, 133–146. [CrossRef] [PubMed]

27. Huysentruyt, K.; Laire, D.; Van Avondt, T.; De Schepper, J.; Vandenplas, Y. Energy and macronutrient intakes and adherence to dietary guidelines of infants and toddlers in belgium. *Eur. J. Nutr.* **2016**, *55*, 1595–1604. [CrossRef] [PubMed]

28. Cochat, P. *Espn Handbook*; European Society for Paediatric Nephrology; Medcom: Lyon, France, 2002.

29. Schwartz, G.J.; Munoz, A.; Schneider, M.F.; Mak, R.H.; Kaskel, F.; Warady, B.A.; Furth, S.L. New equations to estimate gfr in children with ckd. *J. Am. Soc. Nephrol.* **2009**, *20*, 629–637. [CrossRef] [PubMed]

30. Cao, G.; van der Wijst, J.; van der Kemp, A.; van Zeeland, F.; Bindels, R.J.; Hoenderop, J.G. Regulation of the epithelial mg2+ channel trpm6 by estrogen and the associated repressor protein of estrogen receptor activity (rea). *J. Biol. Chem.* **2009**, *284*, 14788–14795. [CrossRef] [PubMed]

31. Nozue, T.; Kobayashi, A.; Kodama, T.; Uemasu, F.; Endoh, H.; Sako, A.; Takagi, Y. Pathogenesis of cyclosporine-induced hypomagnesemia. *J. Pediatr.* **1992**, *120*, 638–640. [CrossRef]

32. Riva, N.; Schaiquevich, P.; Caceres Guido, P.; Halac, E.; Dip, M.; Imventarza, O. Pharmacoepidemiology of tacrolimus in pediatric liver transplantation. *Pediatr. Transplant.* **2017**, *21*. [CrossRef] [PubMed]

33. Hayes, W.; Boyle, S.; Carroll, A.; Bockenhauer, D.; Marks, S.D. Hypomagnesemia and increased risk of new-onset diabetes mellitus after transplantation in pediatric renal transplant recipients. *Pediatr. Nephrol.* **2017**, *32*, 879–884. [CrossRef] [PubMed]

34. Yanik, G.; Levine, J.E.; Ratanatharathorn, V.; Dunn, R.; Ferrara, J.; Hutchinson, R.J. Tacrolimus (fk506) and methotrexate as prophylaxis for acute graft-versus-host disease in pediatric allogeneic stem cell transplantation. *Bone Marrow Transplant.* **2000**, *26*, 161–167. [CrossRef] [PubMed]

35. Nijenhuis, T.; Hoenderop, J.G.; Bindels, R.J. Downregulation of ca(2+) and mg(2+) transport proteins in the kidney explains tacrolimus (fk506)-induced hypercalciuria and hypomagnesemia. *J. Am. Soc. Nephrol.* **2004**, *15*, 549–557. [CrossRef] [PubMed]

36. Freundlich, M. Bone mineral content and mineral metabolism during cyclosporine treatment of nephrotic syndrome. *J. Pediatr.* **2006**, *149*, 383–389. [CrossRef] [PubMed]

37. Ariceta, G.; Rodriguez-Soriano, J.; Vallo, A. Renal magnesium handling in infants and children. *Acta Paediatr.* **1996**, *85*, 1019–1023. [CrossRef] [PubMed]

38. Viering, D.; de Baaij, J.H.F.; Walsh, S.B.; Kleta, R.; Bockenhauer, D. Genetic causes of hypomagnesemia, a clinical overview. *Pediatr. Nephrol.* **2017**, *32*, 1123–1135. [CrossRef] [PubMed]

39. Whang, R. Magnesium deficiency: Pathogenesis, prevalence, and clinical implications. *Am. J. Med.* **1987**, *82*, 24–29. [CrossRef]

40. Agus, Z.S. Mechanisms and causes of hypomagnesemia. *Curr. Opin. Nephrol. Hypertens.* **2016**, *25*, 301–307. [CrossRef] [PubMed]

41. Gheissari, A.; Andalib, A.; Labibzadeh, N.; Modarresi, M.; Azhir, A.; Merrikhi, A. Fractional excretion of magnesium (femg), a marker for tubular dysfunction in children with clinically recovered ischemic acute tubular necrosis. *Saudi J. Kidney Dis. Transpl.* **2011**, *22*, 476–481. [PubMed]

42. Zylka, A.; Gala-Bladzinska, A.; Dumnicka, P.; Ceranowicz, P.; Kuzniewski, M.; Gil, K.; Olszanecki, R.; Kusnierz-Cabala, B. Is urinary ngal determination useful for monitoring kidney function and assessment of cardiovascular disease? A 12-month observation of patients with type 2 diabetes. *Dis. Markers* **2016**, *2016*, 8489543. [CrossRef] [PubMed]

43. Shlipak, M.G.; Mattes, M.D.; Peralta, C.A. Update on cystatin c: Incorporation into clinical practice. *Am. J. Kidney Dis.* **2013**, *62*, 595–603. [CrossRef] [PubMed]

44. Geist, B.K.; Diemling, M.; Staudenherz, A. Glomerular filtration rate and error calculation based on the slope-intercept method with chromium-51 ethylenediaminetetraacetic acid via a new clinical software: Gfrcalc. *Med. Princ. Pract.* **2016**, *25*, 368–373. [CrossRef] [PubMed]

45. Uslu Gokceoglu, A.; Comak, E.; Dogan, C.S.; Koyun, M.; Akbas, H.; Akman, S. Magnesium excretion and hypomagnesemia in pediatric renal transplant recipients. *Ren. Fail.* **2014**, *36*, 1056–1059. [CrossRef] [PubMed]

46. Osorio, J.M.; Bravo, J.; Perez, A.; Ferreyra, C.; Osuna, A. Magnesemia in renal transplant recipients: Relation with immunosuppression and posttransplant diabetes. *Transplant. Proc.* **2010**, *42*, 2910–2913. [CrossRef] [PubMed]

47. Slev, P.R.; Bunker, A.M.; Owen, W.E.; Roberts, W.L. Pediatric reference intervals for random urine calcium, phosphorus and total protein. *Pediatr. Nephrol.* **2010**, *25*, 1707–1710. [CrossRef] [PubMed]

48. Ariceta, G. Clinical practice: Proteinuria. *Eur. J. Pediatr.* **2011**, *170*, 15–20. [CrossRef] [PubMed]

49. Lopez-Sobaler, A.M.; Aparicio, A.; Gonzalez-Rodriguez, L.G.; Cuadrado-Soto, E.; Rubio, J.; Marcos, V.; Sanchidrian, R.; Santos, S.; Perez-Farinos, N.; Dal Re, M.A.; et al. Adequacy of usual vitamin and mineral intake in spanish children and adolescents: Enalia study. *Nutrients* **2017**, *9*, 131. [CrossRef] [PubMed]

50. Manios, Y.; Moschonis, G.; Mavrogianni, C.; Bos, R.; Singh-Povel, C. Micronutrient intakes among children and adults in greece: The role of age, sex and socio-economic status. *Nutrients* **2014**, *6*, 4073–4092. [CrossRef] [PubMed]

51. Affenito, S.G.; Thompson, D.R.; Franko, D.L.; Striegel-Moore, R.H.; Daniels, S.R.; Barton, B.A.; Schreiber, G.B.; Schmidt, M.; Crawford, P.B. Longitudinal assessment of micronutrient intake among african-american and white girls: The national heart, lung, and blood institute growth and health study. *J. Am. Diet. Assoc.* **2007**, *107*, 1113–1123. [CrossRef] [PubMed]

14

Bioaccessibility and Bioavailability of a Marine-Derived Multimineral, Aquamin-Magnesium

Valeria D. Felice [1,2,3,*], Denise M. O'Gorman [4], Nora M. O'Brien [2] and Niall P. Hyland [1,3]

[1]   Department of Pharmacology and Therapeutics and Department of Physiology, University College Cork, T12 K8AF Cork, Ireland; n.hyland@ucc.ie

[2]   School of Food and Nutritional Sciences, University College Cork, T12 K8AF Cork, Ireland; nob@ucc.ie

[3]   APC Microbiome Ireland, University College Cork, T12 K8AF Cork, Ireland

[4]   Marigot Ltd., P43 NN62 Cork, Ireland; denise.ogorman@marigot.ie

*   Correspondence: valeria.felice@marigot.ie

Abstract: Introduction: Magnesium is an essential mineral involved in a range of key biochemical pathways. Several magnesium supplements are present on the market and their degree of bioavailability differs depending on the form of magnesium salt used. Aquamin-Mg is a natural source of magnesium, containing 72 additional trace minerals derived from the clean waters off the Irish coast. However, the in vitro bioaccessibility and bioavailability of Aquamin-Mg in comparison with other supplement sources of magnesium has yet to be tested. **Method:** Aquamin-Mg, magnesium chloride ($MgCl_2$) and magnesium oxide (MgO) were subjected to gastrointestinal digestion according to the harmonized INFOGEST in vitro digestion method and in vitro bioavailability tested using the Caco-2 cell model. Magnesium concentration was measured by atomic absorption spectrophotometry (AAS). **Results:** Magnesium recovery from both Aquamin-Mg and $MgCl_2$ was greater than for MgO. Magnesium from all three sources was transported across the epithelial monolayer with Aquamin-Mg displaying a comparable profile to the more bioavailable $MgCl_2$. **Conclusions:** Our data support that magnesium derived from a marine-derived multimineral product is bioavailable to a significantly greater degree than MgO and displays a similar profile to the more bioavailable $MgCl_2$ and may offer additional health benefits given its multimineral profile.

Keywords: Aquamin; multimineral supplement; magnesium bioavailability

1. Introduction

Magnesium is an essential mineral for the human body and is involved in a wide range of crucial physiological processes [1]. Magnesium can be obtained from the diet, being naturally present in foods such as green leafy vegetables, seeds, beans, whole grains, fish and nuts, amongst others. However, dietary magnesium intake has been shown to be insufficient in the Western population due to industrial food processing that reduces the nutrient contents including magnesium, as well as changes in dietary habits [2]. Deficiency in magnesium dietary intake may lead to hypomagnesemia which has been associated with several disorders including diabetes, osteoporosis and cardiovascular disease [3–5]. Early symptoms of hypomagnesemia are non-specific and include loss of appetite, nausea, vomiting, lethargy, fatigue and weakness with more pronounced hypomagnesemia characterised by increased neuromuscular excitability including muscle cramps, tremor, tetany and generalized seizures [6].

The market currently offers various supplement preparations to reach the recommended magnesium daily intake. These supplements differ in the type of magnesium salt used which can be either organic (i.e., magnesium citrate and magnesium aspartate) or inorganic (i.e., MgO and $MgCl_2$), their dosage and bioavailability. For example, magnesium from $MgCl_2$ has high bioavailability equivalent to organic magnesium supplements such as magnesium lactate and aspartate [7]. Moreover, these three sources of magnesium have significantly greater bioavailability than MgO [7]. Magnesium derived from magnesium hydroxide (Mg(OH)$_2$) (Mablet) has been shown to be absorbed into the circulation and, hence, bioavailable in healthy male adults [8]. In a previous study, the bioavailability of magnesium from formulations containing different combinations of magnesium salts displayed similar bioavailability, however the daily dose of magnesium differed [9].

Aquamin-Mg is a natural source of magnesium in the form of Mg(OH)$_2$ derived from the clean waters off the Irish coast. In addition to magnesium, Aquamin-Mg also contains 72 additional trace minerals (Marigot Ltd., Cork, Ireland, Table 1) with the same profile of Lithothamnion Aquamin which has previously been shown to be a highly bioavailable source of calcium [10].

Here we describe for the first time the in vitro bioaccessibility and bioavailability of Aquamin-Mg in comparison with two commercially available sources of magnesium, MgCl$_2$ and MgO.

Table 1. Mineral composition of Aquamin-Mg. (ppm, parts per million).

Mineral	ppm	Mineral	ppm
Aluminum	461	Molybdenum	1.78
Antimony	<0.5	Neodymium	2.810
Arsenic	1.811	Nickel	<0.5
Barium	1.83	Niobium	<0.5
Beryllium	<0.5	Osmium	0.002
Bismuth	<0.5	Palladium	0.301
Boron	186	Phosphorus	117
Cadmium	0.394	Platinum	0.002
Calcium	23,000	Potassium	88.21
Carbon	10,100	Praseodymium	0.697
Cerium	3.411	Rhenium	0.001
Cesium	0.008	Rhodium	0.010
Chloride	613.4	Rubidium	0.063
Chromium	5.83	Ruthenium	0.135
Cobalt	<0.5	Samarium	0.576
Copper	5.09	Scandium	1.050
Dysprosium	0.829	Selenium	<0.5
Erbium	0.613	Silicon	657
Europium	0.197	Silver	<0.5
Fluoride	1.1	Sodium	1467
Gadolinium	0.770	Strontium	84.7
Gallium	0.163	Sulfur	3335
Germanium	0.020	Tantalum	0.016
Gold	<0.5	Tellurium	<0.5
Hafnium	0.046	Terbium	0.140
Holmium	0.194	Thallium	<0.5
Indium	<0.001	Thorium	0.860
Iodine	9.1	Thulium	0.081
Iridium	0.002	Tin	0.179
Iron	1213	Titanium	18.5
Lanthanum	1.01	Tungsten	2.08
Lead	0.604	Vanadium	16.0
Lithium	<0.5	Ytterbium	0.498
Lutetium	0.116	Yttrium	7.38
Magnesium	404,400	Zinc	2.37
Manganese	486	Zirconium	<0.5
Mercury	0.009		

2. Methods

2.1. Harmonized INFOGEST in Vitro Digestion Protocol

To determine biaccessibility, the amount of magnesium subjected to digestion for each compound was calculated according to the recommended dietary allowance for men (RDA, 420 mg/day). 5.6 mg of magnesium from Aquamin-Mg, $MgCl_2$ and MgO were digested according to the harmonized INFOGEST in vitro digestion method published by Minekus and colleagues [11]. Four to five independent digestions were carried out for each compound (Aquamin-Mg, $MgCl_2$ and MgO). Aquamin-Mg, $MgCl_2$ and MgO were exposed to simulated gastric fluid (composition: 6.9 mM KCl, 0.9 mM KH_2PO_4, 25 mM $NaHCO_3$, 47.2 mM NaCl, 0.1 mM $MgCl_2(H_2O)_6$, 0.5 mM $(NH_4)_2CO_3$). Pepsin and calcium chloride were added to the mixture to achieve a final concentration of 2000 U/mL and 0.075 mM respectively. Hydrochloric acid (HCl, 6 M) was then used to acidify the mixture to pH 3 and water was added to reach a final volume of 20 mL. Samples were then incubated in a stirring water bath at 37 °C and 95 rpm for 2 h. The pH was checked after 1 hour and adjusted if necessary. The simulated intestinal fluid (composition: 6.8 mM KCl, 0.8 mM KH_2PO_4, 85 mM $NaHCO_3$, 38.4 mM NaCl, 0.33 mM $MgCl_2(H_2O)_6$) was then added together with pancreatin (the concentration was based on trypsin activity, 100 U/mL) and bile salts for a final concentration of 10 mM. Calcium chloride was also added to achieve a final concentration of 0.3 mM. Sodium hydroxide (NaOH, 1 M) was used to bring the pH to 7 and the necessary amount of water added to reach a final volume of 20 mL. Samples were incubated in a stirring water bath at 37 °C and 95 rpm for 2 h. The pH was checked after one hour and adjusted if necessary. A control sample containing all reagents included in the digestion protocol except the experimental powders was also subjected to the procedure. Upon completion of the incubation period, aliquots (1 mL) of each sample were frozen in liquid nitrogen. Prior to the analysis, one sample from each treatment was filtered using 0.2 μm cell culture sterile filters. The amount of magnesium recovered from these samples was then compared to non-filtered samples.

2.2. Caco-2 Cell Bioavailability Assay

Caco-2 cells are human epithelial colorectal adenocarcinoma cells that, upon differentiation, express numerous morphological and biochemical characteristics of small intestinal enterocytes. This in vitro model is widely used to study mineral bioavailability from different sources and their transport mechanisms [12].

For Caco-2 bioavailability experiments 60 mg of magnesium derived from Aquamin-Mg, $MgCl_2$ and MgO were subjected to the harmonized INFOGEST in vitro digestion protocol described above (data not shown), and unfiltered samples were used. 60 mg of magnesium was chosen in order to ensure that sufficient concentrations of magnesium could be achieved to perform the Caco-2 experiments. Three independent digestions were carried out for each compound (Aquamin-Mg, $MgCl_2$ and MgO) and these were subsequently used in the Caco-2 bioavailability assay. Caco-2 cells (supplied by the European Collection of Authenticated Cell Cultures (ECACC)) were cultured in Dulbecco's modified eagle's medium (DMEM) supplemented with 1% non-essential amino acids and 10% foetal bovine serum (FBS) and were stored in a humidified incubator at 37 °C and 5% CO_2. For all experiments, cells were seeded at a density of 1×10^5 cells/mL on 6-well Transwell plates with inserts of 24 mm diameter and differentiated for 21 days. Media was changed every other day.

2.3. Bioavailability of Magnesium from Aquamin-Mg, $MgCl_2$ and MgO Using Caco-2 Cells

On the day of the experiment, media was removed from all wells and 1 mL of fresh media was added to the luminal side and 2 mL to the basolateral side of each well. Transepithelial electrical resistance (TEER) was measured to confirm the integrity of the epithelial monolayer. Cells were then incubated with either Aquamin-Mg, $MgCl_2$- or MgO-derived magnesium in the luminal side (concentrations of 25, 50, 100 and 150 μg/mL) for 2 h at 37 °C. Samples from each independent digestion were used in a corresponding independent bioavailability study which was conducted in triplicate. Two controls were included in the assay, a blank sample, only containing media, and a digest sample, containing all reagents included in the digestion protocol except the experimental powders. At the end of the incubation time, TEER values were recorded again to ensure that the treatments did not have any effect on the integrity of the monolayer. Luminal and basolateral samples were collected and stored at 4 °C. Magnesium concentration of luminal and basolateral samples was measured by atomic absorption spectrophotometry (AAS). Three independent experiments were carried out. Each treatment was randomly assigned and was performed in duplicate.

2.4. Atomic Absorption Spectrophotometry (AAS)

The magnesium content of the digested samples, as well as luminal and basolateral samples was determined by AAS. Samples were diluted in Milli-Q water prior to analysis. Lanthanum chloride (0.1%) was also added to eliminate any phosphate interferences. A commercially available magnesium standard (Spectrosol from BDH Chemicals Ltd., Dublin, Ireland) was used. Standard solutions were prepared using Milli-Q water containing lanthanum chloride (0.1%) and ranged from 0 to 1 mg/L.

2.5. Statistical Analyses

Data are expressed as mean ± standard error of the mean (SEM). Statistical analysis was carried out using the Kruskal–Wallis test, followed by Dunn's multiple comparison test for the digestion study. For the bioavailability study, we calculated the residuals of the data to determine whether there were outliers and statistical analysis was performed using one-way analysis of variance (ANOVA) followed by Bonferroni post-hoc test. Values of $p < 0.05$ were considered statistically significant.

3. Results

3.1. Magnesium Recovery from Aquamin-Mg, MgCl$_2$ and MgO Following In Vitro Digestion

Aquamin-Mg-derived magnesium, showed an in vitro bioaccessibility more similar to highly soluble alternative such as MgCl$_2$ than to MgO (Aquamin-Mg, 122.6 ± 4.1 µg/mL, $n = 5$; MgCl$_2$, 115.4 ± 6.0 µg/mL, $n = 4$; MgO, 73.39 ± 10.20 µg/mL, $n = 4$; in unfiltered samples), which is characterised by low solubility (Figure 1, $p < 0.05$ Aquamin-Mg vs. MgO). To determine whether magnesium was lost during filtration for the Caco-2 cell culture experiments, magnesium concentration in filtered samples was also determined and these were lower for all the treatments relative to unfiltered samples (Aquamin-Mg, 99.3 ± 6.2 µg/mL, $n = 5$; MgCl$_2$, 92.2 ± 5.6 µg/mL, $n = 4$; MgO, 64.5 ± 9.3 µg/mL in filtered samples).

Figure 1. Magnesium recovery from Aquamin-Mg, MgCl$_2$ and MgO following in vitro digestion. The percentage of magnesium recovery from Aquamin-Mg was significantly higher than MgO (* $p < 0.5$, $n = 4–5$) in unfiltered samples.

3.2. Transepithelial Electrical Resistance (TEER)

As an indicator of cell viability we measured TEER at the start of each experiment and after treatment. The results from the transepithelial resistance measurements confirmed that after 21 days of culture, Caco-2 cells formed an integral monolayer. Moreover, none of the treatments, at any concentration tested, affected epithelial integrity following 2 h incubation at 37 °C (Figure 2).

Figure 2. Transepithelial electrical resistance in Caco-2 cells following treatment with Aquamin-Mg, MgCl$_2$ and MgO. At time zero (T0) cells were differentiated in an integral monolayer. Transepithelial electrical resistance (TEER) values confirmed that the treatments did not compromise the integrity of the monolayer at any of the concentrations tested following 2 h incubation (T2h) ($n = 3$).

3.3. Bioavailability of Magnesium from Aquamin-Mg, MgCl$_2$ and MgO Using the Caco-2 Cell Model

Digestates were added to the luminal compartment. The reduced amount of magnesium from MgO is reflective of the reduced bioaccessibility (Figure 3a). These results are in accordance with the in vitro digestion data (60 mg; data not shown). When the concentration of magnesium was measured in the basolateral chamber, magnesium derived from Aquamin-Mg and MgCl$_2$ showed the same degree of bioavailability at all the concentrations tested, while only a small amount of magnesium from MgO was transported across the epithelium and thus bioavailable. Both Aquamin-Mg and MgCl$_2$ were significantly more bioavailable than MgO at the highest concentration tested (150 µg/mL) (Figure 3b, Table 2).

Figure 3. Bioavailability of magnesium from Aquamin-Mg, MgCl₂ and MgO using Caco-2 cells. (**a**) Magnesium derived from Aquamin-Mg, MgCl₂ and MgO applied into the luminal side. Following in vitro digestion, the amount of bioaccessible magnesium was significantly higher for Aquamin-Mg and MgCl₂ compared to MgO (*** $p < 0.001$ for Aquamin-Mg vs. MgO at 25 μg/mL, **** $p < 0.0001$ for MgCl₂ vs. MgO at 25 μg/mL and **** $p < 0.0001$ for Aquamin-Mg and MgCl₂ vs. MgO at 50, 100 and 150 μg/mL, $n = 3$); (**b**) Magnesium derived from Aquamin-Mg, MgCl₂ and MgO measured in the basolateral side after 2 h incubation at 37 °C. At the highest concentration tested, magnesium from Aquamin-Mg and MgCl₂ was significantly more bioavailable than MgO (** $p < 0.01$ for Aquamin-Mg and MgCl₂ vs. MgO at 150 μg/mL, $n = 3$).

Table 2. Magnesium derived from Aquamin-Mg, MgCl₂ and MgO measured in the basolateral side after 2 h incubation at 37 °C expressed as μg/mL ($n = 3$).

Magnesium Source	Sample Concentration (μg/mL)	Basolateral Side μg/mL Mean ± Standard Error of the Mean (SEM)
Aquamin-Mg	25	0.37 ± 0.17
	50	0.44 ± 0.16
	100	0.69 ± 0.16
	150	0.89 ± 0.17
MgCl₂	25	0.14 ± 0.06
	50	0.33 ± 0.13
	100	0.51 ± 0.09
	150	0.86 ± 0.13
MgO	25	0.05 ± 0.03
	50	0.08 ± 0.02
	100	0.25 ± 0.01
	150	0.10 ± 0.05

4. Discussion

The aim of these studies was to examine the bioaccessibility and bioavailability of magnesium from Aquamin-Mg compared to $MgCl_2$ and MgO using the Caco-2 cell model. In this model both active saturated and passive non-saturated pathways have been previously identified for magnesium transport [13]. The study from Thongon and Krishnamrain has indeed shown that in Caco-2 monolayers, magnesium transported from the apical to the basolateral side (representing magnesium absorption) against magnesium in the apical solution (representing magnesium concentration) was curvilinear as previously shown in humans [13,14]. Furthermore, the same study has shown that treatment with omeprazole selectively inhibited the non-saturable passive component, without affecting the saturable active component of magnesium transport which was abolished using the Transient Receptor Potential Cation Channel Subfamily M Member 6 (TRPM6) inhibitor Ruthenium Red (RR) [13]. This evidence shows that magnesium can be transported through both a paracellular and a transcellular pathway and that the Caco-2 monolayer is a suitable in vitro model of intestinal magnesium absorption. In the context of our findings, however, we cannot comment on which pathway was responsible for the apical to basolateral transport of magnesium and further research is warranted in order to elucidate these mechanisms. Our results show for the first-time, however, direct evidence that Aquamin-Mg-derived magnesium is highly bioaccessible following in vitro digestion and magnesium is transported across the intestinal epithelium in this well-established in vitro model. Moreover, the degree of bioaccessbility and bioavailability of Aquamin-Mg was comparable to $MgCl_2$ while being superior to MgO.

$MgCl_2$ and MgO represent a high bioavailable and low bioavailable source of magnesium respectively, and our in vitro data are in keeping with in vivo data demonstrating that the mean urinary excretion of magnesium in healthy volunteers was significantly higher for $MgCl_2$ than MgO [7]. Interestingly, in this study, $MgCl_2$ bioavailability was comparable to that of organic magnesium forms such as magnesium aspartate and magnesium lactate [7].

Magnesium in Aquamin-Mg is in the form of $Mg(OH)_2$. However, as well as magnesium, Aquamin-Mg also provides 72 additional trace minerals all derived from sea water (Marigot Ltd., Cork, Ireland, Table 1). In support of $Mg(OH)_2$ as a magnesium supplement, the pharmacokinetic profile of a single oral dose of $Mg(OH)_2$ in healthy male adults showed that the bioavailability of magnesium from $Mg(OH)_2$ was 15% [8]. Moreover, none of the participants recruited reported any side effect following supplementation suggesting that $Mg(OH)_2$ may be a clinically relevant option for oral magnesium supplementation [8]. In a second human study the degree of bioavailability of $Mg(OH)_2$ was compared to other sources of magnesium, including $MgCl_2$ measured as urinary elimination of magnesium [9]. In this study it was found that $Mg(OH)_2$ was required at a higher dose to reach the same level of bioavailability [9].

The solubility of magnesium in the gastrointestinal tract plays a key role in magnesium absorption. Our bioaccessiblity results demonstrate that magnesium from Aquamin-Mg is soluble as $MgCl_2$ and hence potentially available for absorption. Our bioavailability data support that $Mg(OH)_2$, derived from Aquamin-Mg, displays a similar profile and transport characteristics as magnesium derived from $MgCl_2$ at the same concentrations, suggesting that Aquamin-Mg represents a source of magnesium coupled with potential health benefits of a multimineral supplement. Currently, however, as Aquamin-Mg is not formulated as an oral supplement (tablets and capsules), further comparisons with other formulated magnesium supplements were not possible.

Moreover, Aquamin-Mg is composed of multiple minerals and whether these affect its bioaccessibility or bioavailability is difficult to determine.

5. Conclusions

In conclusion, our data suggests that Aquamin-Mg-derived magnesium is bioaccessible and bioavailable to a significantly greater degree than magnesium oxide while displaying a comparable profile to magnesium chloride. Nonetheless, our in vitro results are qualitatively consistent with the clinical study from Firoz and Graber showing that magnesium from $MgCl_2$ has significantly greater bioavailability than MgO. Further research is warranted to investigate the bioaccessibility and bioavailability of Aquamin-Mg in clinical studies.

Author Contributions: V.D.F., N.P.H., N.M.O. and D.M.O. conceived and designed the experiments. D.M.O. provided Aquamin-Mg. V.D.F. performed the experiments and V.D.F. and N.P.H. analysed the data. V.D.F. and N.P.H. wrote the manuscript; N.M.O., and D.M.O., edited the manuscript.

Acknowledgments: Felice has received an Irish Research Council Enterprise Postdoctoral Fellowship. We would like also to acknowledge Marigot Ltd. who provided the mineral-rich algae extract Aquamin and their financial support. Thank you also to O'Callaghan, University College Cork, and Shane O'Connell (Marigot Ltd.), for their help in the preparation of this manuscript.

References

1.   Saris, N.E.; Mervaala, E.; Karppanen, H.; Khawaja, J.A.; Lewenstam, A. Magnesium. An update on physiological, clinical and analytical aspects. *Clin. Chim. Acta* **2000**, *294*, 1–26. [CrossRef]

2.   Marier, J.R. Magnesium content of the food supply in the modern-day world. *Magnesium* **1986**, *5*, 1–8. [PubMed]

3.   Rosique-Esteban, N.; Guasch-Ferré, M.; Hernández-Alonso, P.; Salas-Salvadó, J. Dietary magnesium and cardiovascular disease: A review with emphasis in epidemiological studies. *Nutrients* **2018**, *10*, 168. [CrossRef] [PubMed]

4.   Guerrero-Romero, F.; Jaquez-Chairez, F.O.; Rodríguez-Morán, M. Magnesium in metabolic syndrome: A review based on randomized, double-blind clinical trials. *Magnes. Res.* **2016**, *29*, 146–153. [PubMed]

5.   Castiglioni, S.; Cazzaniga, A.; Albisetti, W.; Maier, J.A.M. Magnesium and osteoporosis: Current state of knowledge and future research directions. *Nutrients* **2013**, *5*, 3022–3033.

6.   Grober, U.; Schmidt, J.; Kisters, K. Magnesium in prevention and therapy. *Nutrients* **2015**, *7*, 8199–8226. [CrossRef] [PubMed]

7.   Firoz, M.; Graber, M. Bioavailability of US commercial magnesium preparations. *Magnes. Res.* **2001**, *14*, 257–262. [PubMed]

8.   Dolberg, M.K.B.; Nielsen, L.P.; Dahl, R. Pharmacokinetic profile of oral magnesium hydroxide. *Basic Clin. Pharmacol. Toxicol.* **2017**, *120*, 264–269. [CrossRef] [PubMed]

9.   Bøhmer, T.; Røseth, A.; Holm, H.; Weberg-Teigen, S.; Wahl, L. Bioavailability of oral magnesium supplementation in female students evaluated from elimination of magnesium in 24-hour urine. *Magnes. Trace Elem.* **1990**, *9*, 272–278.

10. Zenk, J.L.; Frestedt, J.L.; Kuskowski, M.A. Effect of Calcium Derived from Lithothamnion sp. on markers of calcium metabolism in premenopausal women. *J. Med. Food* **2018**, *21*, 154–158. [CrossRef] [PubMed]

11. Minekus, M.; Alminger, M.; Alvito, P.; Balance, S.; Bohn, T.; Bourlieu, C.; Carrière, F.; Boutrou, R.; Corredig, M.; Dupont, D.; et al. A standardised static in vitro digestion method suitable for food—An international consensus. *Food Funct.* **2014**, *5*, 1113–1124. [CrossRef]

12. Glahn, R. The use of Caco-2 cells in defining nutrient bioavailability: Application to iron bioavailability of foods. In *Designing Functional Foods*; McClements, D.J., Decker, E.A., Eds.; Woodhead Publishing: Cambridge, UK, 2009; pp. 340–361.

13. Thongon, N.; Krishnamra, N. Omeprazole decreases magnesium transport across Caco-2 monolayers. *World J. Gastroenterol.* **2011**, *17*, 1574–1583. [CrossRef] [PubMed]

14. Fine, K.D.; Ana, C.A.S.; Porter, J.L.; Fordtran, J.S. Intestinal absorption of magnesium from food and supplements. *J. Clin. Investig.* **1991**, *88*, 396–402. [CrossRef] [PubMed]

15

Inhibition of Mg^{2+} Extrusion Attenuates Glutamate Excitotoxicity in Cultured Rat Hippocampal Neurons

Yutaka Shindo [1], Ryu Yamanaka [1,2], Kohji Hotta [1] and Kotaro Oka [1,3,4,*]

[1] Department of Bioscience and Informatics, Faculty of Science and Technology, Keio University, Yokohama, Kanagawa 223-8522, Japan; shindo@z5.keio.jp (Y.S.); 1024mbmail@gmail.com (R.Y.); khotta@bio.keio.ac.jp (K.H.)

[2] Faculty of Pharmaceutical Sciences, Sanyo-Onoda City University, Sanyo-Onoda, Yamaguchi 756-0884, Japan

[3] Waseda Research Institute for Science and Engineering, Waseda University, Shinjuku, Tokyo 162-8480, Japan

[4] Graduate Institute of Medicine, College of Medicine, Kaohsiung Medical University, Kaohsiung 80708, Taiwan

* Correspondence: oka@bio.keio.ac.jp

Abstract: Magnesium plays important roles in the nervous system. An increase in the Mg^{2+} concentration in cerebrospinal fluid enhances neural functions, while Mg^{2+} deficiency is implicated in neuronal diseases in the central nervous system. We have previously demonstrated that high concentrations of glutamate induce excitotoxicity and elicit a transient increase in the intracellular concentration of Mg^{2+} due to the release of Mg^{2+} from mitochondria, followed by a decrease to below steady-state levels. Since Mg^{2+} deficiency is involved in neuronal diseases, this decrease presumably affects neuronal survival under excitotoxic conditions. However, the mechanism of the Mg^{2+} decrease and its effect on the excitotoxicity process have not been elucidated. In this study, we demonstrated that inhibitors of Mg^{2+} extrusion, quinidine and amiloride, attenuated glutamate excitotoxicity in cultured rat hippocampal neurons. A toxic concentration of glutamate induced both Mg^{2+} release from mitochondria and Mg^{2+} extrusion from cytosol, and both quinidine and amiloride suppressed only the extrusion. This resulted in the maintenance of a higher Mg^{2+} concentration in the cytosol than under steady-state conditions during the ten-minute exposure to glutamate. These inhibitors also attenuated the glutamate-induced depression of cellular energy metabolism. Our data indicate the importance of Mg^{2+} regulation in neuronal survival under excitotoxicity.

Keywords: magnesium; excitotoxicity; fluorescence imaging; neuroprotection

1. Introduction

Magnesium plays important roles in the nervous system [1,2]. Elevation of the Mg^{2+} concentration in cerebrospinal fluid (CSF) increases synapse formation, enhances recognition and learning abilities in rats [3], and causes neural stem cell proliferation in mice [4]. Further, a deficiency of Mg^{2+} in the brain is implicated in neuronal diseases, and some researchers have reported lower Mg^{2+} concentrations than normal in the brain of patients with neurodegenerative diseases [5,6]. In rats, significant loss of dopaminergic neurons in the substantia nigra, similar to the loss seen in Parkinson's disease, was elicited merely by feeding them a low-magnesium diet for two generations [7]. In contrast, Mg^{2+} supplementation or overexpression of the Mg^{2+} channel have neuro-protective effects on cellular and animal models of Parkinson's [8–10] and Alzheimer's diseases [11]. These evidences show that Mg^{2+} is intricately involved in nervous system functioning and neuroprotection.

At the cellular level, Mg^{2+} is essential for maintaining enzymatic activities and energy metabolism, and its intracellular concentration is regulated by a number of ion channels and transporters on cell and organelle membranes [12–16]. Recent researches have revealed that Mg^{2+} also has more active roles in regulating intracellular signal transduction [17], cellular metabolism [18,19], and cell division [20]. These studies indicate that the concentration changes of Mg^{2+} is in a small range from 0.5 mM to 1.2 mM but essential for cellular functions. In neurons, the most widely known role of Mg^{2+} is the extracellular blockade and regulation of N-methyl-D-aspartate (NMDA) receptors, which occurs under physiologically normal extracellular concentrations [21,22]. In addition, intracellular Mg^{2+} is thought to play an indispensable role in neuronal functions [1]. Previously, we demonstrated that some neurotransmitters, as well as neuronal excitation itself, elicit changes in the intracellular Mg^{2+} concentration ($[Mg^{2+}]_i$) in cultured neurons [23–26]. In particular, glutamate induced interesting changes in $[Mg^{2+}]_i$. Although it is the most abundant neurotransmitter in the mammalian brain, excessive accumulation of glutamate around neurons induces neuronal cell death in a phenomenon known as excitotoxicity [27]. Toxic concentration of extracellular glutamate induced the release of Mg^{2+} from mitochondria, which is triggered by excessive Ca^{2+} accumulation in the mitochondria, leading to the increase in $[Mg^{2+}]_i$ [26]. Subsequently, the $[Mg^{2+}]_i$ turns to decrease. Given that Mg^{2+} deficiency is involved in neuronal diseases, the decreasing $[Mg^{2+}]_i$ phase likely has detrimental effects on neuronal survival, and thus plays a key role in excitotoxicity. However, the mechanism causing the decreasing $[Mg^{2+}]_i$ phase and its effect on excitotoxicity has not yet been elucidated.

In this study, we examined whether changes in $[Mg^{2+}]_i$ are involved in neuronal cell death via excitotoxicity in rat hippocampal neurons. We investigated the mechanisms involved in the phase in which the transient $[Mg^{2+}]_i$ increase in response to glutamate is reversed, and the effects of $[Mg^{2+}]_i$ on cellular energy metabolism. Quinidine and amiloride were used to inhibit cellular Mg^{2+} extrusion. Because those inhibitors are not specific for Mg^{2+} transport, it is important to confirm that both inhibitors show similar effects and that the effects were mediated via the changes in $[Mg^{2+}]_i$. Glutamate excitotoxicity results from continuous activation of the NMDA receptors on neurons, which leads to excessive Ca^{2+} influx into the cytosol and overload in the mitochondria, resulting in depolarization of the mitochondrial membrane potential and the release of cell death signals [27,28]. Mitochondria begin to release apoptosis signals within 10–20 min in response to toxic concentrations of glutamate [27]. Therefore, the Mg^{2+} transient elicited during the first 10 min of exposure to the glutamate stimulus may affect intracellular signals prior to the release of cell death signals under excitotoxicity. We investigated the hypothesis that the intracellular Mg^{2+} homeostasis and the intracellular Mg^{2+} regulatory system are key to cell protection in neuronal pathology.

2. Materials and Methods

2.1. Ethical Approval

All animal procedures were approved by the ethics committee of Keio University (permit number 09106-(7)). All methods were carried out in accordance with the relevant guidelines and regulations.

2.2. Dissociation Culture of Rat Hippocampal Neurons

The primary cultures of hippocampal neurons were prepared from day 18 embryonic Wistar rats (Charles River Laboratories Japan, Tokyo, Japan). Extracted hippocampi were dissociated using a dissociation kit (Sumitomo Bakelite, Tokyo, Japan). Isolated hippocampal neurons were plated on glass bottom dishes (Iwaki, Tokyo, Japan) coated with poly-D-lysine (PDL; Sigma-Aldrich, St. Louis, MO, USA) for fluorescence imaging or in 96-well plates for MTT assay, and cultured in neurobasal medium (Thermo Fisher Scientific, Waltham, MA, USA) supplemented with B-27 (Thermo Fisher Scientific, Waltham, MA, USA), 2 mM L-glutamine, 50 U/mL penicillin, and 50 µg/mL streptomycin (Nacalai Tesque, Kyoto, Japan). The neurons were cultured at 37 °C in a humidified atmosphere of 5% CO_2 for 7–9 days. Neuronal culture and synaptic formation among neurons were confirmed by immunofluorescence imaging of a neuron marker, βIII-tubulin (Sigma-Aldrich, St. Louis, MO, USA), and a synapse marker, synapsin I (Abcam, Cambridge, UK) (Figure S1).

2.3. MTT Assay

The MTT assay was conducted to measure cell viability. Neurons at the concentration of 8×10^3 cells/well were cultured on 96-well plates for 7 days. Neurons cultured in 96-well plates were incubated in culture medium with or without an inhibitor of Mg^{2+} extrusion (quinidine at 200 μM or amiloride at 500 μM; Sigma-Aldrich) and/or an inhibitor of mechanistic target of rapamycin (mTOR) (Torin1 at 2.5 μM; Chem Scene, Monmouth Junction, NJ, USA) for 10 min. Next, 100 μM glutamate with 10 μM glycine or control culture medium was applied and cells were incubated for 10 min. The culture medium containing inhibitor and/or glutamate was then replaced with normal culture medium, and the neurons were incubated for 24 h. The neurons were then incubated in culture medium containing 0.5 mg/mL MTT (Nacalai Tesuque). The culture medium was removed and 100 μL of dimethyl sulfoxide (DMSO; Nacalai Tesuque) was added to each well to dissolve the precipitate, and absorbance at 570 nm was measured using a microplate reader, Fluoroskan Ascent FL (Thermo Fisher Scientific). Cell viability in the treatment cultures is expressed as a proportion of cell viability in the control cultures.

2.4. Simultaneous Fluorescence Imaging of Intracellular Mg^{2+} and Ca^{2+}

Changes in $[Mg^{2+}]_i$ and intracellular Ca^{2+} concentration ($[Ca^{2+}]_i$) were measured by simultaneous imaging using the probes KMG-104-AM [29] and Fura-Red-AM (Thermo Fisher Scientific), respectively. KMG-104 is sufficiently selective to measure the Mg^{2+} signal without interference from the Ca^{2+} signal [29,30]. Neurons cultured on glass-bottom dishes were washed with Hanks' balanced salt solution (HBSS; NaCl 137 mM, KCl 5.4 mM, $CaCl_2$ 1.3 mM, $MgCl_2$ 0.5 mM, $MgSO_4$ 0.4 mM, Na_2HPO_4 0.3 mM, KH_2PO_4 0.4 mM, $NaHCO_3$ 4.2 mM, D-glucose 5.6 mM, HEPES 10 mM, pH adjusted to 7.4 with NaOH) and incubated in HBSS containing 5 μM KMG-104-AM, 10 μM Fura-Red-AM and 0.02% pluronic F-127 (Thermo Fisher Scientific) at 37 °C for 30 min. The neurons were then washed twice and incubated in HBSS, in HBSS without $CaCl_2$ (nominally Ca^{2+}-free HBSS) for measurements under Ca^{2+}-free conditions, for 15 min at 37 °C to allow for complete hydrolysis of the acetoxymethyl (AM) ester.

Fluorescence measurements were performed using fluorescence microscope, ECLIPSE TE300 (Nikon, Tokyo, Japan) equipped with 10× and 20× objective lenses, S Fluor (Nikon). Excitation light with a wavelength of approximately 488 nm was selected from a 150W Xe lamp using a monochrometer unit (Hamamatsu photonics, Shizuoka, Japan). The fluorescence signals that passed through a 510 nm dichroic mirror were separated using a 590 nm dichroic mirror and detected with a CCD camera, HiSCA (Hamamatsu photonics) using a 535/55 nm band pass filter for KMG-104 and a 600 nm long-pass filter for Fura-Red, respectively. Time-lapse images were acquired every 5 sec. Fluorescence intensity (F) was calculated as the mean intensity in a region of interest (ROI) containing the entire cell body by using Aquacosmos software (Hamamatsu photonics). The values of F recorded during time-lapse imaging were normalized by the initial fluorescence intensity (F_0) of each cell. The KMG-104 data were presented and analyzed as F/F_0. Since a decrease in the fluorescence intensity of Fura-Red indicates an increase in $[Ca^{2+}]$, the Fura-Red data were presented and analyzed as F_0/F.

2.5. Fluorescence Imaging of Mitochondrial Membrane Potential

Mitochondrial membrane potential was measured using tetramethylrhodamine ethyl ester (TMRE; Thermo Fisher Scientific). The neurons were washed with HBSS and then incubated for 20 min in HBSS containing 25 nM TMRE. Next, the dye was diluted to 2.5 nM in HBSS, and the neurons were incubated for an additional 10 min to equilibrate the dye. For measurements under high Mg^{2+} conditions, cells were stained and further incubated in HBSS with 8 mM Mg^{2+}.

Fluorescence of the TMRE was measured using the fluorescence microscope, ECLIPSE TE300. Excitation light with a wavelength of approximately 560 nm was selected from a 150W Xe lamp using the monochrometer unit. The fluorescence signals that passed through a 580 nm dichroic mirror and a

600 nm long-pass filter were detected with the CCD camera. F was calculated as the mean fluorescence intensity in a ROI containing the entire cell body. The values of F recorded during time-lapse imaging were normalized by the F_0 of each cell, and the data were presented and analyzed as F/F_0.

2.6. Fluorescence Imaging of Intracellular ATP

To compare intracellular ATP concentrations, genetically encoded ATP sensor, ATeam [31], was induced in neurons using an adeno-associated virus (AAV) vector. 30 µL of the AAV vector were added to every dish and neurons were incubated for 3–7 days to ensure sufficient expression of the sensor protein. After washing the cells twice with HBSS, or with HBSS with 8 mM Mg^{2+} for measurements under high Mg^{2+} conditions, the fluorescence was measured.

Fluorescence imaging of the neurons was performed using a confocal laser scanning microscope system, FV-1000 (Olympus, Tokyo, Japan) with a 40× oil-immersion objective lens. ATeam was excited at 440 nm from a diode laser. The fluorescence signals were separated using a 510 nm dichroic mirror and observed at 460–500 nm for cyan fluorescent protein (CFP) and 515–615 nm for yellow fluorescent protein (YFP). Fluorescence intensity was calculated as the mean intensity in a ROI containing the entire cell body. The intracellular ATP levels are represented by the YFP to CFP fluorescence ratio (ATeam ratio).

2.7. Statistical Analysis

For multiple testing, analysis of variance (ANOVA) was performed, and then Dunnett's test was used to compare the control group with the other groups or Tukey's test was used to compare all possible combinations of groups, assuming parametric distribution. $p < 0.05$ was considered significantly different.

3. Results

3.1. Inhibitors of Mg^{2+} Extrusion Attenuated the Excitotoxicity

Previous studies have indicated that cells express several Mg^{2+} extrusion mechanisms, and quinidine, amiloride, and imipramine are used to inhibit these Mg^{2+} extrusion mechanism [32,33]. Because these inhibitors are not specific for Mg^{2+} transport, we checked whether both quinidine and amiloride have similar effect on neurons. First, we examined whether inhibitors of Mg^{2+} extrusion mechanisms had an effect on cell viability under excitotoxic conditions. A combination of 100 µM glutamate and 10 µM glycine was used as an excitotoxic glutamate stimulus. It has been demonstrated that even 10 min of exposure to toxic concentrations of glutamate induces, to some extent, neuronal cell death 24 h after the stimulation [27]. Here, we aimed to assess the impact of the glutamate stimulus for 10 min on cell viability 24 h after the stimulus and to evaluate the effects of inhibition of Mg^{2+} extrusion on it. We therefore replaced the culture medium for a fresh one not containing glutamate or inhibitors after ten-minute exposure to glutamate stimulus in the presence or absence of an inhibitor to assess the effects of the glutamate stimulus and the inhibition of Mg^{2+} extrusion only during the ten-minute glutamate stimulus. Then, the cell viability after 24 h was measured with MTT assay (Figure 1a). The ten-minute exposure to glutamate stimulus induced cell death in approximately 40% of the neurons after 24 h (controls with glutamate stimulus in Figure 1b,c). This experimental condition, which induces 40% cell death, was adopted in this study because it is easy to assess the effect of inhibitors on cell viability, whether to accelerate or suppress the toxicity. Both inhibitors partially attenuated this decrease in cell viability, while exposure to the inhibitors for 20 min without glutamate stimulus had no effect on viability (Figure 1b,c).

Figure 1. Inhibitors of Mg^{2+} extrusion attenuated excitotoxicity. (**a**) Experimental procedure of the MTT assay for measuring the effect of a ten-minute glutamate stimulus. Comparison of cell viability in the presence or absence of quinidine (200 μM) (**b**) or amiloride (500 μM) (**c**) ($n = 30$ for each). Error bars indicate SEM. * indicates $p < 0.05$ among all possible combinations by Tukey's test. N.S. indicates no statistically significant difference.

3.2. The Inhibitors Suppressed the Decreasing Phase of the Glutamate-Induced Mg^{2+} Transient

To confirm the effects of the inhibitors on cellular ion transports immediately after the application of glutamate stimulus, $[Mg^{2+}]_i$ and $[Ca^{2+}]_i$ were simultaneously visualized using KMG-104 and Fura-Red, respectively. The glutamate stimulus elicited a gradual increase in $[Mg^{2+}]_i$ and a steep increase in $[Ca^{2+}]_i$, after which $[Mg^{2+}]_i$ began to decrease. Within 10 min, $[Mg^{2+}]_i$ in the control was below the initial concentration (Figure 2a). Quinidine (200 μM) and amiloride (500 μM) partially suppressed both the $[Mg^{2+}]_i$ decrease and the $[Ca^{2+}]_i$ increase, but did not suppress the $[Mg^{2+}]_i$ increase (Figure 2a,b). Distributions of the increases in $[Mg^{2+}]_i$ and $[Ca^{2+}]_i$ were different (Figure 2b). In addition, no morphological changes such as cell body rounding or neurite fragmentation were observed, indicating that the neurons are still alive at 10 min. Quinidine enhanced the $[Mg^{2+}]_i$ increase (Figure 2c), and both quinidine and amiloride suppressed the Mg^{2+} decrease (Figure 2d). This indicates that glutamate stimulus simultaneously induced both Mg^{2+} mobilization and Mg^{2+} extrusion, which restricts amplitude of the increase in $[Mg^{2+}]_i$. As a result, neurons maintained a higher $[Mg^{2+}]_i$ level in the presence of the inhibitors than that in the control during the ten-minute exposure to glutamate stimulus. The inhibitors also partially attenuated the $[Ca^{2+}]_i$ peak observed within 1 min of the addition of the glutamate stimulus (Figure 2e). Following the initial peak, while the neurons in the control exhibited a further gradual increase in $[Ca^{2+}]_i$ to a level higher than the initial peak, in the presence of the inhibitors, $[Ca^{2+}]_i$ showed plateau after 4 min and did not exceed the initial peak level (Figure 2a middle panel,b,f). This was probably due to suppression of the Ca^{2+} influx via the voltage-gated Ca^{2+} channels (VGCC) by the higher $[Mg^{2+}]_i$ [34].

Figure 2. Inhibitors of Mg^{2+} extrusion suppressed the decreasing phase of the glutamate-induced Mg^{2+} transient. (**a**) Time-courses of $[Mg^{2+}]_i$ (upper) and $[Ca^{2+}]_i$ (middle) responses to the glutamate stimulus, and the correlation between them (bottom) in the presence or absence of inhibitor (blue: control, $n = 52$ cells; red: with quinidine at 200 μM, $n = 48$ cells; green: with amiloride at 500 μM, $n = 64$ cells; from 5 replicates each). Mg^{2+} and Ca^{2+} were simultaneously measured in the same neurons. Data are presented as the average (solid line) ± SEM (shaded area). The glutamate stimulus (100 μM glutamate with 10 μM glycine) was applied at 0 min (dotted line). The period 0–1 min is shaded orange. (**b**) Pseudo-colored images showing representative responses of Mg^{2+} and Ca^{2+} in each condition. Scale bars, 20 μm. Comparisons of amplitudes of increase in KMG-104 signal ($[Mg^{2+}]_i$) (**c**), decrease in KMG-104 signal ($[Mg^{2+}]_i$) (**d**), initial peak in Fura-red signal ($[Ca^{2+}]_i$) (**e**), and further changes in Fure-red signal ($[Ca^{2+}]_i$) after the initial peak (**f**) among the conditions extracted from the data shown in (**a**). Error bars indicate SEM. * indicates $p < 0.05$ compared with control by Dunnett's test. (**g**) Scatter plot of maximum values of $[Mg^{2+}]_i$ and $[Ca^{2+}]_i$ within the first minute (orange area in Figure 2a) and their regression lines (blue: control; red: with quinidine; green: with amiloride). p values were determined from the correlation coefficient and the number of plots.

Under all three conditions, the changes in $[Mg^{2+}]_i$ and $[Ca^{2+}]_i$ were well correlated with each other immediately after the application of glutamate stimulus, and the correlation coefficient decreased with time (Figure 2a bottom panel). To further analyze the relationship between the $[Ca^{2+}]_i$ increase and the increasing phase of $[Mg^{2+}]_i$, we examined the correlation of the $[Mg^{2+}]_i$ and $[Ca^{2+}]_i$ maxima observed within 1 min of glutamate stimulus (Figure 2g). These correlated well in control neurons, because the increase in $[Mg^{2+}]_i$ is triggered by the increase in $[Ca^{2+}]_i$ as previously shown [26]. In the presence of the inhibitors, these maxima were still correlated, and although their regression lines shifted upward, they were almost parallel with each other (Figure 2g). This indicates that the inhibitors attenuated the $[Ca^{2+}]_i$ response, without affecting the Mg^{2+} response, immediately after the stimulus.

3.3. Neurons Extruded Mg^{2+} in Response to the Glutamate Stimulus

Next, we investigated whether the Ca^{2+} signal is a prerequisite for the Mg^{2+} extrusion. To do this, glutamate-induced responses were observed in nominally Ca^{2+}-free conditions. Under this conditions, there was only a small $[Ca^{2+}]_i$ response, and the $[Mg^{2+}]_i$ increase was completely abolished. However the decrease in $[Mg^{2+}]_i$ remained (Figure 3a). Combined with Figure 2g, this suggests that the $[Mg^{2+}]_i$ increasing phase is Ca^{2+}-dependent event. Both quinidine and amiloride suppressed this Mg^{2+} decrease to a similar extent (Figure 3b). Quinidine abolished the small $[Ca^{2+}]_i$ increase evoked by the glutamate stimulus, and amiloride partially attenuated it (Figure 3c). This suggests that both inhibitors affect the glutamate-induced Ca^{2+} mobilization other than Ca^{2+} influx from extracellular medium. This might have some contribution to the attenuation of glutamate-induced Ca^{2+} response by these inhibitors shown in Figure 2. These results also indicate that the decrease in $[Mg^{2+}]_i$ does not require the preceding $[Mg^{2+}]_i$ and $[Ca^{2+}]_i$ increases. This means that the $[Mg^{2+}]_i$-decreasing phase is not a homeostatic cellular response attempting to maintain a normal $[Mg^{2+}]_i$, but rather a glutamate-induced activation of Mg^{2+} extrusion via channels and/or transporters, and that this occurs in response to a neuronal excitation or an intracellular signal other than Ca^{2+}. Taken together, these results indicate that glutamate stimulus induces both Ca^{2+}-dependent Mg^{2+} release from the mitochondria and Mg^{2+} extrusion from the cytosol, simultaneously.

Figure 3. The Mg^{2+} and Ca^{2+} increases were not required for Mg^{2+} extrusion. (**a**) Time-courses of $[Mg^{2+}]_i$ (upper) and $[Ca^{2+}]_i$ (bottom) response to glutamate stimulus in nominally Ca^{2+}-free conditions in the presence or absence of inhibitor (blue: control, $n = 60$ cells; red: with quinidine at 200 μM, $n = 52$ cells; green: with amiloride at 500 μM, $n = 54$ cells, from 5 replicates each). Data are presented as the average (solid line) $\pm$ SEM (shaded area). Comparison of decrease in KMG-104 signal ($[Mg^{2+}]_i$) (**b**) and increase in Fura-red signal ($[Ca^{2+}]_i$) (**c**) at 10 min after application of the glutamate stimulus extracted from the data shown in (**a**). Error bars indicate SEM. * indicates $p < 0.05$ compared with control by Dunnett's test.

3.4. Effect of the Inhibition of the Mg^{2+} Extrusion on Cellular Energy Metabolism

Next, we investigated whether inhibitors of Mg^{2+} extrusion had any effect on cellular energy metabolism. Since mitochondria play a central role in neuronal ATP synthesis, changes in mitochondrial membrane potential during glutamate stimulus were measured. In response to the glutamate stimulus, mitochondrial membrane potential decreased gradually (Figure 4a). It was still decreasing at 10 min, indicating the neurons still alive at this point. Quinidine partially attenuated this decrease, but amiloride had no effect on it (Figure 4b). Thus, although these inhibitors attenuated the glutamate-induced $[Ca^{2+}]_i$ increase to the same extent (Figure 2), amiloride did not suppress the depolarization of mitochondrial membrane potential. To further confirm the contribution of Mg^{2+} for maintenance of mitochondrial membrane potential, glutamate stimulus-induced changes in the mitochondrial membrane potential under high Mg^{2+} conditions were compared to those under normal conditions. High Mg^{2+} partially attenuated the decrease in mitochondrial membrane potential (Figure 4c,d), presumably by keeping $[Mg^{2+}]_i$ high. This supports the idea that Mg^{2+} has a protective effect on depolarization of mitochondrial membrane potential.

Figure 4. Changes in mitochondrial membrane potential in response to glutamate stimulus. (**a**) Time-courses of changes in mitochondrial membrane potential in response to the glutamate stimulus (blue: control, $n = 90$ cells; red: with quinidine at 200 μM, $n = 89$ cells; green: with amiloride at 500 μM, $n = 100$ cells, from 5 replicates each). Data are presented as the average (solid line) ± SEM (shaded area). (**b**) Comparison of decreases in mitochondrial membrane potential after 10 min extracted from the data shown in (**a**). Error bars indicate SEM. * indicates $p < 0.05$ compared with control by Dunnett's test. (**c**) Time-courses of changes in mitochondrial membrane potential in response to the glutamate stimulus (blue: control, $n = 75$ cells; yellow: under high Mg^{2+} (8 mM) condition, $n = 80$ cells, from 5 replicates each). Data are presented as the average (solid line) ± SEM (shaded area). (**d**) Comparison of decreases in mitochondrial membrane potential after 10 min extracted from the data shown in (**c**). Error bars indicate SEM. * indicates $p < 0.05$ by t-test.

We also investigated whether the inhibition of Mg^{2+} extrusion and the resulting high $[Mg^{2+}]_i$ lead to the maintenance of cellular ATP concentrations during the excitotoxicity process. Intracellular ATP concentrations were compared using a genetically encoded ATP sensor, ATeam [31]. The presence of quinidine or amiloride did not affect ATP levels in steady-state neurons, but both inhibitors partially attenuated the decrease in ATP levels evoked by the glutamate stimulus (Figure 5a). High Mg^{2+} also suppressed the glutamate-induced decrease in ATP level (Figure 5b). These results suggest that the high $[Mg^{2+}]_i$ resulting from the inhibition of Mg^{2+} extrusion contributes to the maintenance of intracellular ATP levels.

Figure 5. Inhibitors of Mg^{2+} extrusion attenuated the glutamate-induced decrease in intracellular ATP level. (**a**) Comparison of intracellular ATP levels (YFP/CFP ratio of ATeam) before and 10 min after application of the glutamate stimulus in the presence or absence of inhibitor (n = 10, 16, 18 cells from 6 replicates for each). Error bars indicate SEM. * indicates $p < 0.05$ among all possible combinations by Tukey's test. N.S. indicates no statistically significant difference. (**b**) Comparison of decrease in ATeam ratio induced by glutamate stimulus in 10 min under control and high Mg^{2+} (8 mM) conditions (control: n = 32 cells from 9 replicates; High Mg^{2+}: n = 34 cells from 11 replicates). Error bars indicate SEM. * indicates $p < 0.05$ by t-test.

3.5. Involvement of mTOR in the Attenuation of Excitotoxicity by Mg^{2+}

In the previous study, we demonstrated that increase in $[Mg^{2+}]_i$ activates mTOR in cultured hippocampal neurons [23]. mTOR is an important signal implicated in the regulation of energy metabolism, cell growth and cell death [35,36]. We therefore examined the effect of mTOR inhibitor, Torin1, on the glutamate-induced neuronal cells death and its attenuation by the inhibitors of Mg^{2+} extrusion, according to the procedure shown in Figure 1a. While torin1 did not enhance the toxicity of glutamate stimulus, it abolished the attenuation of the toxicity by quinidine or amiloride (Figure 6). This suggests that the mTOR signal is involved in the attenuation of excitotoxicity by increasing $[Mg^{2+}]_i$.

Figure 6. Inhibitor of mTOR abolished the attenuation of excitotoxicity by inhibiting Mg^{2+} extrusion. Comparison of cell viability 24 h after ten-minute glutamate stimulus with or without inhibitor of mTOR (Torin1: 2.5 μM) and/or inhibitors of Mg^{2+} extrusion (Quinidine: 200 μM, Amiloride: 500 μM) (n = 12, 9, 12, 12, 12, 12 for each). Error bars indicate SEM. * indicates $p < 0.05$ among all possible combinations by Tukey's test. N.S. indicates no statistically significant difference.

4. Discussion

In this study, we demonstrated that inhibitors of Mg^{2+} extrusion attenuate glutamate excitotoxicity in cultured rat hippocampal neurons (Figure 1). A toxic concentration of glutamate induced Mg^{2+} extrusion from neurons, which was suppressed by both quinidine and amiloride (Figures 2 and 3). These inhibitors also attenuated the glutamate-induced depression of cellular energy metabolism (Figure 5). The protective effect of those inhibitors against excitotoxicity was abolished by inhibition of mTOR (Figure 6). While quinidine and amiloride partially attenuated the glutamate-evoked $[Ca^{2+}]_i$ response (Figure 2e,f), in particular, mobilization of Ca^{2+} from other than extracellular medium (Figure 3), they did not suppress the increasing phase of the $[Mg^{2+}]_i$ transient (Figure 2c), in spite of its Ca^{2+}-dependency (Figures 2g and 3). Amiloride also had no effect on the glutamate-induced mitochondrial depolarization (Figure 4), despite attenuating the cytosolic Ca^{2+} increase (Figure 2e,f). Given that the depolarization of mitochondrial membrane potential is a critical event in the process of excitotoxicity [27], the partial attenuation of the $[Ca^{2+}]_i$ increase by the amiloride does not affect glutamate excitotoxicity. Therefore, the neuroprotective effect of the inhibitors is probably due to the maintenance of high $[Mg^{2+}]_i$ during the glutamate stimulus. This idea is also supported by the results that glutamate-induced decrease in mitochondrial membrane potential and cytosolic ATP level were partially attenuated under high Mg^{2+} conditions (Figure 4c,d and Figure 5b), presumably by keeping $[Mg^{2+}]_i$ high. Our data therefore indicate the importance of Mg^{2+} regulation in neuronal cell death and survival.

One of the key roles of Mg^{2+} in ensuring cell survival involves the regulation of mitochondrial functions [37]. It affects enzymatic activities in the tricarboxylic acid (TCA) cycle in mitochondria; thus, a decrease in mitochondrial Mg^{2+} concentration results in a downregulation of mitochondrial membrane potential and ATP synthesis [38–40]. On the other hand, extra-mitochondrial Mg^{2+} suppresses mitochondrial Ca^{2+} uptake [41] which depolarizes mitochondrial membrane potential. Either or both of these processes might contribute to the attenuation of mitochondrial membrane potential depolarization by quinidine (Figure 4) and the suppression of the decrease in ATP levels caused by quinidine and amiloride (Figure 5). The idea that elevated $[Mg^{2+}]_i$ contributes to the maintenance of cellular ATP levels was also supported by our previous work [42]. Although amiloride did not inhibit the depolarization of mitochondrial membrane potential (Figure 4), it did suppress the decrease in ATP levels and cell death (Figures 1 and 5). This suggests that Mg^{2+} affects not only mitochondrial functions but also other mechanisms that are involved in maintaining the cellular ATP concentration and cell viability.

One of the ways in which Mg^{2+} might do this is by regulating intracellular signal transductions [17]. In particular, mTOR is considered an important downstream target of Mg^{2+} [18,19,43]. The mTOR pathway is implicated in the regulation of cellular metabolism and proliferation [36]. In pancreatic cancer cells, overexpression of SLC41A1, a membrane protein for Mg^{2+} extrusion [32], and the resulting low $[Mg^{2+}]_i$, inhibited the Akt/mTOR pathway and cancer proliferation [44]. In cultured hippocampal neurons, $[Mg^{2+}]_i$ within the physiological concentration range is correlated with mTOR activity [23]. These findings strongly suggest that Mg^{2+} is a key regulator of mTOR and mTOR-related signal transductions. Inhibition of the Akt/mTOR pathway in cultured neurons in response to toxic concentrations of glutamate has been reported [45]. This inhibition might result from the glutamate-induced decrease in $[Mg^{2+}]_i$ demonstrated in this study (Figures 2 and 3). The fact that the Akt/mTOR signal is also involved in regulation of both cellular ATP synthesis and also apoptotic signals [35,46,47] would explain why maintaining a high $[Mg^{2+}]_i$ prevent neuronal cell death. In this study, we showed that inhibition of mTOR abolished the attenuation of glutamate excitotoxicity by inhibiting Mg^{2+} extrusion (Figure 6). This suggests that maintaining high $[Mg^{2+}]_i$ protect neurons against excitotoxicity via the mTOR signal.

As discussed above and summarized in Figure 7, Mg^{2+} is a key factor in saving neurons from neurodegenerative diseases. Since inhibition of cellular Mg^{2+} extrusion and resulting maintenance of high $[Mg^{2+}]_i$ protect cells from neurodegenerative disorders, the Mg^{2+} extrusion mechanisms might be a therapeutic target for neuronal diseases. Among Mg^{2+} channels and transporters, SLC41A1 is considered to be the major transporter for cellular Mg^{2+} extrusion [32,48], while it was also suggested that cells has several different mechanisms for extruding cytosolic Mg^{2+} [49]. Preventing cellular Mg^{2+} loss by inhibiting such transporters might delay the progression of neurodegeneration. Because Mg^{2+} is a broad-spectrum regulator of cellular metabolisms and signaling, change in $[Mg^{2+}]_i$ affects multiple aspects of the process of excitotoxicity, even though it is not a main signal for inducing neuronal cell death (Figure 7). In present study, we have demonstrated that keeping Mg^{2+} inside cells is important for neuronal survival under conditions of cellular stress. It may protect neurons from neurodegeneration also in vivo because it has been reported that gain-of-function mutation in SLC41A1, that leads to enhanced Mg^{2+} release from cytosol, and mutation in a Mg^{2+} and Ca^{2+} permeable channel, TRPM7, that attenuates cellular Mg^{2+} uptake, are associated with the pathogenesis of neurodegenerative diseases in human brain [50,51]. To support this, further studies on Mg^{2+} dynamics in vivo are needed. Our results demonstrated in this study suggest the potential of cellular Mg^{2+} homeostasis and the Mg^{2+} transport system for therapy and the prevention of neurodegenerative diseases.

Figure 7. Schematic of roles of Mg^{2+} in excitotoxicity. The transport and effects of Mg^{2+} and mTOR demonstrated in this study are shown in red. In this study, we demonstrated that glutamate stimulus induces not only Mg^{2+} released from mitochondria but also Mg^{2+} extrusion from the cytosol, and quinidine and amiloride inhibit it. Maintaining Mg^{2+} in neurons suppressed glutamate-induced decrease in cellular ATP level and also attenuated neuronal cell death via mTOR signaling pathway. Dotted lines indicate pathways that are still obscure whether they are direct or indirect effects. The effects of Mg^{2+} demonstrated previous studies are shown in blue, and the main excitotoxic signals are shown in green.

Author Contributions: Data curation, Y.S.; Formal analysis, Y.S. and R.Y.; Funding acquisition, K.O.; Project administration, K.O.; Supervision, K.O.; Writing—original draft, Y.S.; Writing—review & editing, R.Y., K.H. and K.O. All authors have read and agreed to the published version of the manuscript.

Acknowledgments: We thank H. Imamura and H. Noji for providing the ATeam plasmid.

References

1. Yamanaka, R.; Shindo, Y.; Oka, K. Magnesium Is a Key Player in Neuronal Maturation and Neuropathology. *Int. J. Mol. Sci.* **2019**, *20*, 3439. [CrossRef]

2. Kirkland, A.; Sarlo, G.; Holton, K. The Role of Magnesium in Neurological Disorders. *Nutrients* **2018**, *10*, 730. [CrossRef]

3. Slutsky, I.; Abumaria, N.; Wu, L.J.; Huang, C.; Zhang, L.; Li, B.; Zhao, X.; Govindarajan, A.; Zhao, M.G.; Zhuo, M.; et al. Enhancement of Learning and Memory by Elevating Brain Magnesium. *Neuron* **2010**, *65*, 165–177. [CrossRef] [PubMed]

4. Jia, S.; Liu, Y.; Shi, Y.; Ma, Y.; Hu, Y.; Wang, M.; Li, X. Elevation of Brain Magnesium Potentiates Neural Stem Cell Proliferation in the Hippocampus of Young and Aged Mice. *J. Cell. Physiol.* **2016**, *231*, 1903–1912. [CrossRef] [PubMed]

5.   Andrási, E.; Páli, N.; Molnár, Z.; Kösel, S. Brain aluminum, magnesium and phosphorus contents of control and Alzheimer-diseased patients. *J. Alzheimer's Dis.* **2005**, *7*, 273–284.

6.   Yasui, M.; Kihira, T.; Ota, K. Calcium, magnesium and aluminum concentrations in Parkinson's disease. *Neurotoxicology* **1992**, *13*, 593–600. [PubMed]

7.   Oyanagi, K.; Kawakami, E.; Kikuchi-Horie, K.; Ohara, K.; Ogata, K.; Takahama, S.; Wada, M.; Kihira, T.; Yasui, M. Magnesium deficiency over generations in rats with special references to the pathogenesis of the parkinsonism-dementia complex and amyotrophic lateral sclerosis of Guam. *Neuropathology* **2006**, *26*, 115–128. [CrossRef]

8.   Hashimoto, T.; Nishi, K.; Nagasao, J.; Tsuji, S.; Oyanagi, K. Magnesium exerts both preventive and ameliorating effects in an in vitro rat Parkinson disease model involving 1-methyl-4-phenylpyridinium (MPP$^+$) toxicity in dopaminergic neurons. *Brain Res.* **2008**, *1197*, 143–151. [CrossRef]

9.   Shen, Y.; Dai, L.; Tian, H.; Xu, R.; Li, F.; Li, Z.; Zhou, J.; Wang, L.; Dong, J.; Sun, L. Treatment of Magnesium-L-Threonate Elevates the Magnesium Level in the Cerebrospinal Fluid and Attenuates Motor Deficits and Dopamine Neuron Loss in a Mouse Model of Parkinson's disease. *Neuropsychiatr. Dis. Treat.* **2019**, *15*, 3143–3153. [CrossRef]

10. Shindo, Y.; Yamanaka, R.; Suzuki, K.; Hotta, K.; Oka, K. Altered expression of Mg^{2+} transport proteins during Parkinson's disease-like dopaminergic cell degeneration in PC12 cells. *Biochim. Biophys. Acta Mol. Cell Res.* **2016**, *1863*, 1979–1984. [CrossRef]

11. Li, W.; Yu, J.; Liu, Y.; Huang, X.; Abumaria, N.; Zhu, Y.; Huang, X.; Xiong, W.; Ren, C.; Liu, X.G.; et al. Elevation of brain magnesium prevents synaptic loss and reverses cognitive deficits in Alzheimer's disease mouse model. *Mol. Brain* **2014**, *7*, 1–20. [CrossRef] [PubMed]

12. Romani, A.M.P. Cellular magnesium homeostasis. *Arch. Biochem. Biophys.* **2011**, *512*, 1–23. [CrossRef] [PubMed]

13. de Baaij, J.H.F.; Hoenderop, J.G.J.; Bindels, R.J.M. Magnesium in Man: Implications for Health and Disease. *Physiol. Rev.* **2015**, *95*, 1–46. [CrossRef] [PubMed]

14. Kubota, T.; Shindo, Y.; Tokuno, K.; Komatsu, H.; Ogawa, H.; Kudo, S.; Kitamura, Y.; Suzuki, K.; Oka, K. Mitochondria are intracellular magnesium stores: Investigation by simultaneous fluorescent imagings in PC12 cells. *Biochim. Biophys. Acta Mol. Cell Res.* **2005**, *1744*, 19–28. [CrossRef]

15. Quamme, G.A. Molecular identification of ancient and modern mammalian magnesium transporters. *Am. J. Physiol. Physiol.* **2010**, *298*, C407–C429. [CrossRef]

16. Nadler, M.J.S.; Hermosura, M.C.; Inabe, K.; Perraud, A.-L.; Zhu, Q.; Stokes, A.J.; Kurosaki, T.; Kinet, J.-P.; Penner, R.; Scharenberg, A.M.; et al. LTRPC7 is a Mg·ATP-regulated divalent cation channel required for cell viability. *Nature* **2001**, *411*, 590–595. [CrossRef]

17. Li, F.Y.; Chaigne-Delalande, B.; Kanellopoulou, C.; Davis, J.C.; Matthews, H.F.; Douek, D.C.; Cohen, J.I.; Uzel, G.; Su, H.C.; Lenardo, M.J. Second messenger role for Mg^{2+} revealed by human T-cell immunodeficiency. *Nature* **2011**, *475*, 471–476. [CrossRef]

18. Feeney, K.A.; Hansen, L.L.; Putker, M.; Olivares-Yañez, C.; Day, J.; Eades, L.J.; Larrondo, L.F.; Hoyle, N.P.; O'Neill, J.S.; van Ooijen, G. Daily magnesium fluxes regulate cellular timekeeping and energy balance. *Nature* **2016**, *532*, 375–379. [CrossRef]

19. Rubin, H. The logic of the Membrane, Magnesium, Mitosis (MMM) model for the regulation of animal cell proliferation. *Arch. Biochem. Biophys.* **2007**, *458*, 16–23. [CrossRef]

20. Maeshima, K.; Matsuda, T.; Shindo, Y.; Imamura, H.; Tamura, S.; Imai, R.; Kawakami, S.; Nagashima, R.; Soga, T.; Noji, H.; et al. A Transient Rise in Free Mg^{2+} Ions Released from ATP-Mg Hydrolysis Contributes to Mitotic Chromosome Condensation. *Curr. Biol.* **2018**, *28*, 444–451.e6. [CrossRef]

21. Slutsky, I.; Sadeghpour, S.; Li, B.; Liu, G. Enhancement of Synaptic Plasticity through Chronically Reduced Ca^{2+} Flux during Uncorrelated Activity. *Neuron* **2004**, *44*, 835–849. [CrossRef]

22. Nowak, L.; Bregestovski, P.; Ascher, P.; Herbet, A.; Prochiantz, A. Magnesium gates glutamate-activated channels in mouse central neurones. *Nature* **1984**, *307*, 462–465. [CrossRef] [PubMed]

23. Yamanaka, R.; Shindo, Y.; Hotta, K.; Suzuki, K.; Oka, K. GABA-Induced Intracellular Mg^{2+} Mobilization Integrates and Coordinates Cellular Information Processing for the Maturation of Neural Networks. *Curr. Biol.* **2018** *28*, 3984–3991.e5. [CrossRef] [PubMed]

24. Yamanaka, R.; Shindo, Y.; Hotta, K.; Suzuki, K.; Oka, K. NO/cGMP/PKG signaling pathway induces magnesium release mediated by mitoK ATP channel opening in rat hippocampal neurons. *FEBS Lett.* **2013**,

    587, 2643–2648. [CrossRef] [PubMed]

25. Yamanaka, R.; Shindo, Y.; Karube, T.; Hotta, K.; Suzuki, K.; Oka, K. Neural depolarization triggers Mg^{2+} influx in rat hippocampal neurons. *Neuroscience* **2015**, *310*, 731–741. [CrossRef] [PubMed]

26. Shindo, Y.; Fujimoto, A.; Hotta, K.; Suzuki, K.; Oka, K. Glutamate-induced calcium increase mediates magnesium release from mitochondria in rat hippocampal neurons. *J. Neurosci. Res.* **2010**, *88*, 3125–3132. [CrossRef]

27. Abramov, A.Y.; Duchen, M.R. Mechanisms underlying the loss of mitochondrial membrane potential in glutamate excitotoxicity. *Biochim. Biophys. Acta Bioenerg.* **2008**, *1777*, 953–964. [CrossRef]

28. Rueda, C.B.; Llorente-Folch, I.; Traba, J.; Amigo, I.; Gonzalez-Sanchez, P.; Contreras, L.; Juaristi, I.; Martinez-Valero, P.; Pardo, B.; del Arco, A.; et al. Glutamate excitotoxicity and Ca^{2+}-regulation of respiration: Role of the Ca^{2+} activated mitochondrial transporters (CaMCs). *Biochim. Biophys. Acta Bioenerg.* **2016**, *1857*, 1158–1166. [CrossRef]

29. Komatsu, H.; Iwasawa, N.; Citterio, D.; Suzuki, Y.; Kubota, T.; Tokuno, K.; Kitamura, Y.; Oka, K.; Suzuki, K. Design and Synthesis of Highly Sensitive and Selective Fluorescein-Derived Magnesium Fluorescent Probes and Application to Intracellular 3D Mg^{2+} Imaging. *J. Am. Chem. Soc.* **2004**, *126*, 16353–16360. [CrossRef]

30. Trapani, V.; Farruggia, G.; Marraccini, C.; Iotti, S.; Cittadini, A.; Wolf, F.I. Intracellular magnesium detection: Imaging a brighter future. *Analyst* **2010**, *135*, 1855–1866. [CrossRef]

31. Imamura, H.; Huynh Nhat, K.P.; Togawa, H.; Saito, K.; Iino, R.; Kato-Yamada, Y.; Nagai, T.; Noji, H. Visualization of ATP levels inside single living cells with fluorescence resonance energy transfer-based genetically encoded indicators. *Proc. Natl. Acad. Sci. USA* **2009**, *106*, 15651–15656. [CrossRef] [PubMed]

32. Kolisek, M.; Nestler, A.; Vormann, J.; Schweigel-Röntgen, M. Human gene SLC41A1 encodes for the Na^+/Mg^{2+} exchanger. *Am. J. Physiol. Physiol.* **2012**, *302*, C318–C326. [CrossRef] [PubMed]

33. Cefaratti, C.; Romani, A.; Scarpa, A. Characterization of two Mg^{2+} transporters in sealed plasma membrane vesicles from rat liver. *Am. J. Physiol. Physiol.* **1998**, *275*, C995–C1008. [CrossRef] [PubMed]

34. Brunet, S.; Scheuer, T.; Catterall, W.A. Cooperative regulation of Cav12 channels by intracellular Mg^{2+}, the proximal C-terminal EF-hand, and the distal C-terminal domain. *J. Gen. Physiol.* **2009**, *134*, 81–94. [CrossRef]

35. Zheng, X.; Boyer, L.; Jin, M.; Kim, Y.; Fan, W.; Bardy, C.; Berggren, T.; Evans, R.M.; Gage, F.H.; Hunter, T. Alleviation of neuronal energy deficiency by mTOR inhibition as a treatment for mitochondria-related neurodegeneration. *eLife* **2016**, *5*, 1–23. [CrossRef]

36. Saxton, R.A.; Sabatini, D.M. mTOR Signaling in Growth, Metabolism, and Disease. *Cell* **2017**, *168*, 960–976. [CrossRef]

37. Pilchova, I.; Klacanova, K.; Tatarkova, Z.; Kaplan, P.; Racay, P. The Involvement of Mg^{2+} in Regulation of Cellular and Mitochondrial Functions. *Oxid. Med. Cell. Longev.* **2017**, *2017*, 6797460. [CrossRef]

38. Yamanaka, R.; Tabata, S.; Shindo, Y.; Hotta, K.; Suzuki, K.; Soga, T.; Oka, K. Mitochondrial Mg^{2+} homeostasis decides cellular energy metabolism and vulnerability to stress. *Sci. Rep.* **2016**, *6*, 30027. [CrossRef]

39. Panov, A.; Scarpa, A. Mg^{2+} Control of Respiration in Isolated Rat Liver Mitochondria. *Biochemistry* **1996**, *35*, 12849–12856. [CrossRef]

40. Rodríguez-Zavala, J.S.; Moreno-Sánchez, R. Modulation of Oxidative Phosphorylation by Mg^{2+} in Rat Heart Mitochondria. *J. Biol. Chem.* **1998**, *273*, 7850–7855. [CrossRef]

41. Boelens, A.D.; Pradhan, R.K.; Blomeyer, C.A.; Camara, A.K.S.; Dash, R.K.; Stowe, D.F. Extra-matrix Mg^{2+} limits Ca^{2+} uptake and modulates Ca^{2+} uptake–independent respiration and redox state in cardiac isolated mitochondria. *J. Bioenerg. Biomembr.* **2013**, *45*, 203–218. [CrossRef] [PubMed]

42. Shindo, Y.; Yamanaka, R.; Suzuki, K.; Hotta, K.; Oka, K. Intracellular magnesium level determines cell viability in the MPP^+ model of Parkinson's disease. *Biochim. Biophys. Acta Mol. Cell Res.* **2015**, *1853*, 3182–3191. [CrossRef] [PubMed]

43. Trapani, V.; Wolf, F.I. Dysregulation of Mg^{2+} homeostasis contributes to acquisition of cancer hallmarks. *Cell Calcium* **2019**, *83*, 102078. [CrossRef] [PubMed]

44. Xie, J.; Cheng, C.; Zhu, X.Y.; Shen, Y.H.; Song, L.B.; Chen, H.; Chen, Z.; Liu, L.M.; Meng, Z.Q. Magnesium transporter protein solute carrier family 41 member 1 suppresses human pancreatic ductal adenocarcinoma through magnesium-dependent Akt/mTOR inhibition and bax-associated mitochondrial apoptosis. *Aging (Albany NY)* **2019**, *11*, 2681–2698. [CrossRef]

45. Pomytkin, I.; Krasil'nikova, I.; Bakaeva, Z.; Surin, A.; Pinelis, V. Excitotoxic glutamate causes neuronal insulin resistance by inhibiting insulin receptor/Akt/mTOR pathway. *Mol. Brain* **2019**, *12*, 112. [CrossRef]

46. Sponder, G.; Abdulhanan, N.; Fröhlich, N.; Mastrototaro, L.; Aschenbach, J.R.; Röntgen, M.; Pilchova, I.; Cibulka, M.; Racay, P.; Kolisek, M. Overexpression of Na$^+$/Mg^{2+} exchanger SLC41A1 attenuates pro-survival signaling. *Oncotarget* **2018**, *9*, 5084–5104. [CrossRef]

47. Hung, Y.P.; Teragawa, C.; Kosaisawe, N.; Gillies, T.E.; Pargett, M.; Minguet, M.; Distor, K.; Rocha-Gregg, B.L.; Coloff, J.L.; Keibler, M.A.; et al. Akt regulation of glycolysis mediates bioenergetic stability in epithelial cells. *eLife* **2017**, *6*, 1–25. [CrossRef]

48. Schäffers, O.J.M.; Hoenderop, J.G.J.; Bindels, R.J.M.; de Baaij, J.H.F. The rise and fall of novel renal magnesium transporters. *Am. J. Physiol. Physiol.* **2018**, *314*, F1027–F1033. [CrossRef]

49. Cefaratti, C.; Romani, A.M.P. Functional characterization of two distinct Mg^{2+} extrusion mechanisms in cardiac sarcolemmal vesicles. *Mol. Cell. Biochem.* **2007**, *303*, 63–72. [CrossRef]

50. Kolisek, M.; Sponder, G.; Mastrototaro, L.; Smorodchenko, A.; Launay, P.; Vormann, J.; Schweigel-Röntgen, M. Substitution pA350V in Na$^+$/Mg^{2+} Exchanger SLC41A1, Potentially Associated with Parkinson's Disease, Is a Gain-of-Function Mutation. *PLoS ONE* **2013**, *8*, e71096. [CrossRef]

51. Hermosura, M.C.; Nayakanti, H.; Dorovkov, M.V.; Calderon, F.R.; Ryazanov, A.G.; Haymer, D.S.; Garruto, R.M. A TRPM7 variant shows altered sensitivity to magnesium that may contribute to the pathogenesis of two Guamanian neurodegenerative disorders. *Proc. Natl. Acad. Sci. USA* **2005**, *102*, 11510–11515. [CrossRef] [PubMed]

16

Changes of Blood Pressure and Hemodynamic Parameters after Oral Magnesium Supplementation in Patients with Essential Hypertension

Nikolina Banjanin * and Goran Belojevic

Institute of Hygiene and Medical Ecology, Faculty of Medicine, University of Belgrade, 11000 Belgrade, Serbia; goran.belojevic@med.bg.ac.rs
* Correspondence: nikolina.banjanin@med.bg.ac.rs

Abstract: The objective of this study was to examine the changes of blood pressure and hemodynamic parameters after oral magnesium supplementation in patients with essential hypertension. The single-arm non-blinded intervention study comprised 48 patients (19 men; 29 women) whose antihypertensive therapy was not changed for at least one month. The participants were asked to consume (daily at home) 300 mg of oral magnesium-oxide supplementation product for one month and to have their blood pressure and hemodynamic parameters (thoracic fluid content, stroke volume, stroke index, cardiac output, cardiac index, acceleration index, left cardiac work index and systemic vascular resistance index, heart rate) measured in the hospital before and after the intervention. Measurements were performed with impedance cardiography. After magnesium supplementation, systolic and diastolic pressures were significantly decreased (mean $\pm$ standard deviation (SD)/mmHg/from 139.7 ± 15.0 to 130.8 ± 13.4 and from 88.0 ± 10.4 to 82.2 ± 9.0, respectively; both $p < 0.001$). The two significant hemodynamic changes were the decrease of systemic vascular resistance index (dyn s m^2/cm^5) and left cardiac work index (kg m/m^2)/mean $\pm$ SD from 2319.3 ± 753.3 to 2083.0 ± 526.9 and from 4.8 ± 1.4 to 4.4 ± 0.9, respectively; both $p < 0.05$. The observed hemodynamic changes may explain lowering blood pressure after magnesium supplementation.

Keywords: magnesium; dietary supplements; hypertension; systemic vascular resistance; cardiac output

1. Introduction

Magnesium is an important cation for the activity of many enzymes related to energy metabolism, e.g., serine racemase [1], ATP diphosphohydrolase [2] or myosin ATPase [3]. In addition, elevated levels of serum magnesium may lead to smooth muscle relaxation and vasodilatation due to antagonistic action on calcium receptors and channels [4]. On the other hand, the reduction of extracellular magnesium causes vasospasm, particularly important pathogenic factor for sudden death in ischemic heart disease [5] and for glaucoma and diabetic retinopathy [6]. Elevated extracellular magnesium leads to decrease of blood pressure through stimulated production of prostacyclin in endothelial cells and vascular smooth muscle cells [7] and the inhibition of norepinephrine release from nerve endings [8].

An intervention study of a 6-month supplementation with magnesium aspartate hydrochloride among patients on a diuretic therapy for hypertension showed a significant reduction of both systolic and diastolic blood pressure [9]. On the other hand, a double-blind randomized study reported no effect of a three-month magnesium supplementation on blood pressure when compared with placebo treatment [10]. A recent meta-analysis of randomized double-blind placebo controlled trials showed that a daily supplementation with a dose of 300 mg magnesium of at least one month duration significantly reduced blood pressure [11]. The discrepancies in the presented studies may be explained by the differences regarding the study designs, study protocols, ways, form or duration of supplement application, age and race of participants, patients' compliance, the instruments of measurement and the inclusion and exclusion criteria.

Due to conflicting results there is a lack of definitive conclusion and consensus on the effectiveness of magnesium in the treatment of hypertension. Besides blood pressure there is a need for further investigation of the effects of magnesium on other hemodynamic parameters that may explain the Mg-hypertension relationship. The aim of this intervention study was to examine the changes of blood pressure and hemodynamic parameters after oral magnesium supplementation in patients with essential hypertension. We hypothesized that magnesium supplementation would lead to lowering blood pressure and other compatible hemodynamic changes.

2. Materials and Methods

This study was performed in the collaboration between the Institute of Hygiene with Medical Ecology, Faculty of Medicine, and the Multidisciplinary Center for Polyclinic Diagnostics, Assessment and Treatment of Blood Pressure Disorders, Clinic for Cardiology, Clinical Center of Serbia. The study has been registered by The Iranian Registry of Clinical Trials (www.irct.ir; Registration number: IRCT2017081535716N1). All subjects signed their informed consent for inclusion before they participated in the study. The study was conducted in accordance with the declaration of Helsinki, and the protocol was approved by the Ethics Committee of the Clinical Center of Serbia, Belgrade (code 1322/1) and by the Ethics Committee of the Faculty of Medicine, University of Belgrade, Serbia (code 29/VII-16).

The investigation was designed as a single-arm non-blinded intervention study due to an expected limited pool of patients that would fulfill all inclusion and exclusion criteria [12]. The recruitment of patients was performed from September to November 2014 and comprised all patients aged 24–65 years with essential hypertension who came for a regular blood pressure check-up. Among them, only patients whose antihypertensive therapy was not changed for at least one month were eligible for the intervention study. The patients were not allowed to change their blood pressure medication during the trial. The exclusion criteria for participation in the study were: renal diseases, gastrointestinal diseases, diabetes mellitus, diseases of adrenal, thyroid and parathyroid glands, angina pectoris, myocardial infarction, coronary revascularization, congestive heart failure, aortic coarctation, food and drug allergy, pregnancy and lactation, transitory ischemic attack and oral intake of magnesium supplements in the previous month.

The minimum sample size of 43 patients was calculated based on previously reported clinically significant reduction of mean values of systolic and diastolic pressure of 3 mmHg and 2 mmHg, respectively, and effect size of 0.44 after magnesium supplementation [13]. The calculation was performed online using the input values of a power of 80% and a two sided level of significance of 5% [14].

The eligible participants ($n = 68$, 27 men and 41 women) were asked to consume 300 mg of oral magnesium-oxide supplementation product for one month and to have their blood pressure and hemodynamic parameters measured in hospital settings at baseline and at the end of the intervention. The participants were given a dietary supplement ("Magnezijum 300 Direkt", Hermes Arzneimittel GmbH, Wolfratshausen, Germany) which is approved by the Ministry of Health of the Republic of Serbia (Number: 1708/2011). All participants were informed how to use this product, were warned not to exceed the daily recommended dose, and were advised not to change their dietary habits. The participants did not report adverse effects that might be related to magnesium supplementation. They were not informed about the expected changes of blood pressure and hemodynamic parameters after magnesium supplementation.

At baseline, the participants underwent a detailed medical examination and completed a questionnaire that included personal data (age, gender), duration of hypertension (years), hypertension in the family (coded as: 1-any family member diagnosed with hypertension; 0-none), physical activity of at least 30 min most days per week (coded as: 1-Yes; 0-No) and smoking habits (coded as: 0-non-smoker;1-current smoker; 2-ex-smoker). Data on antihypertensive treatment were obtained from patient's medical records. Antihypertensive treatment included: ACE inhibitors (23 patients; 48%); calcium channel blockers (24;50); thiazide diuretics (24;50); beta blockers (35;73) and angiotensin II receptor blockers (10;21). At follow-up after one month, all participants were invited for medical examination. Despite being called several times, 20 participants did not return for check-up (8 men and 12 women), but they did not report adverse effects of magnesium supplementation as the reason. The statistical analysis revealed that the non-responders were significantly younger than the responders (mean age of the non-responders 37.75 ± 12.45 years) with non-significantly shorter duration of hypertension (mean duration of hypertension among the non-responders 5.39 ± 5.19 years). The final sample comprised 48 persons, 19 men and 29 women, aged 47.40 ± 11.30 years, range 24 to 65 years. This sample size was considered sufficient according to afore mentioned calculation.

Average daily magnesium intake from food and drinks was obtained using a 24-h recall questionnaire. The participants were very carefully asked about food and drinks they consumed during 24 h prior to the interview. The questions referred to food types and amounts, time and place of consumption, how the food was prepared (fried, fresh, baked or cooked) and what was used to prepare the food (salt, oil, sugar etc.). A trained physician conducted the interview with the participants. Magnesium intake from food and drinks was calculated from all foodstuffs consumed the previous day using Serbian food tables [15]. Serum magnesium concentration was measured both at baseline and follow up using the photometric method [16]. Blood samples were taken at the central laboratory of the Clinical Center of Serbia between 8 and 9 a.m., after a morning fast. The laboratory is an accredited institution with a strict quality control standards for all laboratory analyses.

Participants had their weight and height measured by a trained physician. Body height was measured to the nearest 0.5 cm. Body weight was measured on a digital scale (TANITA Inner Scan Body Composition Monitor BC-543) to the nearest 0.1 kg. Participants were in light clothes and barefoot. Body mass index (BMI) was calculated as body weight (in kilograms) divided by squared body height (in meters).

Both at baseline and at follow-up participants had their systolic, diastolic and mean arterial blood pressure measured with impedance cardiography (ICG) by CardioScreen® 2000 (Medis. Medizinische Messtechnik GmbH, Ilmenau, Germany). A cuff was placed on patient's left upper arm.

We also used ICG for measurements of hemodynamic parameters at baseline and follow-up. ICG electrodes measure the change in thorax impedance during the flow of the alternating current through the thorax. The following parameters were measured: thoracic fluid content (the electrical conductivity of the chest, L/kOhm), acceleration index (the acceleration of blood in the ascending aorta and the aortic arch, $L/100/s^2$) and heart rate (beats per minute). The following parameters were calculated: stroke volume (the amount of blood pumped by the left ventricle each beat, mL) and cardiac output (stroke volume multiplied by heart rate, L/min). With reference to body surface area the following parameters were calculated: stroke index (stroke volume related to the body surface, mL/m^2), cardiac index (cardiac output related to the body surface, $L/(min\ m^2)$, systemic vascular resistance index (the resistance to the blood flow through the arterial system the heart works against, $dyn\ s\ m^2/cm^5$) and left cardiac work index (an expression for the work of the left ventricle, $kg\ m/m^2$). DuBois formula was used to calculate the body surface area [17].

Descriptive statistic was presented as mean values and standard deviation for numeric variables, or as percent's (relative numbers) for categorical variables. All investigated parameters were tested by Kolmogorov-Smirnov test and almost all observed distributions corresponded to the normal distribution. The differences between men and women were tested with Student's t-test for parametric variables and with Mann-Whitney U-test and Chi-square test for non-parametric data. The differences between baseline and follow-up were tested with paired-samples t-test. Probability level of less than 0.05 was accepted as significant. Statistical analyses were performed using SPSS 15.0 for Windows software (SPSS Inc., Chicago, IL, USA, 1989–2006).

3. Results

Men and women were of similar age, and had similar body mass index, blood pressure levels, and shared smoking habits, engagement in physical activity and magnesium intake from food and water and serum magnesium concentrations. Men and women had similar duration of hypertension, and had similar family history of hypertension. These results support further analysis regardless of gender (Table 1).

Table 1. Baseline characteristics of the investigated population by gender.

Parameters	Men	Women	Total	p Value
Gender (%)	19 (39.6)	29 (60.4)	48 (100.0)	NS ($p > 0.05$) *
Age (years)	43.79 ± 11.11	49.76 ± 10.98	47.40 ± 11.30	NS **
Body mass index (kg/m^2)	27.03 ± 2.48	25.94 ± 5.36	26.38 ± 4.42	NS **
Duration of hypertension (years)	9.50 ± 9.75	7.75 ± 6.99	8.44 ± 8.14	NS ***
Hypertension in the family (%)	15 (83.3)	25 (92.6)	40 (88.9)	NS *
Current smoker (%)	7 (36.8)	9 (31.0)	16 (33.3)	NS *
Regular physical activity (%)	10 (52.6)	18 (64.3)	28 (59.6)	NS *
Systolic pressure (mmHg)	140.74 ± 11.14	139.09 ± 17.26	139.74 ± 15.03	NS **
Diastolic pressure (mmHg)	87.37 ± 11.43	88.50 ± 9.83	88.05 ± 10.39	NS **
Mg intake from food (mg/day)	196.30 ± 114.74	158.73 ± 50.19	173.60 ± 82.99	NS ***
Mg intake from water (mg/day)	12.69 ± 6.44	15.55 ± 8.13	14.42 ± 7.56	NS ***
Total Mg intake (mg/day)	208.89 ± 115.66	174.28 ± 51.72	187.98 ± 83.72	NS ***
Serum magnesium concentration (mmol/L)	0.86 ± 0.05	0.85 ± 0.06	0.85 ± 0.05	NS **

* Chi-square test; ** Student's t-test; *** Mann–Whitney U-test. NS (not significant)

There was no significant difference between serum magnesium concentrations at baseline and at follow-up (mean ± SD = 0.858 ± 0.054 and 0.847 ± 0.070 mmol/L, respectively; $p = 0.432$). The range of serum magnesium concentrations at baseline and at follow-up was 0.74–0.94 and 0.69–0.96 mmol/L, respectively.

Magnesium supplementation lead to significant decrease in systolic, diastolic and mean arterial blood pressure. Mean systolic pressure was decreased by 8.97 ± 2.01 mmHg; mean diastolic pressure was decreased by 5.87 ± 1.49 mmHg; mean arterial pressure was decreased by 8.06 ± 1.67 mmHg (Table 2).

Table 2. Changes of blood pressure after magnesium supplementation in patients with essential hypertension ($N = 48$).

Parameters	At Baseline	At Follow-Up	95% Confidence Interval of the Difference	p Value *
Systolic pressure (mmHg)	139.74 ± 15.03	130.77 ± 13.42	4.92–13.02	<0.001
Diastolic pressure (mmHg)	88.05 ± 10.39	82.19 ± 9.00	2.88–8.86	<0.001
Mean pressure (mmHg)	102.13 ± 12.07	94.07 ± 10.11	4.70–11.42	<0.001

* Paired-samples t-test.

After one month of supplementation, thoracic fluid content, stroke index, cardiac index acceleration index and heart rate remained stable. On the other hand, systemic vascular resistance index and left cardiac work index were significantly decreased following a month of magnesium supplementation (Table 3). Mean change of left cardiac work index equaled 0.439 ± 0.19 kg m/m^2, whereas mean change of systemic vascular resistance index was 236.29 ± 93.49 dyn s m^2/cm^5.

Table 3. Changes of hemodynamic parameters after magnesium supplementation in patients with essential hypertension ($N = 48$).

Parameters	At Baseline	At Follow-Up	95% Confidence Interval of the Difference	p Value *
Thoracic fluid content (L/kOhm)	38.75 ± 8.95	36.57 ± 6.09	-0.67–5.04	0.131
Stroke volume (mL)	101.74 ± 27.90	99.26 ± 24.13	-10.18–15.13	0.686
Stroke index (mL/m^2)	48.77 ± 11.31	48.44 ± 11.09	-5.62–6.28	0.905
Cardiac output (L/min)	6.93 ± 1.42	6.76 ± 1.29	-0.58–0.93	0.636
Cardiac index (L/(min m^2))	3.61 ± 0.95	3.56 ± 0.64	-0.21–0.30	0.727
Acceleration index (L/100/s^2)	105.96 ± 39.64	104.88 ± 40.27	-8.98–11.13	0.831
Left cardiac work index (kg m/m^2)	4.83 ± 1.42	4.39 ± 0.91	0.05–0.82	0.026
Systemic vascular resistance index (dyn s m^2/cm^5)	2319.30 ± 753.31	2083.01 ± 526.95	47.87–424.71	0.015
Heart rate (beat/min)	71.56 ± 11.82	69.55 ± 9.06	-0.83–4.85	0.162

* Paired-samples t-test.

4. Discussion

We show a reduction of blood pressure after a one-month magnesium supplementation in hypertensive patients. This effect is compatible with a reduction in two hemodynamic parameters: systemic vascular resistance and left cardiac work.

Our results are in accordance with a meta-analysis of 22 trials which showed that the intake of magnesium supplements exceeding 370 mg daily has a bigger effectiveness in the reduction of systolic and diastolic blood pressures in hypertensive patients than the dose lower than 370 mg daily. The study found that the average reduction of systolic blood pressure was 3–4 mmHg and diastolic 2–3 mmHg after the consumption of magnesium supplements lasting from 3 to 24 weeks (average duration 11.3 weeks) [13]. Another review reported that oral magnesium supplements at a dosage from 10 to 15 mmol per day may reduce blood pressure in hypertensive patients on antihypertensive therapy [18].Additionally, our study points out the changes in hemodynamic parameters after magnesium supplementation that are compatible with lowering blood pressure. But, the results of the studies on the association between magnesium intake and blood pressure are not fully congruent. For example, a double-blind randomized study was conducted in patients with essential hypertension. When treatment with 40 mmol (972 mg) magnesium aspartate supplementation daily was compared with placebo treatment for three months no effect of magnesium supplementation on blood pressure was found [10]. However, this study had a small sample size of 13 patients. Another experimental study conducted in the US showed that magnesium supplementation for 16 weeks in dose of 14 mmol (336 mg) of magnesium had no blood pressure-lowering effect in normotensive women who reported low habitual intake of this mineral in comparison with placebo group [19].

An important magnesium function, the vasodilatation of peripheral arteries [20], may explain the lowering of systemic vascular resistance in our study. Magnesium may achieve its vasodilatatory effect through its impact on: intracellular calcium concentration [21], production of prostacyclin [7], and sensitivity to angiotensin II [22].

Serum magnesium concentration was not significantly changed after magnesium supplementation in our study. This finding is congruent with other intervention studies of a similar duration [23,24]. A significant raise of serum magnesium concentration after a seven-week magnesium supplementation may be expected only in participants with hypomagnesemia (concentrations lower than 0.70 mmol/L) [23] but in our sample the lowest serum magnesium concentration at baseline was 0.74 mmol/L. But, in longer intervention studies of a median duration of 12 weeks a significant elevation of serum magnesium concentrations after magnesium supplementation may be expected even in patients with baseline median serum magnesium concentrations of 0.785 mmol/L [25].

There are several limitations of this study. First, a single-arm non-blinded design was chosen because of a limited pool of patients. We consider that a placebo effect was alleviated by the fact that although the patients knew they were given magnesium supplementation they were not informed about the expected changes in blood pressure and hemodynamic parameters. Second, we did not control the possible effect of thiazide diuretics on magnesium excretion in some patients. Third, we did not check for magnesium concentration in a 24 h urine sample at baseline and at follow-up. Fourth, the intervention period of our study was limited to thirty days. In further investigations it would be useful to examine the effects of different duration (shorter and longer than in our study) of magnesium supplementation on blood pressure and hemodynamic parameters. Fifth, the study was conducted in persons with essential hypertension; the hemodynamic changes in persons with diabetes or kidney diseases would be of great importance for understanding the mechanisms of action of magnesium supplementation. The strength of this study is the use of ICG, which objectively measures both blood pressure and hemodynamic parameters that may explain blood pressure changes after magnesium supplementation.

5. Conclusions

In conclusion, oral magnesium supplementation probably had a positive effect on blood pressure reduction in patients with essential hypertension. The decrease in systemic vascular resistance and left cardiac work may explain the reduction of blood pressure after magnesium supplementation.

Author Contributions: N.B. designed the study, collected data, and wrote the first draft; N.B. and G.B. performed statistical analysis, wrote the manuscript, revised and approved the final version of manuscript and prepared the paper for submission.

References

1.   Bruno, S.; Margiotta, M.; Marchesani, F.; Paredi, G.; Orlandi, V.; Faggiano, S.; Ronda, L.; Campanini, B.; Mozzarelli, A. Magnesium and calcium ions differentially affect human serine racemase activity and modulate its quaternary equilibrium toward a tetrameric form. *Biochim. Biophys. Acta* **2017**, *1865*, 381–387. [CrossRef] [PubMed]

2.   Sinha, P.; Paswan, R.K.; Kumari, A.; Kumar, S.; Bimal, S.; Das, P.; Lal, C.S. Magnesium-Dependent Ecto-ATP Diphosphohydrolase Activity in *Leishmania donovani. Curr. Microbiol.* **2016**, *73*, 811–819. [CrossRef] [PubMed]

3.   Ge, J.; Huang, F.; Nesmelov, Y.E. Metal cation controls phosphate release in the myosin ATPase. *Protein Sci.* **2017**, *26*, 2181–2186. [CrossRef] [PubMed]

4.   Odom, M.J.; Zuckerman, S.L.; Mocco, J. The role of magnesium in the management of cerebral vasospasm. *Neurol. Res. Int.* **2013**, *2013*, 943914. [CrossRef] [PubMed]

5.   Turlapaty, P.D.; Altura, B.M. Magnesium deficiency produces spasms of coronary arteries: Relationship to etiology of sudden death ischemic heart disease. *Science* **1980**, *208*, 198–200. [CrossRef] [PubMed]

6.   Agarwal, R.; Iezhitsa, L.; Agarwal, P. Pathogenetic role of magnesium deficiency inophthalmic diseases. *Biometals* **2014**, *27*, 5–18. [CrossRef] [PubMed]

7.   Satake, K.; Lee, J.D.; Shimizu, H.; Uzui, H.; Mitsuke, Y.; Yue, H.; Ueda, T. Effects of magnesium on prostacyclin synthesis and intracellular free calcium concentration in vascular cells. *Magnes. Res.* **2004**, *17*, 20–27. [PubMed]

8.   Shimosawa, T.; Takano, K.; Ando, K.; Fujita, T. Magnesium inhibits norepinephrine release by blocking N-type calcium channels at peripheral sympathetic nerve endings. *Hypertension* **2004**, *44*, 897–902. [CrossRef] [PubMed]

9.   Dyckner, T.; Wester, P.O.; Widman, L. Effects of peroral magnesium on plasma and skeletal muscle electrolytes in patients on long-term diuretic therapy. *Int. J. Cardiol.* **1988**, *19*, 81–87. [CrossRef]

10. Zemel, P.C.; Zemel, M.B.; Urberg, M.; Douglas, F.L.; Geiser, R.; Sowers, J.R. Metabolic and hemodynamic effects of magnesium supplementation in patients with essential hypertension. *Am. J. Clin. Nutr.* **1990**, *51*, 665–669. [CrossRef] [PubMed]

11. Zhang, X.; Li, Y.; Del Gobbo, L.C.; Rosanoff, A.; Wang, J.; Zhang, W.; Song, Y. Effects of Magnesium Supplementation on Blood Pressure: A Meta-Analysis of Randomized Double-Blind Placebo-Controlled Trials. *Hypertension* **2016**, *68*, 324–333. [CrossRef] [PubMed]

12. Evans, S.R. Clinical trial structures. *J. Exp. Stroke Transl. Med.* **2010**, *3*, 8–18. [CrossRef] [PubMed]

13. Kass, L.; Weekes, J.; Carpenter, L. Effect of magnesium supplementation on blood pressure: a meta-analysis. *Eur. J. Clin. Nutr.* **2012**, *66*, 411–418. [CrossRef] [PubMed]
14. Dhand, N.K.; Khatkar, M.S. Statulator: An Online Statistical Calculator. Sample Size Calculator for Comparing Two Paired Means 2014. Available online: http://statulator.com/SampleSize/ss2PM.html (accessed on 10 April 2018).
15. Jokić, N. *Calorics in Daily Life 5000 Groceries-Dishes and Natural Mineral Waters*, 1st ed.; Institute for Textbooks: Belgrade, Serbia, 2007; ISBN 978-86-17-14449-2. (In Serbian)
16. Wong, H.K.C. Fully automated procedure for serum magnesium. *Clin. Chem.* **1975**, *21*, 169. [PubMed]
17. DuBois, D.; DuBois, E.F. A formula to estimate the approximate surface area if height and weight be known. *Arch. Intern. Med.* **1916**, *17*, 863–871. [CrossRef]
18. Rosanoff, A. Importance of magnesium dose in the treatment of hypertension. In *Advances in Magnesium Research: New Data*; Porr, P.J., Nechifor, M., Durlach, J., Eds.; Éditions John Libbey Eurotext: Montrouge, France, 2006; pp. 97–103. ISBN 2-7420-0606-0.
19. Sacks, F.M.; Willett, W.C.; Smith, A.; Brown, L.E.; Rosner, B.; Moore, T.J. Effect on blood pressure of potassium, calcium, and magnesium in women with low habitual intake. *Hypertension* **1998**, *31*, 131–138. [CrossRef] [PubMed]
20. Gröber, U.; Schmidt, J.; Kisters, K. Magnesium in Prevention and Therapy. *Nutrients* **2015**, *7*, 8199–8226. [CrossRef] [PubMed]
21. D'Angelo, E.K.; Singer, H.A.; Rembold, C.M. Magnesium relaxes arterial smooth muscle by decreasing intracellular Ca^{2+} without changing intracellular Mg^{2+}. *J. Clin. Investig.* **1992**, *89*, 1988–1994. [CrossRef] [PubMed]
22. Altura, B.M.; Turlapaty, P.D. Withdrawal of magnesium enhances coronary arterial spasms produced by vasoactive agents. *Br. J. Pharmacol.* **1982**, *77*, 649–659. [CrossRef] [PubMed]
23. Nielsen, F.H.; Johnson, L.K.; Zeng, H. Magnesium supplementation improves indicators of low magnesium status and inflammatory stress in adults older than 51 years with poor quality sleep. *Magnes. Res.* **2010**, *23*, 158–168. [CrossRef] [PubMed]
24. Asemi, Z.; Karamali, M.; Jamilian, M.; Foroozanfard, F.; Bahmani, F.; Heidarzadeh, Z.; Benisi-Kohansal, S.; Surkan, P.J.; Esmaillzadeh, A. Magnesium supplementation affects metabolic status and pregnancy outcomes in gestational diabetes: A randomized, double-blind, placebo-controlled trial. *Am. J. Clin. Nutr.* **2015**, *102*, 222–229. [CrossRef] [PubMed]
25. Costello, R.B.; Elin, R.J.; Rosanoff, A.; Wallace, T.C.; Guerrero-Romero, F.; Hruby, A.; Lutsey, P.L.; Nielsen, F.H.; Rodriguez-Moran, M.; Song, Y.; et al. Perspective: The Case for an Evidence-Based Reference Interval for Serum Magnesium: The Time Has Come. *Adv. Nutr.* **2016**, *7*, 977–993. [CrossRef] [PubMed]

17

Magnesium Status and Stress: The Vicious Circle Concept Revisited

Gisèle Pickering [1], **André Mazur** [2], **Marion Trousselard** [3]⬤, **Przemyslaw Bienkowski** [4], **Natalia Yaltsewa** [5], **Mohamed Amessou** [6]⬤, **Lionel Noah** [6,*] and **Etienne Pouteau** [6]

[1] Plateforme d'Investigation Clinique/CIC Inserm 1405, University Hospital CHU,
    63000 Clermont-Ferrand, France; gisele.pickering@uca.fr
[2] INRAE, UNH, Unité de Nutrition Humaine, Université Clermont Auvergne,
    63001 Clermont-Ferrand, France; andre.mazur@inrae.fr
[3] Independent Regulatory Board for Auditors (IRBA), 91220 Bretigny-sur-Orge, France;
    marion.trousselard@gmail.com
[4] Department of Psychiatry, Warsaw Medical University, 02-091 Warsaw, Poland; pbienko@yahoo.com
[5] Department of General Medicine, The Yaroslavl State Medical University Institute
    of Postgraduate Education, 150000 Yaroslavl, Russia; yaltzewa@yandex.ru
[6] Medical Affairs Department, Consumer HealthCare, Sanofi, Gentilly, 94250 Paris, France;
    Mohamed.Amessou@sanofi.com (M.A.); Etienne.Pouteau@sanofi.com (E.P.)
* Correspondence: Lionel. Noah@sanofi.com

Abstract: Magnesium deficiency and stress are both common conditions among the general population, which, over time, can increase the risk of health consequences. Numerous studies, both in pre-clinical and clinical settings, have investigated the interaction of magnesium with key mediators of the physiological stress response, and demonstrated that magnesium plays an inhibitory key role in the regulation and neurotransmission of the normal stress response. Furthermore, low magnesium status has been reported in several studies assessing nutritional aspects in subjects suffering from psychological stress or associated symptoms. This overlap in the results suggests that stress could increase magnesium loss, causing a deficiency; and in turn, magnesium deficiency could enhance the body's susceptibility to stress, resulting in a magnesium and stress vicious circle. This review revisits the magnesium and stress vicious circle concept, first introduced in the early 1990s, in light of recent available data.

Keywords: stress; magnesium; hypomagnesemia; magnesium deficiency; vicious circle; dietary intake; magnesium supplementation

1. Introduction

Stress, often intended as a psychological response to external stressors, has become a common issue of modern life [1]. From a neurobiology perspective, stress is an adaptive system that continuously assesses and interacts physically, physiologically, or psychosocially, with the environment. When this stress system is overloaded, negative health outcomes could result [2]. Magnesium is a fundamental nutrient, the role of which in human health is widely recognized [3]. Today, magnesium deficiency is also a common condition among the general population [4], and given its importance in the functioning of many reactions of the human body, this deficiency can increase the risk of physical and mental health illness over time. Of note, symptoms of magnesium deficiency and stress are very similar, the most common being fatigue, irritability, and mild anxiety [5–7]; further symptoms are shown in Table 1.

Table 1. Symptoms of magnesium deficiency and symptoms of stress.

Most Frequently Reported Symptoms of Stress [6,7]	Symptoms of Magnesium Deficiency [5,8]
Fatigue	**Tiredness**
Irritability or anger	**Irritability**
Feeling nervous	**Mild anxiety/nervousness**
Lack of energy	**Muscle weakness**
Upset stomach	**Gastrointestinal spasms**
Muscle tension	**Muscle cramps**
Headache	**Headache**
Sadness/depression	Mild sleep disorders
Chest pain/hyperventilation	Nausea/vomiting

Note: Similar symptoms are highlighted in bold.

The idea of a bidirectional relationship between magnesium and stress was first introduced by Galland and Seelig, in the early 1990s [9,10] and then referred to as the vicious circle. This vicious circle implies that stress can increase magnesium loss, causing a deficiency; in turn, magnesium deficiency can enhance the body's susceptibility to stress [10].

Taking into account the increasing prevalence of stress in modern societies [11], and its related consequences to health, this review revisits the magnesium and stress vicious circle concept, with a focus on the role of magnesium on the body's response to stress and the pathways that regulate such a response. In particular, the scope of this article was to assess the evidence available on the need of an adequate intake of magnesium, and strengthen the hypothesis that a revision of the current recommended intake of magnesium is needed for the general population when exposed to stress, in order to reduce associated health risks.

2. Magnesium: Biological Role and Dietary Needs

2.1. Biological Role of Magnesium and Homeostasis

Magnesium is an essential mineral for humans [12]. Being the second most abundant intracellular cation [5], magnesium is involved in almost all major metabolic and biochemical processes [13]. It acts as a cofactor in hundreds of enzymatic reactions [13], its primary functions including protein and nucleic acid synthesis, regulation of metabolic pathways, neuronal transmission, neuromuscular function, and regulation of cardiac rhythm [8,14,15]. In addition, magnesium is a naturally occurring calcium channel blocker, is involved in the maintenance of electrolyte balance (e.g., regulation of sodium–potassium ATPase activity), and plays a key role in membrane excitability [5,12].

It is estimated that an adult human body contains around 21–28 g of magnesium, 50–60% of which is stored in the bones, with the remainder distributed in soft tissues such as muscles [14,16]. Magnesium is also an essential component of the extracellular fluid (ECF) and the cerebrospinal fluid (CSF) in the central nervous system [17,18]. Magnesium enters the brain through the blood–brain barrier which maintains the passage of nutrients and electrolytes for the ECF homeostasis, and is actively transported by choroidal epithelial cells into the CSF [17,18]. Although little has been revealed about the exact mechanisms of magnesium transport into the brain, it is known that magnesium concentration is higher in the CSF than in plasma [19]. Under conditions of deficiency, magnesium levels still decline in the CSF, but slower when compared to the changes observed in plasma magnesium levels [19]. Experimental studies have shown that in magnesium-deficient animals, the brain uptake of magnesium is almost doubled compared to normal-fed controls [20] and CFS magnesium concentration was readily repleted, showing that magnesium is an essential mineral for the brain homeostasis [19,20].

Only 1% of the total magnesium is extracellular and 0.3% of this circulates in serum in three different forms [21]: Free (unbound; 60%), which represents the biologically active form; albumin-bound (30%); or in a complex with other ions (10%) [13].

Magnesium homeostasis is tightly regulated and relies on the dynamic balance between intestinal absorption, kidney excretion, and storage in bones (Figure 1) [22]. Magnesium is mainly absorbed in the distal parts of the small intestine [22], and mostly stored in bones [22], where it serves as a reservoir to maintain the equilibrium with its extracellular concentration [22]. The kidneys play a critical part in magnesium homeostasis by eliminating its excess [22].

Figure 1. Magnesium homeostasis. Figure adapted from Jahnen–Dechent, 2012 [17]. Data from Elin, 1988 [19] and deBaaij, 2015 [8]. Mg, magnesium.

Many factors can affect magnesium balance: A diet high in sodium, calcium, and protein [5,23–25], the consumption of caffeine and alcohol [5,13,26], and the use of certain medicines such as diuretics, proton-pump, and inhibitors or antibiotics [13,26,27], which can all cause lower magnesium retention. In healthy individuals, some physiological conditions such as pregnancy [28,29], menopause [30], or ageing [31,32] are associated with changes in the need for magnesium. Pathological conditions, particularly those affecting the absorption and the elimination of nutrients (e.g., diabetes, renal function impairment, and physiological stress), may also result in significant magnesium loss or malabsorption [4,5,26,33,34]. Studies on hereditary forms of magnesium deficiency have contributed to the identification of both recessive and dominant genetic disorders directly affecting the transport of magnesium at a cellular level [35]. Although mutated transporting-proteins mainly contribute to renal wasting or intestinal malabsorption of magnesium, the mechanisms at the molecular level remain to be elucidated [8,36]. Notably, several studies showed that lower magnesium levels are involved in the course of several mental disorders, especially depression [37]. A summary of the factors affecting magnesium homeostasis is presented in Table 2.

Table 2. Factors contributing to magnesium deficiency.

Diet related
Inadequate magnesium intake [5,13,26]
High protein diet [5,25]
High sodium diet [5,25]
High calcium diet [5,23–25]
High caffeine intake [5]
Alcohol dependence [5,13,26]
Lifestyle
Sports [25,38–40]
Sleep quality and quantity [41,42]
Chronic stress [43,44]
Pharmacological related
Diuretics, e.g., furosemide [13,26,27]
Proton-pump inhibitors, e.g., omeprazole [13,27]
Cisplatin [13,26,27]
Antibiotics, e.g., gentamicin [13,27]
Physiological conditions
Pregnancy [28,29]
Ageing [31,32]
Menopause [30]
Pathological conditions
Genetic disorders [8,35,36]
Type 2 diabetes mellitus [4,5]
Gastrointestinal disorders [5,26]
Kidney failure [5,33]
Cardiovascular diseases [5,45]
Metabolic syndrome [5,34]
Osteoporosis [15,25,33]

2.2. Food Sources, Current Recommended Intakes and Safety

Nuts, legumes, whole cereals, and fruits have the highest magnesium content of all foods [16]. Coffee or cocoa-based products may also contain significant amounts of magnesium, while fish, meats, and milk have an intermediate amount [46,47]. Drinking water, especially harder water, can also be rich in magnesium salts [48]. The source of dietary magnesium varies widely according to gender, age, and dietary habits. For example, French adults in 2016 obtained more than 21% of their magnesium from hot beverages including coffee, 9% from bread, and 6% from vegetables [47], whereas in a sample of American adults, the main sources of magnesium were vegetables (13%), milk (7%) and meat (7%) [49]. In a sample of Polish adults, dietary magnesium requirements were mostly maintained by the consumption of cereal products (11.8–15.3%) [50], and milk or dairy products (10.9%) [51]. A study investigating the Italian diet found that cereals (27%) are the primary source of magnesium in adults [52].

Over time, public health agencies have reviewed and established recommendations for dietary intake of magnesium (and other nutrients). These include the estimated average requirement (EAR), which represents the average daily intake that satisfies the nutritional requirement of 50% of the population considered; and the recommended dietary allowance (RDA), which is the daily intake that meets the requirement of 97.5% of the same population [15,53]. Values are set on the basis of dietary balance experiments and/or results from clinical studies and meta-analyses [54–57].

Dietary balance studies performed in the 1980s in the USA concluded that the EAR for magnesium was 310–330 in men and 255–265 mg/day in women [55–57]. As a consequence, in 1997, the Standing Committee on the Scientific Evaluation of Dietary Reference Intakes (for the USA and Canada) set an RDA of 400–420 and 310–320 mg/day for men and women, respectively [58]. Nowadays, nutrient requirements and dietary guidelines are available in every country. For instance, in Poland, the RDA for magnesium is 400–420 for men and 310–320 mg/day for women [59], and in Russia, it is 300 mg/day for both men and women [60]. The European Food Safety Agency (EFSA) did not consider the available scientific evidence strong enough to determine RDAs, and has suggested an "adequate intake" of 350 and 300 mg/day for men and women, respectively [16]. Within the EU, national governmental bodies have set local RDAs. In 2015, the Japanese Ministry of Health, Labor and Welfare updated the dietary reference intake guidelines and set the RDA at 320–340 and 220–230 mg/day for adult men and women, respectively [61]. Recommended intakes are summarized by country in Table 3.

Table 3. Current magnesium recommended dietary allowances (RDAs) across countries.

Country	Magnesium, mg/day	
	Men	Women
Italy [62]	240	240
Russia [60]	300	300
Japan [61]	320–340	220–230
Poland [59]	400–420	310–320
USA and Canada [58]	400–420	310–320
France [63]	420	360

Values shown refer to adult population only (≥19 years).

Studies have consistently shown that the dietary magnesium intake is often inadequate across different countries [5,64]. In 2005, King et al. reported that approximately 60% of Americans do not reach the recommended daily intake of magnesium through their diet [65]. In the USA, between 2003–2006, the average intakes of magnesium from food were 268 for men and 234 mg for women, which meant that 63% of men and 69% of women did not meet the EAR [66]. These results were confirmed and supported by the Dietary Guidelines Advisory Committee, which, in 2015, concluded that magnesium is an under-consumed nutrient for many Americans [46].

In Europe, the situation is similar. The National Diet and Nutrition Survey conducted in the UK between 2014–2016 showed that men's mean dietary intake in magnesium was 302 and women's was 238 mg/day [67]. In France in 2007, the mean daily dietary intake was 323 in men and 263 mg in women and more than two-thirds of the French adult population (67.4% of men and 76.7% of women, aged 18 to 54) had an inadequate magnesium intake [68]. Furthermore, in Spain, the Anthropometry, Intake and Energy Balance in Spain (ANIBES) study revealed that the mean consumption of magnesium in the population was 222 mg/day, indicating that 79% of the population had an intake below 80% of the national RDA [69]. The Mediterranean Healthy Eating, Ageing, and Lifestyle (MEAL) observational study conducted in Italy found that the dietary intake of magnesium was adequate both in men (397) and women (390 mg/day), with cereals, dairy products, and legumes being the main food sources [70]. Lastly, an analysis based on national surveys conducted across European countries showed that the mean magnesium intake among adults (18–60 years old) in Poland was 396 in men and 264 mg/day in women; [71] whereas German adults had the highest mean intake magnesium, 522 in men and 418 mg/day in women [71].

When there is a need for optimizing the magnesium status, a variety of oral supplements are available. Magnesium supplementation is considered well-tolerated, with diarrhea typically being the main manifestation of an excessive intake [72]. The upper limit for magnesium supplementation in healthy adults is 350 mg/day [73]. Normally, an increased renal filtration can reverse a wide range of serum magnesium concentration to normal levels. However, serious adverse effects have been reported for serum magnesium concentration exceeding 1.74–2.61 mmol/L. Symptoms of magnesium toxicity include hypotension, nausea, flushing of the face, retention of urine, and lethargy, and may progress to difficulty breathing, extreme hypotension, irregular heartbeat, and cardiac arrest [72].

2.3. Magnesium Deficiency: Causes and Health Consequences

In clinical practice, measurement of serum magnesium levels is the most common means of assessing nutrient status [13], with normal values considered to be within the 0.7–1.0 mmol/L range [74,75]. Hypomagnesemia is clinically defined when serum concentrations drop below 0.7 mmol/L [8]. Severe hypomagnesemia (<0.4 mmol/L) is rare and occurs mostly in serious pathological conditions [76]. Symptoms may include neuromuscular dysfunction (muscular weakness, tremors, seizures or tetany); cardiovascular signs (electrocardiographic abnormalities and arrhythmias); and hypokalemia and hypocalcemia [13]. However, mild hypomagnesemia (0.5–0.7 mmol/L) is common and estimated to affect around 2.5–15% of the population [4,26]. In the majority of cases, magnesium deficiency is not identified, as low serum levels are compensated by the release of magnesium from the bone reservoir [48]. In addition, mild deficiency can remain undetected as it often occurs with nonspecific symptoms such as irritability, nervousness, mild anxiety, muscle contractions, weakness, fatigue, and digestive troubles [26]. In addition, it has been suggested that chronic latent magnesium deficiency could start developing below 0.85 mmol/L with a potential impact on human health [12,77]. A recent study by Noah et al. found that nearly half (~44%) of the subjects screened for stress had chronic latent magnesium deficiency (defined as serum magnesium <0.85 mmol/L) [78]. Moreover, subclinical, chronic magnesium depletion may contribute to various dysfunctions and diseases and the scientific literature is rich in studies highlighting the association between low dietary magnesium intake and a higher risk of type 2 diabetes, cardiovascular diseases, osteoporosis, and metabolic syndrome [8,79,80].

Several factors contribute to magnesium deficiency (Table 2). Dietary surveys point to an inadequate magnesium intake from food. Surveys conducted in different countries have consistently showed a substantial inadequate intake of magnesium from food in the general population, particularly in young adults, those over 70 years of age [81], and in women [71]. Of note, over the past 60 years, intensive farming practices have caused a significant depletion of the mineral content of the soil [82–84], including a decrease in magnesium of up to 30% [85,86]. Additionally, western diets typically have a greater proportion of processed food, where several products are mostly refined, with magnesium being depleted by up to 80–90% in the process [5,8]. Factors and behaviors associated with the western lifestyle, including intense sport and physical activity [38], poor sleep quality and quantity [41], and psychological stress [43,44], can also induce magnesium loss. Magnesium deficiency is linked to many health conditions, from those affecting its metabolism, such as gastrointestinal diseases, type 2 diabetes, alcohol dependence, or kidney failure [5,26], to genetic disorders [35]. A growing body of evidence also suggests that chronic stress may cause magnesium loss/deficiency [43]. Numerous studies have shown lower magnesium levels associated with different neurological and psychiatric disorders, particularly depression and post-traumatic stress disorder [87,88] but also anxiety disorders, attention deficit hyperactivity disorder, and bipolar disorder [37,89]. Although evidence on a causal factor between mental disorders and magnesium deficiency has yet to be confirmed, stress appears as a key component in the relationship between mental health illness and magnesium deficiency.

3. Stress

Stress is commonly described as a trigger that evokes a physiological and psychological response of the body [90]. Over the past decades, the understanding of stress biology has largely evolved. Stress is no longer considered as a temporary response to occasional threats, but rather an ongoing and adaptive system that enables an individual to assess, cope, and predict constantly changing conditions. However, the capacity of this stress system is limited and can be overloaded, resulting in poor health outcomes, particularly those related to mental illness like depression or cognitive deficits [2].

Stress not only affects the mental health status of an individual, but it is also characterized by a physical response of the body that, depending on the type and length of exposure, may lead to short-term effects (e.g., increased blood pressure, increased heart and respiration rates, increased alertness) [91], or long-term effects (e.g., impaired hippocampal neurogenesis, cognitive and memory disorders) [92].

The following sections summarize widely recognized theoretical models of stress and describe possible physiological roles of magnesium in the stress response. Here, the term "stress model" refers to a theoretical framework used to predict outcomes and to explain specific processes.

3.1. Neurobiological Stress and Allostatic Load Model

In the 1950s, Selye proposed the general adaptation syndrome model to describe stress as the reaction of the body to emergency situations [93]. This theory divides the response to stressful stimuli into three phases: (1) Alarm: Upon perceiving a stressor, the body reacts with a "fight-or-flight" response, the sympathetic nervous system (SNS) is stimulated, and the body's resources are mobilized to meet the threat. (2) Resistance: The body resists and compensates as the parasympathetic nervous system (PNS) attempts to return many physiological functions to normal levels, while the body remains on alert and focuses resources against the stressor. (3) Exhaustion: If the stressor continues beyond the body's capacity, the resources are depleted and the body becomes susceptible to disease (distress) [91,93].

A more contemporary concept, which better describes the cumulative impact of stressor exposure on health outcomes, is that of allostasis. Allostasis is the process by which constant changes allow an organism to achieve and maintain normal functions, thus reflecting the ability of the body to adapt to daily situations like exercising or hunger, effectively [94]. However, this continual maintenance costs the body energy and resources, and over time, may lead to symptoms of allostatic load—the functional and structural damage caused by "the wear and tear" of the body's resources in response to stress [95]. Therefore, the response to a new stressor depends on the body's resources available following the previous stress response [96]. The allostatic load is characterized by a cumulative effect, which becomes greatest when stress is chronic or intense [96].

The hypothalamic–pituitary–adrenal (HPA) axis and the autonomic nervous system (comprising SNS and PNS) have been identified as the mediators of this neurobiological stress model [90,91,95]. First, corticotrophin-releasing factor (CRF) is secreted from the paraventricular nucleus in the hypothalamus; the subsequent secretion of adrenocorticotropic hormone (ACTH) from the anterior pituitary stimulates the release of glucocorticoids (mainly cortisol) from the adrenal cortex [97]. Noradrenaline (NA) and adrenaline are also released from the sympathetic nerves and the adrenal medulla, and together with the glucocorticoids regulate the stress response [90,91]. Cortisol also interacts with the serotonergic pathway, adjusting the release of serotonin (5-hydroxytryptamine or 5-HT) neurotransmitter in response to acute or chronic stressors [98]. Serotoninergic neurons modulate the stress response either via direct neurotransmission to the hypothalamus, or by stimulation of noradrenergic neurons [97]. In addition to the regulation through feedback mechanisms, the HPA axis is also modulated by other central systems, particularly by the inhibitory action of the γ-aminobutyric acid (GABA), and the excitatory effect of glutamate [99].

In this neurobiological model, cortisol is a well-known mediator of the stress response. The nocturnal cortisol urinary excretion in apparently healthy subjects reflects the basal tone of the HPA axis [100]; conversely, the blood cortisol concentration measured in a challenging environment is a sign of stress activity [101]. It has been shown that cortisol coordinates the central response to stress at several levels [102], and indirectly influences mechanisms of neuroprotection [103]. Neurotrophic factor production, represented by the brain-derived neurotrophic factor (BNDF), intervenes in allostasis through protecting neurons [104]. Normally, BNDF promotes neuronal survival and plasticity [104]; however, changes in BNDF expression have been reported following exposure to stressful stimuli. An increase of BNDF has been observed in response to moderate stress [105], whereas a decrease has been associated with high levels of stress [106]. Furthermore, increasing evidence shows a link between cortisol responses and oxidant elevation [107]. The accumulation of free radicals and other reactive oxygen species is also a sign of allostatic load, resulting from the imbalance between cellular metabolic activities and antioxidant defense mechanisms [108,109].

Noteworthy, magnesium interacts with all these stress mediators [17,110–112], overall serving an inhibitory function in the regulation and central neurotransmission of the stress response (details of these interactions are summarized in chapter 6).

3.2. Generalized Unsafety Theory of Stress (GUTS) Model

Conventional theories of stress have historically focused on the assumption that stress is a response to an actual environmental threat (either internal or external to the body), making it difficult to explain the relation between stress and disease. In contrast, GUTS is a new psychological and cognitive theoretical model proposed by Brosschot in 2016 [113] that revises and expands the stress theory by focusing on safety instead of threat, and by including risk factors that have hitherto not been attributed to stress [113]. Based on neurobiological and evolutionary evidence, GUTS hypothesizes that stressors are not necessary for a chronic stress response to occur but the perception of an unsafe state is enough. In GUTS, PNS is the key system controlling the stress response (particularly the vagus nerve and the prefrontal cortex activity) [113]. Of note, preclinical data suggest that magnesium may be important for the functionality of these central systems. An excess of magnesium or magnesium deficiency have been shown to modulate the autonomic nervous system, but further research is still needed [114–116].

The GUTS model suggests that the default stress response can be chronically activated in various situations, three of which are particularly susceptible to health risks. (1) Reduced body capacity: In compromised physical conditions, e.g., obesity or aging, the brain perceives the body as inadequate to be able to "fight-or-flight", and therefore maintains a state of general alarm, or unsafety [117]. (2) Compromised social network: Being part of a group is a fundamental aspect of survival for social animals and humans, and isolation is one of the main conditions in which safety is lacking [117]. Interestingly, there is evidence that patients suffering from metabolic syndrome [118] or congestive heart failure [5] (both conditions of reduced body capacity as described in GUTS) exhibit lower serum magnesium concentration. (3) Perceived aversive environment: In cases of specific stressors (e.g., work stressors), a neutral daily environment (e.g., an office working environment) can be perceived as unsafe [117]. The GUTS model suggests that repetitive negative thinking may result in the impairment of key systems controlling the stress response [119]; however, the relationship between general unsafety and magnesium status is to be elucidated yet.

4. Evidence of the Impact of Stress on Magnesium Homeostasis

Initially, the shift from intracellular to extracellular magnesium following a stressor exposure plays a protective and regulatory role [90]. Normally, magnesium inhibits the glutamatergic transmission while promoting GABA activity, resulting in a mostly inhibitory effect at the central level [42]. Magnesium also tends to diminish the stress response mediated by catecholamines and glucocorticoids. However, a chronic stressor exposure may result in a depletion of various resources as described by Selye, including magnesium [42,93]. The progressive loss of magnesium from the reservoir in bone can eventually compromise its physiological inhibitory action and lead to an over-activation of the HPA axis and neuronal hyperactivity [120]. The impact of stress on magnesium status has been extensively investigated in both animal and human studies [42,121].

Pre-clinical evidence. Animal studies have shown a transient hypermagnesemia in the short-term period after the exposure to acute stress stimuli [122–125]. A series of experiments conducted on cats by Classen et al. showed that stimuli such as withdrawal of blood, infusion of catecholamines, or potassium poisoning all caused an increase of blood magnesium concentration [122]. This increase was not influenced by pre-treatment with an adrenergic blocking agent (e.g., reserpine), suggesting that other mechanisms rather than catecholamines are responsible for the change in magnesium levels [122]. Similarly, a shift of magnesium from erythrocytes to serum was reported in different studies investigating the effect of acute noise on magnesium-deficient guinea pigs [123] and rats. As a consequence, a net renal excretion of magnesium occurs, leaving the animal magnesium deficient.

Mild hypomagnesemia can be observed in response to mid- or long-term exposure to stress. A study conducted on guide dog candidates at different levels of a training program (elementary, intermediate, and advanced) showed the effects of temperature and physical stress on serum magnesium levels. First, it was demonstrated that serum magnesium levels were significantly lower in winter than in summer (average temperature was 6 and 29 °C, respectively), suggesting an impact of seasonality on magnesium homeostasis. Thereafter, it was noticed that physical exercise had a greater impact on serum magnesium levels of dog candidates in the elementary class compared to more trained ones. These results were lastly confirmed by a third experiment, assessing both the impact of physical stress and temperature on serum magnesium levels and finding that serum magnesium levels after exercise were significantly lower in winter than in summer. [126]. The impact of physical stressors was assessed also in another study conducted on rats. A greater serum magnesium reduction was observed in those administered with ethanol and then exposed to restraint stress, compared to control rats facing the same restraint test but receiving water [127]. An additional study conducted by Heroux et al. on rats fed with a magnesium-deficient diet and kept at low temperature (6 °C) for about 17 months found that the studied animals were capable of adapting to cold stress despite suboptimal magnesium intake; initial signs of magnesium deficiency (including skin sores, reduced growth rate, lower levels of magnesium in most organs) gradually disappeared after two months. However, regardless this adaptation, the long-term stress resistance (measured as cold resistance at −20 °C) of magnesium-deficient rats was reported to decline over time when compared to controls [128]. Lastly, exposure to cold (2–5 °C) and a deficient dietary intake of magnesium significantly reduced plasma magnesium in sheep, whereas no effect was observed in normally fed sheep [129].

Clinical evidence. To help elucidate the stress hormone-induced magnesium deficiency and its clinical relevance, Whyte et al. investigated the effect produced by the infusion of adrenaline on plasma magnesium concentrations [130]. They found that magnesium levels were significantly reduced not only during the infusion time but also an hour after test cessation, without any sign of recovery [130]. A variety of tests have demonstrated that magnesium levels, both in serum and urine, are affected by the exposure to stress stimuli. Significant reductions in plasma and total magnesium concentrations were reported in a 3-month analysis on young adults exposed to either chronic or sub-chronic stressful conditions (e.g., acts of intolerance or fear of military actions) [43]. A similar effect was also seen in a study investigating the effect of temporary (one day) and chronic (one month) sleep deprivation on magnesium levels; in a group of otherwise healthy men, chronic sleep restriction was associated with greater reductions in erythrocyte magnesium concentrations [131]. University students during an exam period reported an increase in anxiety that was also associated with an increased urinary excretion of magnesium [44]. In a similar study conducted on college students during the 4 weeks following an examination period, erythrocyte magnesium content was found to be significantly depleted [132]. Interestingly, the variations in blood and urine magnesium levels were confirmed by Mocci et al. who studied the effect of noise on catecholamines and magnesium serum and urinary excretions on healthy men [133]. Mocci and his study group also noted how the timing for the change to occur was very different between the two variables, with serum magnesium increasing a few hours after the exposure to the noise (probably reflecting extracellular flux immediately after the stress), and urine excretion reaching a peak in a few hours but lasting up two days [133]. A similar result was reported by Ising et al. on a study investigating the effect of traffic noise on workers' performance. Under noise stress (7 h), a decrease in erythrocyte magnesium levels was observed, followed by an increase of serum levels and urine excretion of magnesium [134]. The impact of acute stress on transient hypermagnesemia was noted also under physical stress. Short- and long-term exercise (20 min versus 1 h, respectively) had a different influence on the plasma magnesium levels: an increase of plasma magnesium was reported after short-term exercise but not after long-term exercise. However, after both physical tests, magnesium levels dropped below the pre-exercise values [135]. A summary of the pre-clinical and clinical evidence is shown in Table 4.

Table 4. Summary of the pre-clinical and clinical evidence supporting the impact of stress on magnesium homeostasis.

	Evidence of the Impact of Stress on Magnesium Homeostasis		
	Population Tested	**Stress Stimulus**	**Impact on Magnesium**
Pre-clinical	Cats (N = 30)	Withdrawal of blood; infusion of catecholamines; potassium poisoning	↑Blood Mg [122]
	Guinea pigs (41)	Noise	↑Serum Mg, ↓Erythrocytes Mg [123]
	Rats (88)	Noise	↑Serum Mg, ↓Erythrocytes Mg [124]
	Rats	Noise	↓Serum Mg, ↓Erythrocytes Mg
	Dogs	Physical exercise, temperature	↓Serum Mg [126]
	Rats	Ethanol/Restraint stress	↓Serum Mg [127]
	Rats	Cold	↓Tissue content of Mg [129]
	Sheep	Dietary Mg restriction, cold	↓Plasma Mg [129]
Clinical	Adults (N = 8)	Adrenaline infusion	↓Plasma Mg [130]
	Young adults (N = 35)	Chronic or sub-chronic psychological stress	↓Plasma Mg [43]
	Healthy men (N = 16)	Chronic sleep deprivation	↓Erythrocyte Mg [131]
	Young adults (N = 35)	University exams	↑Urinary Mg [44]
	Young adults (N = 30)	University exams	↓Erythrocyte Mg [132]
	Young adults (N = 25)	Noise	↑Urinary Mg ↑Serum Mg [133]
	Healthy men (56)	Noise	↑Serum Mg, ↓Erythrocytes Mg; ↑Urinary Mg [134]
	Healthy men	Short- and long-term physical exercise	↑Plasma Mg [135]

Mg, magnesium; ↑, increase; ↓, decrease.

5. Evidence of the Impact of Magnesium Status on Stress Susceptibility

Pre-clinical evidence. The relationship between magnesium deficiency and stress-related behavior is well documented. In 1986, Caddell et al. reported an increase of circulating catecholamines following the exposure of magnesium-deficient rats to a noise stress test [136]. The relationship between low serum magnesium concentrations and the increased release of catecholamines in the central nervous system was then confirmed in studies conducted on mice selected for low (MGL) and high (MGH) blood magnesium. The simple selection of genetic traits inducing low blood magnesium was found to significantly affect the metabolism of NA but not that of other neurotransmitters [137]. MGL mice not only showed higher NA levels (17% in the brain; 200% in urine) but also a more restless behavior and higher rectal temperature, all signs of an exaggerated stress response [138]. In a different study also conducted on MGL and MGH mice, both fed with the same magnesium-rich diet, the number of stress-induced gastric ulcers through the immobilization test was higher in the magnesium-deficient mice [139]. Besides the noradrenergic hyperactivity in basal magnesium deficiency conditions, dietary magnesium restrictions have also been associated with an upregulation of the stress system via increases in CRH and ACTH levels [140]. Experimental data indicate that magnesium-deficient rats exhibit more anxiety- and depression-like behavior compared with controls [42,138]. For example, in the light–dark test (often used to screen for anxiolytic and antidepressant drugs) [141], mice with magnesium deficiency showed a net preference for the darker compartment [42,140,141]. Similarly, in the forced swimming test, magnesium-deficient rats spent more time immobile compared with their controls [142,143]. Dietary magnesium deficiency in laboratory animals was also associated with stress-like behavior in the open field test. Rats with a reduced dietary magnesium content tended to visit the bright and central area less frequently [142,143], even when motivated by the presence of food, showing a psychological stress caused by the open space [140].

Clinical evidence. Results in human studies are consistent with animal findings and show low magnesium status in stressed/depressed populations. In a study investigating the potential benefit of magnesium supplementation in Russian women who suffered from chronic emotional stress, Akarachkova et al. found that at baseline the majority of women were suffering from symptoms like irritability, fatigue, and sleep disorders, and 60% presented magnesium deficiency [144]. In other studies, subclinical chronic magnesium deficiency was found in up to 45% of the stressed subjects enrolled [78,145,146]. Nielsen et al. found that out of 96 American adults complaining of sleep disorders, a potential source of stress, 58% were consuming less than the EAR for magnesium and had higher levels of C-reactive protein (CRP), an indicator of inflammatory stress [145]. Lastly, it is generally recognized that chronic stress and magnesium deficiency may influence an individual's susceptibility to depressive disorders [147]. In a group of Australian patients experiencing depression and/or anxiety, the analysis of their nutrition status showed that 22% of participants did not meet magnesium EAR. Furthermore, magnesium intake (expressed as % EAR) was negatively correlated with stress, depression, and total Depression Anxiety Stress Scale (DASS) scores [148].

A summary of the pre-clinical and clinical evidence supporting a relation between magnesium status and stress is shown in Table 5.

Table 5. Summary of the pre-clinical and clinical evidence supporting magnesium status on stress susceptibility. [a] Only symptoms shown in ≥70% of women at baseline are reported.

Evidence of the Impact of Magnesium Status on Stress Susceptibility				
	Population Tested	Mg Status	Stress Stimulus	Impact on Stress Mediator/Stress
Pre-clinical	Rats (N = 84)	Mg-deficient	Noise	↑Catecholamines (NA, adrenaline, dopamine) [136]
	Mice (N = 120)	Mg-deficient	Genetic selection	↑NA [137]
	Mice (N = 80)	Mg-deficient	Genetic selection; forced swimming test; four-plate test	↑NA [138]
	Mice (N = 100)	Mg-deficient	Genetic selection; immobilization test	↑Gastric ulcers [139]
	Mice (N = 20/test)	Dietary Mg restriction	Hyperthermia; open field test; light/dark test; hyponeophagia test	↑CRH; ↑ACHT [140]
	Mice	Mg-deficient	Light/dark test	Depression-like behavior [42,140]
	Rats	Dietary Mg restriction	Forced swimming test	Depression-like behavior [142,143]
	Rats	Dietary Mg restriction	Open field test	Stress/anxiety [142,143]
Clinical	Women (N = 100)	Mg-deficient	-	Chronic emotional stress; irritability; fatigue; sleep disturbance; headache [a] [144]
	Adults (N = 264)	Mg-deficient	-	Severe stress [78,145,146]
	Adults (N = 100)	Mg-deficient	Poor sleep quality	↑CRP [145]
	Adults (N = 109)	Mg-deficient	-	Depression/anxiety [148]

ACHTH, adrenocorticotropic hormone; CRH, corticotrophin-releasing hormone; CRP, C-reactive protein; Mg, magnesium; NA, noradrenaline; ↑, increase.

6. Proposed Model for the Vicious Circle of Stress and Magnesium Deficiency

Over the years, a growing body of evidence has consistently shown that magnesium acts on several key physiological steps involved in the response to stressful stimuli.

- Magnesium and HPA. *5-HT transmission:* Magnesium directly enhances the interaction between 5-HT and its membrane receptor, and it promotes the cellular transmission of the serotoninergic signal (Figure 2A) [90]. Additionally, magnesium is a cofactor of tryptophan hydroxylase, the enzyme involved in 5-HT synthesis [90]. Glutamatergic transmission: Magnesium inhibits the glutamate directly and indirectly by blocking the glutamate N-methyl-D-aspartate (NMDA) receptor and by enhancing its reuptake in the synaptic vesicles through stimulation of the sodium–potassium ATPase, respectively (Figure 2B) [42]. GABA transmission: A GABA-agonistic activity of magnesium has been observed, although the mechanism has not yet been elucidated,

(Figure 2B) [42]. *Cortisol:* Magnesium indirectly reduces the release of ACTH by modulating the neurotransmission pathways, and therefore decreases cortisol levels in the body [42];

- Magnesium and neuroprotection. Studies on the antidepressant effects of magnesium have shown the positive impact of this mineral on the expression of BNDF in the brain [149,150];
- Magnesium and oxidative stress. Magnesium may be involved in suppressing the production of free radicals in various tissues including the brain [17], and several laboratory studies have shown that magnesium-deficient animals are more at risk of oxidative stress [112,151].

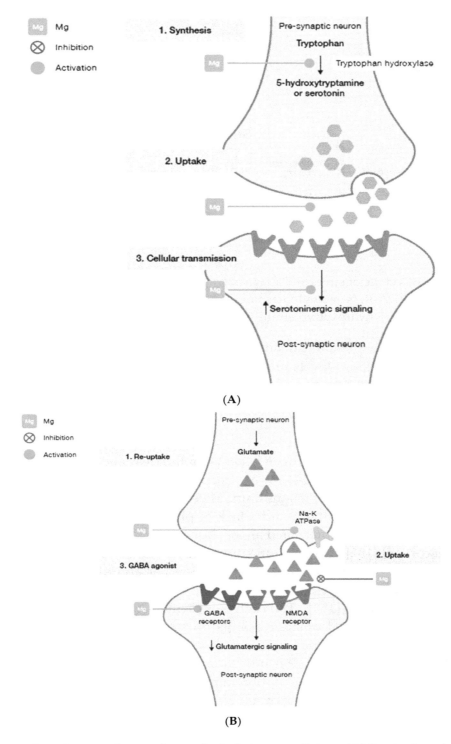

Figure 2. Interaction of magnesium and neurological stress mediators. (**A**) Serotoninergic transmission. (**B**) Glutamatergic and GABAergic transmission. GABA, γ-aminobutyric acid; Mg, magnesium; NMDA, N-methyl-D-aspartate.

In response to a stressful stimulus, stress hormones are released, causing an increase of magnesium extracellular levels [90]. As a consequence, higher magnesium concentrations are excreted through the kidneys [133]. When the stressor persists over time, this mechanism may contribute to magnesium cation depletion and deficiency [42,130], and trigger the stress and magnesium vicious circle as illustrated in Figure 3.

Figure 3. The vicious circle of stress and magnesium. GABAA-R, γ-aminobutyric acid-A receptor; Mg, magnesium; NMDA-R, N-methyl-D-aspartate receptor; NA, noradrenaline; SNS, sympathetic nervous system, 5HT-R, 5-hydroxytryptamine receptor.

Comprehensively, both pre-clinical and clinical studies' results point to the bi-directional relationship between magnesium levels and stress: Magnesium deficiency can induce symptoms and increase susceptibility to stress, and acute and chronic stress can precipitate magnesium deficiency [10,104,106].

7. Magnesium Supplementation

Magnesium supplementation has proven benefits for the treatment of symptoms of psychological daily stress (fatigue, irritability, sleep) [144]. It has been shown that subjects with mental and physical stress can benefit from a daily intake of magnesium. Male students experiencing common stress factors such as sleep deprivation, malnutrition, and a lack of physical activity, and receiving magnesium 250 mg/day for four weeks not only presented an increase in erythrocyte magnesium content but also a reduction of serum cortisol [152]. Magnesium supplementation of 400 mg/day was associated with a clear improvement of the heart rate variability, measured as an indicator of the parasympathetic and vagal systems' response to stress, in subjects who were asked to complete moderate muscle endurance training once weekly [153]. The daily supplementation with 300 mg (combined or not with vitamin B6, 30 mg) provided positive results on stress relief [154], particularly on subjects who reported severe stress levels at baseline, with a reduction in Depression Anxiety Stress Scale scores of up to 45% from baseline [154]. It is interesting to note that several studies investigating the potential benefit of magnesium supplementation in populations with symptoms of stress reported a subclinical chronic magnesium deficiency or a low magnesium status at baseline in the majority of the subjects enrolled [37,78,144–146]. Nevertheless, despite several studies reporting an association between magnesium deficiency and stress, the effect of magnesium supplementation on stress has been less documented than its effects on depression [37,155] and anxiety disorders [156]; therefore, further investigation is still needed on stress symptoms. A possible limiting factor to the performance of such studies could be the difficulty of setting up optimal experimental conditions for studying the effect of stress; however, this challenge may be overcome in future analyses by focusing on well-defined conditions (e.g., psychological stress), and by using robust and validated tools to assess stress (such as DASS scores).

8. Conclusions: Implications in Terms of Dietary Magnesium Needs

Over the past decades, increasing evidence, as shown in the present narrative review, has investigated and supported the link between magnesium deficiency and increased susceptibility to stress disorders, and further suggested that stress itself can lead to magnesium depletion. Magnesium is an essential element involved in reactions regulating the body's stress response at several levels. Severe magnesium deficiency is rare, but chronic latent deficiency appears to be common among the general population and even more among those suffering from a number of chronic diseases or stress [5]. Although the current intake of magnesium through our diet seems sufficient to avoid overt signs of magnesium deficiency in the majority of the population, it might not be adequate to provide optimal health and risk reduction of chronic diseases [5]. Stress is also an increasing condition worldwide and its effects can negatively impact health outcomes. Noteworthy, magnesium intake has been found negatively correlated with subjective stress in some populations [148], and magnesium supplementation has shown benefits in stressed but otherwise healthy subjects [153,154]. Additionally, magnesium intake is safe with limited side-effects in cases of chronic overconsumption [72].

To conclude, while there is good evidence from animal and human studies of the bi-directional link between magnesium and stress, further research is needed to better understand the impact of this correlation and the benefit of magnesium supplementation on general health. Additional studies should apply standard methodologies (e.g., magnesium load test) to evaluate the magnesium status in well-characterized stressed population. These studies would help to demonstrate the increased need of magnesium supplementation during stress periods, and further strengthen our initial hypothesis. Further, in line with the GUTS model, repetitive negative thinking could be considered as a cognitive indicator of stress and evaluated in relation to blood magnesium levels in a cohort of subjects exposed to chronic stress. Given the strong association of stress with mental and physical diseases, these studies are fundamental to further support adequate magnesium dietary needs.

Author Contributions: Conceptualization, M.A., L.N.; writing—original draft preparation, and writing—review and editing, G.P., A.M., M.T., P.B., N.Y., M.A., L.N., E.P.; supervision, project administration, funding acquisition, A.M., L.N. All authors have read and agreed to the published version of the manuscript.

Acknowledgments: Editorial support was provided by Martina Klinger Sikora and Mark Davies of inScience Communications, Springer Healthcare Ltd., UK.

References

1. Kessler, R.C.; Aguilar-Gaxiola, S.; Alonso, J.; Chatterji, S.; Lee, S.; Ormel, J.; Üstün, T.B.; Wang, P.S. The global burden of mental disorders: An update from the WHO World Mental Health (WMH) Surveys. *Epidemiol. Psichiatr. Soc.* **2009**, *18*, 23–33. [CrossRef] [PubMed]
2. McEwen, B.S.; Akil, H. Revisiting the Stress Concept: Implications for Affective Disorders. *J. Neurosci.* **2020**, *40*, 12–21. [CrossRef] [PubMed]
3. Konrad, M.; Schlingmann, K.P.; Gudermann, T. Insights into the molecular nature of magnesium homeostasis. *Am. J. Physiol. Renal. Physiol.* **2004**, *286*, F599–F605. [CrossRef] [PubMed]
4. Pham, P.C.; Pham, P.M.; Pham, S.V.; Miller, J.M.; Pham, P.T. Hypomagnesemia in patients with type 2 diabetes. *Clin. J. Am. Soc. Nephrol.* **2007**, *2*, 366–373. [CrossRef]
5. DiNicolantonio, J.J.; O'Keefe, J.H.; Wilson, W. Subclinical magnesium deficiency: A principal driver of cardiovascular disease and a public health crisis. *Open Heart* **2018**, *5*, e000668. [CrossRef]
6. American Psychological Association. Stress Effects on the Body. Available online: https://www.apa.org/helpcenter/stress (accessed on 30 June 2020).
7. American Psychological Association. Understanding Chronic Stress. Available online: https://www.apa.org/

helpcenter/understanding-chronic-stress.aspx (accessed on 30 June 2020).

8.   De Baaij, J.H.; Hoenderop, J.G.; Bindels, R.J. Magnesium in man: Implications for health and disease. *Physiol. Rev.* **2015**, *95*, 1–46. [CrossRef]

9.   Galland, L. Magnesium, stress and neuropsychiatric disorders. *Magnes. Trace Elem.* **1991**, *10*, 287–301.

10.   Seelig, M.S. Consequences of magnesium deficiency on the enhancement of stress reactions; preventive and therapeutic implications (a review). *J. Am. Coll. Nutr.* **1994**, *13*, 429–446. [CrossRef]

11.   American Psychological Association. 2015 Stress in America. Available online: https://www.apa.org/news/press/releases/stress/2015/snapshot (accessed on 10 August 2020).

12.   Costello, R.; Wallace, T.C.; Rosanoff, A. Magnesium. *Adv. Nutr.* **2016**, *7*, 199–201. [CrossRef]

13.   Reddy, S.T.; Soman, S.S.; Yee, J. Magnesium Balance and Measurement. *Adv. Chronic Kidney Dis.* **2018**, *25*, 224–229. [CrossRef] [PubMed]

14.   Glasdam, S.M.; Glasdam, S.; Peters, G.H. The Importance of Magnesium in the Human Body: A Systematic Literature Review. *Adv. Clin. Chem.* **2016**, *73*, 169–193. [CrossRef] [PubMed]

15.   Bergman, C.; Gray-Scott, D.; Chen, J.J.; Meacham, S. What is next for the Dietary Reference Intakes for bone metabolism related nutrients beyond calcium: Phosphorus, magnesium, vitamin D, and fluoride? *Crit Rev Food Sci. Nutr.* **2009**, *49*, 136–144. [CrossRef] [PubMed]

16.   EFSA Panel on Dietetic Products Nutrition and Allergies (NDA). Scientific Opinion on Dietary Reference Values for magnesium. *EFSA J.* **2015**, *13*, 4186. [CrossRef]

17.   Yamanaka, R.; Shindo, Y.; Oka, K. Magnesium Is a Key Player in Neuronal Maturation and Neuropathology. *Int. J. Mol. Sci.* **2019**, *20*, 3439. [CrossRef] [PubMed]

18.   Ghabriel, M.N.; Vink, R. Magnesium transport across the blood-brain barriers. In *Magnesium in the Central Nervous System*; Nechifor, M., Vink, R., Eds.; The University of Adelaide Press: Adelaide, Australia, 2011; pp. 59–74. [CrossRef]

19.   Morris, M.E. Brain and CSF magnesium concentrations during magnesium deficit in animals and humans: Neurological symptoms. *Magnes. Res.* **1992**, *5*, 303–313. [PubMed]

20.   Chutkow, J.G. Uptake of magnesium into the brain of the rat. *Exp. Neurol.* **1978**, *60*, 592–602. [CrossRef]

21.   Jahnen-Dechent, W.; Ketteler, M. Magnesium basics. *Clin. Kidney J.* **2012**, *5*, i3–i14. [CrossRef]

22.   Ross, C.A.; Caballero, B.; Cousins, R.J.; Tucker, K.L.; Ziegler, T.R. *Modern Nutrition in Health and Disease*, 11th ed.; Lippincott Williams & Wilkins: Baltimore, MD, USA, 2014; pp. 159–175.

23.   Clarkson, E.M.; Warren, R.L.; McDonald, S.J.; de Wardener, H.E. The effect of a high intake of calcium on magnesium metabolism in normal subjects and patients with chronic renal failure. *Clin. Sci.* **1967**, *32*, 11–18.

24.   Norman, D.A.; Fordtran, J.S.; Brinkley, L.J.; Zerwekh, J.E.; Nicar, M.J.; Strowig, S.M.; Pak, C.Y. Jejunal and ileal adaptation to alterations in dietary calcium: Changes in calcium and magnesium absorption and pathogenetic role of parathyroid hormone and 1,25-dihydroxyvitamin D. *J. Clin. Investig.* **1981**, *67*, 1599–1603. [CrossRef]

25.   Johnson, S. The multifaceted and widespread pathology of magnesium deficiency. *Med. Hypotheses* **2001**, *56*, 163–170. [CrossRef]

26.   Ayuk, J.; Gittoes, N.J. Contemporary view of the clinical relevance of magnesium homeostasis. *Ann. Clin. Biochem.* **2014**, *51*, 179–188. [CrossRef] [PubMed]

27.   Gröber, U. Magnesium and Drugs. *Int. J. Mol. Sci.* **2019**, *20*, 2094. [CrossRef] [PubMed]

28.   Dalton, L.M.; DM, N.F.; Gaydadzhieva, G.T.; Mazurkiewicz, O.M.; Leeson, H.; Wright, C.P. Magnesium in pregnancy. *Nutr. Rev.* **2016**, *74*, 549–557. [CrossRef] [PubMed]

29.   Morton, A. Hypomagnesaemia and pregnancy. *Obstet. Med.* **2018**, *11*, 67–72. [CrossRef] [PubMed]

30.   Parazzini, F.; Di Martino, M.; Pellegrino, P. Magnesium in the gynecological practice: A literature review. *Magnes. Res.* **2017**, *30*, 1–7. [CrossRef]

31.   Seelig, M.S.; Preuss, H.G. Magnesium metabolism and perturbations in the elderly. *Geriatr. Nephrol. Urol.* **1994**, *4*, 101–111. [CrossRef]

32.   Lo Piano, F.; Corsonello, A.; Corica, F. Magnesium and elderly patient: The explored paths and the ones to be explored: A review. *Magnes. Res.* **2019**, *32*, 1–15. [CrossRef]

33.   Swaminathan, R. Magnesium metabolism and its disorders. *Clin. Biochem. Rev.* **2003**, *24*, 47–66.

34.   Guerrero-Romero, F.; Rodríguez-Morán, M. Low serum magnesium levels and metabolic syndrome. *Acta Diabetol.* **2002** *39*, 209–213. [CrossRef]

35. Viering, D.H.H.M.; de Baaij, J.H.F.; Walsh, S.B.; Kleta, R.; Bockenhauer, D. Genetic causes of hypomagnesemia, a clinical overview. *Pediatr. Nephrol.* **2017**, *32*, 1123–1135. [CrossRef]

36. Naderi, A.S.A.; Reilly, R.F. Hereditary etiologies of hypomagnesemia. *Nat. Clin. Pract. Nephrol.* **2008**, *4*, 80–89. [CrossRef] [PubMed]

37. Botturi, A.; Ciappolino, V.; Delvecchio, G.; Boscutti, A.; Viscardi, B.; Brambilla, P. The Role and the Effect of Magnesium in Mental Disorders: A Systematic Review. *Nutrients* **2020**, *12*, 1661. [CrossRef] [PubMed]

38. Nielsen, F.H.; Lukaski, H.C. Update on the relationship between magnesium and exercise. *Magnes. Res.* **2006**, *19*, 180–189. [PubMed]

39. Laires, M.J.; Monteiro, C. Exercise and Magnesium. In *New Perspectives in Magnesium Research: Nutrition and Health*; Nishizawa, Y., Morii, H., Durlach, J., Eds.; Springer: London, UK, 2007; pp. 173–185. [CrossRef]

40. Warburton, D.E.R.; Welsh, R.C.; Haykowsky, M.J.; Taylor, D.A.; Humen, D.P. Biochemical changes as a result of prolonged strenuous exercise. *Br. J. Sports Med.* **2002**, *36*, 301. [CrossRef]

41. Ikonte, C.J.; Mun, J.G.; Reider, C.A.; Grant, R.W.; Mitmesser, S.H. Micronutrient Inadequacy in Short Sleep: Analysis of the NHANES 2005–2016. *Nutrients* **2019**, *11*, 2335. [CrossRef]

42. Murck, H. Magnesium and affective disorders. *Nutr. Neurosci.* **2002**, *5*, 375–389. [CrossRef]

43. Cernak, I.; Savic, V.; Kotur, J.; Prokic, V.; Kuljic, B.; Grbovic, D.; Veljovic, M. Alterations in magnesium and oxidative status during chronic emotional stress. *Magnes. Res.* **2000**, *13*, 29–36.

44. Grases, G.; Pérez-Castelló, J.A.; Sanchis, P.; Casero, A.; Perelló, J.; Isern, B.; Rigo, E.; Grases, F. Anxiety and stress among science students. Study of calcium and magnesium alterations. *Magnes. Res.* **2006**, *19*, 102–106.

45. Classen, H.G. Systemic stress, magnesium status and cardiovascular damage. *Magnesium* **1986**, *5*, 105–110.

46. United States Department of Health and Human Services. *Scientific Report of the 2015 Dietary Guidelines Advisory Committee—Advisory Report to the Secretary of Health and Human Services and the Secretary of Agriculture*; USDA Agricoltural Research Service: Washngton, DC, USA, 2015.

47. Agence Nationale de Sécurité Sanitaire de L'alimentation de L'environnement et du Travail (ANSES). *TANSES-CIQUAL French Food Composition Table, Version 2017*; ANSES: Maisons-Alfort, France, 2017.

48. Costello, R.B.; Elin, R.J.; Rosanoff, A.; Wallace, T.C.; Guerrero-Romero, F.; Hruby, A.; Lutsey, P.L.; Nielsen, F.H.; Rodriguez-Moran, M.; Song, Y.; et al. Perspective: The Case for an Evidence-Based Reference Interval for Serum Magnesium: The Time Has Come. *Adv. Nutr.* **2016**, *7*, 977–993. [CrossRef]

49. Ford, E.S.; Mokdad, A.H. Dietary Magnesium Intake in a National Sample of U.S. Adults. *J. Nutr.* **2003**, *133*, 2879–2882. [CrossRef] [PubMed]

50. Winiarska-Mieczan, A.; Zaricka, E.; Kwiecień, M.; Kwiatkowska, K.; Baranowska-Wójcik, E.; Danek-Majewska, A. Can Cereal Products Be an Essential Source of Ca, Mg and K in the Deficient Diets of Poles? *Biol. Trace Elem. Res.* **2020**, *195*, 317–322. [CrossRef] [PubMed]

51. Górska-Warsewicz, H.; Rejman, K.; Laskowski, W.; Czeczotko, M. Milk and Dairy Products and Their Nutritional Contribution to the Average Polish Diet. *Nutrients* **2019**, *11*, 1771. [CrossRef] [PubMed]

52. Lombardi-Boccia, G.; Aguzzi, A.; Cappelloni, M.; Di Lullo, G.; Lucarini, M. Total-diet study: Dietary intakes of macro elements and trace elements in Italy. *Br. J. Nutr.* **2003**, *90*, 1117–1121. [CrossRef] [PubMed]

53. Nielsen, F.H. The Problematic Use of Dietary Reference Intakes to Assess Magnesium Status and Clinical Importance. *Biol. Trace Elem. Res.* **2019**, *188*, 52–59. [CrossRef] [PubMed]

54. Dong, J.Y.; Xun, P.; He, K.; Qin, L.Q. Magnesium intake and risk of type 2 diabetes: Meta-analysis of prospective cohort studies. *Diabetes Care* **2011**, *34*, 2116–2122. [CrossRef] [PubMed]

55. Schwartz, R.; Apgar, B.J.; Wien, E.M. Apparent absorption and retention of Ca, Cu, Mg, Mn, and Zn from a diet containing bran. *Am. J. Clin. Nutr.* **1986**, *43*, 444–455. [CrossRef]

56. Lakshmanan, F.L.; Rao, R.B.; Kim, W.W.; Kelsay, J.L. Magnesium intakes, balances, and blood levels of adults consuming self-selected diets. *Am. J. Clin. Nutr.* **1984**, *40*, 1380–1389. [CrossRef]

57. Greger, J.L.; Baier, M.J. Effect of dietary aluminum on mineral metabolism of adult males. *Dev. Med. Child Neurol.* **1983**, *38*, 411–419. [CrossRef]

58. Standing Commitee on the Scientific Evaluation of Dietary Reference Intakes Institute of Medicine. Dietary reference intakes for calcium, phosphorus, magnesium, vitamin D, and fluoride. In *Dietary Reference Intakes for Calcium, Phosphorus, Magnesium, Vitamin D, and Fluoride*; National Acedemies Press, Ed.; The National Academies Press: Washington, DC, USA, 1997; pp. 190–249.

59. Jarosz, M. *Nutritional Guidelines for the Polish Population*; National Food and Nutrition Institute, Ed.; National

Food and Nutrition Institute: Warsaw, Poland, 2017.

60. Tutel'ian, V.A. Norms of physiological requirements in energy and nutrients in various groups of population in Russian Federation. *Vopr. Pitan.* **2009**, *78*, 4–15.

61. Ministry of Health Labour and Welfare. *Dietary Reference Intakes for Japanese*; Japan Government Printing Office, Ed.; Ministry of Health Labour and Welfare: Tokyo, Japan, 2015.

62. Società Italiana di Nutrizione Umana-SINU. LARN—Livelli di Assunzione di Riferimento per la Popolazione Italiana: MINERALI. Assunzione Raccomandata per la Popolazione (PRI in Grassetto) e Assunzione Adeguata (AI in Corsivo): Valori su Base Giornaliera. Available online: https://sinu.it/2019/07/09/minerali-assunzione-raccomandata-per-la-popolazione-pri-e-assunzione-adeguataai/ (accessed on 30 June 2020).

63. Agence Nationale de Sécurité Sanitaire de L'alimentation de L'environnement et du Travail (ANSES). Avis de l'ANSES. In *Actualisation des Repères du PNNS: Élaborationdes Références Nutritionnelles*; ANSES, Ed.; ANSES: Maisons-Alfort, France, 2016.

64. Vormann, J. Magnesium: Nutrition and metabolism. *Mol. Asp. Med.* **2003**, *24*, 27–37. [CrossRef]

65. King, D.E.; Mainous, A.G., 3rd; Geesey, M.E.; Woolson, R.F. Dietary magnesium and C-reactive protein levels. *J. Am. Coll. Nutr.* **2005**, *24*, 166–171. [CrossRef] [PubMed]

66. Bailey, R.L.; Fulgoni, V.L., 3rd; Keast, D.R.; Dwyer, J.T. Dietary supplement use is associated with higher intakes of minerals from food sources. *Am. J. Clin. Nutr.* **2011**, *94*, 1376–1381. [CrossRef] [PubMed]

67. Public Health England. *Official Statistics NDNS: Results from Years 7 and 8 (Combined). Results of the National Diet and Nutrition Survey (NDNS) Rolling Programme for 2014 to 2015 and 2015 to 2016*; Public Health England: England, UK, 2018.

68. Agence Nationale de Sécurité Sanitaire de L'alimentation de L'environnement et du Travail (ANSES). *Avis de l'ANSES relatif à l'évaluation des apports en vitamines et minéraux issus de l'alimentation non enrichie, de l'alimentation enrichie et des compléments alimentaires dans la population Française: estimation des aApports usuels, des prévalences d'inadéquation et des risques de dépassement des limites de sécurité (Saisine n° 2012-SA-0142)*; ANSES, Ed.; ANSES: Maisons-Alfort, France, 2015.

69. Olza, J.; Aranceta-Bartrina, J.; González-Gross, M.; Ortega, R.M.; Serra-Majem, L.; Varela-Moreiras, G.; Gil, Á. Reported Dietary Intake, Disparity between the Reported Consumption and the Level Needed for Adequacy and Food Sources of Calcium, Phosphorus, Magnesium and Vitamin D in the Spanish Population: Findings from the ANIBES Study. *Nutrients* **2017**, *9*, 168. [CrossRef]

70. Castiglione, D.; Platania, A.; Conti, A.; Falla, M.; D'Urso, M.; Marranzano, M. Dietary Micronutrient and Mineral Intake in the Mediterranean Healthy Eating, Ageing, and Lifestyle (MEAL) Study. *Antioxidants* **2018**, *7*, 79. [CrossRef]

71. Mensink, G.B.; Fletcher, R.; Gurinovic, M.; Huybrechts, I.; Lafay, L.; Serra-Majem, L.; Szponar, L.; Tetens, I.; Verkaik-Kloosterman, J.; Baka, A.; et al. Mapping low intake of micronutrients across Europe. *Br. J. Nutr.* **2013**, *110*, 755–773. [CrossRef]

72. National Institute of Health, Office of Dietary Supplements. Magnesium. Available online: https://ods.od.nih.gov/factsheets/Magnesium-HealthProfessional/#en1 (accessed on 10 August 2020).

73. Institute of Medicine. *Dietary Reference Intakes for Calcium, Phosphorus, Magnesium, Vitamin D, and Fluoride*; The National Academies Press: Washington, DC, USA, 1997; p. 448. [CrossRef]

74. Spätling, L.; Classen, H.G.; Külpmann, W.R.; Manz, F.; Rob, P.M.; Schimatschek, H.F.; Vierling, W.; Vormann, J.; Weigert, A.; Wink, K. Diagnosing magnesium deficiency. Current recommendations of the Society for Magnesium Research. *Fortschr. Med. Orig.* **2000**, *118* (Suppl. 2), 49–53.

75. Lowenstein, F.W.; Stanton, M.F. Serum magnesium levels in the United States, 1971–1974. *J. Am. Coll. Nutr.* **1986**, *5*, 399–414. [CrossRef]

76. Topf, J.M.; Murray, P.T. Hypomagnesemia and hypermagnesemia. *Rev. Endocr. Metab. Disord.* **2003**, *4*, 195–206. [CrossRef]

77. Elin, R.J. Assessment of magnesium status for diagnosis and therapy. *Magnes. Res.* **2010**, *23*, S194–S198. [CrossRef]

78. Noah, L.; Pickering, G.; Mazur, A.; Dubray, C.; Hitier, S.; Dualé, C.; Pouteau, E. Impact of magnesium supplementation, in combination with vitamin B6, on stress and magnesium status: Secondary data from a randomised controlled trial. *Magnes. Res. J.* **2020**, *33*, 45–57.

79. Rosanoff, A.; Weaver, C.M.; Rude, R.K. Suboptimal magnesium status in the United States: Are the health consequences underestimated? *Nutr. Rev.* **2012** *70*, 153–164. [CrossRef] [PubMed]

80. Meyer, T.E.; Verwoert, G.C.; Hwang, S.J.; Glazer, N.L.; Smith, A.V.; van Rooij, F.J.; Ehret, G.B.; Boerwinkle, E.; Felix, J.F.; Leak, T.S.; et al. Genome-wide association studies of serum magnesium, potassium, and sodium concentrations identify six Loci influencing serum magnesium levels. *PLoS Genet.* **2010**, *6*, e1001045. [CrossRef] [PubMed]

81. Moshfegh, A.; Goldman, J.; Ahuja, J.; Rhodes, D.; LaComb, R. *What We Eat in America, NHANES 2005–2006. Usual Nutrient Intakes from Food and Water Compared to 1997 Dietary Reference Intakes for Vitamid D, Calcium, Phosphorus, and Magnesium*; United States Department of Agriculture, Agricultural Research Service, Eds.; 2009. Available online: https://www.ars.usda.gov/ARSUserFiles/80400530/pdf/0506/usual_nutrient_intake_vitD_ca_phos_mg_2005-06.pdf (accessed on 30,June 2020).

82. Guo, W.; Nazim, H.; Liang, Z.; Yang, D. Magnesium deficiency in plants: An urgent problem. *Crop J.* **2016**, *4*, 83–91. [CrossRef]

83. Cakmak, I. Magnesium in crop production, food quality and human health. *Plant Soil* **2013**, *368*, 1–4. [CrossRef]

84. Workinger, J.L.; Doyle, R.P.; Bortz, J. Challenges in the Diagnosis of Magnesium Status. *Nutrients* **2018**, *10*, 1202. [CrossRef]

85. Worthington, V. Nutritional quality of organic versus conventional fruits, vegetables, and grains. *J. Altern. Complement. Med.* **2001**, *7*, 161–173. [CrossRef]

86. Thomas, D. The mineral depletion of foods available to us as a nation (1940–2002)—A Review of the 6th Edition of McCance and Widdowson. *Nutr. Health* **2007**, *19*, 21–55. [CrossRef]

87. Du, J.; Zhu, M.; Bao, H.; Li, B.; Dong, Y.; Xiao, C.; Zhang, G.Y.; Henter, I.; Rudorfer, M.; Vitiello, B. The Role of Nutrients in Protecting Mitochondrial Function and Neurotransmitter Signaling: Implications for the Treatment of Depression, PTSD, and Suicidal Behaviors. *Crit. Rev. Food Sci. Nutr.* **2016**, *56*, 2560–2578. [CrossRef]

88. Fromm, L.; Heath, D.L.; Vink, R.; Nimmo, A.J. Magnesium Attenuates Post-Traumatic Depression/Anxiety Following Diffuse Traumatic Brain Injury in Rats. *J. Am. Coll. Nutr.* **2004**, *23*, 529S–533S. [CrossRef]

89. Veronese, N.; Solmi, M. Impaired Magnesium Status and Depression. In *Handbook of Famine, Starvation, and Nutrient Deprivation: From Biology to Policy*; Preedy, V.R., Patel, V.B., Eds.; Springer: Berlin/Heidelberg, Germany, 2019; pp. 1861–1872. [CrossRef]

90. Cuciureanu, M.; Vink, R. Magnesium and stress. In *Magnesium in the Central Nervous System*; Vink, R., Nechifor, M., Eds.; University of Adelaide Press: Adelaide, Australia, 2011.

91. Chrousos, G.P. Stress and disorders of the stress system. *Nat. Rev. Endocrinol.* **2009**, *5*, 374–381. [CrossRef] [PubMed]

92. Yaribeygi, H.; Panahi, Y.; Sahraei, H.; Johnston, T.P.; Sahebkar, A. The impact of stress on body function: A review. *EXCLI J.* **2017**, *16*, 1057–1072. [CrossRef] [PubMed]

93. Selye, H. Stress and the general adaptation syndrome. *Br. Med. J.* **1950**, *1*, 1383–1392. [CrossRef] [PubMed]

94. Clark, M.S.; Bond, M.J.; Hecker, J.R. Environmental stress, psychological stress and allostatic load. *Psychol. Health Med.* **2007**, *12*, 18–30. [CrossRef] [PubMed]

95. McEwen, B.S. Protective and damaging effects of stress mediators. *N. Engl. J. Med.* **1998**, *338*, 171–179. [CrossRef]

96. McEwen, B.S. Protection and damage from acute and chronic stress: Allostasis and allostatic overload and relevance to the pathophysiology of psychiatric disorders. *Ann. N. Y. Acad Sci* **2004**, *1032*, 1–7. [CrossRef]

97. Carrasco, G.A.; Van de Kar, L.D. Neuroendocrine pharmacology of stress. *Eur. J. Pharm.* **2003**, *463*, 235–272. [CrossRef]

98. Lanfumey, L.; Mongeau, R.; Cohen-Salmon, C.; Hamon, M. Corticosteroid-serotonin interactions in the neurobiological mechanisms of stress-related disorders. *Neurosci. Biobehav. Rev.* **2008**, *32*, 1174–1184. [CrossRef]

99. Herman, J.P.; Mueller, N.K.; Figueiredo, H. Role of GABA and glutamate circuitry in hypothalamo-pituitary-adrenocortical stress integration. *Ann. N. Y. Acad. Sci.* **2004**, *1018*, 35–45. [CrossRef]

100. Nakamura, J.; Yakata, M. Two-cycle liquid-chromatographic quantitation of cortisol in urine. *Clin. Chem.* **1982**, *28*, 1497–1500. [CrossRef]

101. Singh, A.; Petrides, J.S.; Gold, P.W.; Chrousos, G.P.; Deuster, P.A. Differential hypothalamic-pituitary-adrenal axis reactivity to psychological and physical stress. *J. Clin. Endocrinol. Metab.* **1999**, *84*, 1944–1948. [CrossRef] [PubMed]

102. Ullmann, E.; Perry, S.W.; Licinio, J.; Wong, M.-L.; Dremencov, E.; Zavjalov, E.L.; Shevelev, O.B.; Khotskin, N.V.; Koncevaya, G.V.; Khotshkina, A.S.; et al. From Allostatic Load to Allostatic State—An Endogenous Sympathetic Strategy to Deal With Chronic Anxiety and Stress? *Front. Behav. Neurosci.* **2019**, *13*. [CrossRef] [PubMed]

103. de Assis, G.G.; Gasanov, E.V. BDNF and Cortisol integrative system—Plasticity vs. degeneration: Implications of the Val66Met polymorphism. *Front. Neuroendocrinol.* **2019**, *55*. [CrossRef] [PubMed]

104. Karatsoreos, I.N.; McEwen, B.S. Psychobiological allostasis: Resistance, resilience and vulnerability. *Trends Cogn. Sci.* **2011**, *15*, 576–584. [CrossRef]

105. Wallingford, J.K.; Deurveilher, S.; Currie, R.W.; Fawcett, J.P.; Semba, K. Increases in mature brain-derived neurotrophic factor protein in the frontal cortex and basal forebrain during chronic sleep restriction in rats: Possible role in initiating allostatic adaptation. *Neuroscience* **2014**, *277*, 174–183. [CrossRef]

106. Yuluğ, B.; Ozan, E.; Gönül, A.S.; Kilic, E. Brain-derived neurotrophic factor, stress and depression: A minireview. *Brain Res. Bull.* **2009**, *78*, 267–269. [CrossRef]

107. Colaianna, M.; Schiavone, S.; Zotti, M.; Tucci, P.; Morgese, M.G.; Bäckdahl, L.; Holmdahl, R.; Krause, K.-H.; Cuomo, V.; Trabace, L. Neuroendocrine profile in a rat model of psychosocial stress: Relation to oxidative stress. *Antioxid. Redox. Signal* **2013**, *18*, 1385–1399. [CrossRef]

108. Kapczinski, F.; Vieta, E.; Andreazza, A.C.; Frey, B.N.; Gomes, F.A.; Tramontina, J.; Kauer-Sant'anna, M.; Grassi-Oliveira, R.; Post, R.M. Allostatic load in bipolar disorder: Implications for pathophysiology and treatment. *Neurosci. Biobehav. Rev.* **2008**, *32*, 675–692. [CrossRef]

109. Danhof-Pont, M.B.; van Veen, T.; Zitman, F.G. Biomarkers in burnout: A systematic review. *J. Psychosom. Res.* **2011**, *70*, 505–524. [CrossRef]

110. Pochwat, B.; Szewczyk, B.; Sowa-Kucma, M.; Siwek, A.; Doboszewska, U.; Piekoszewski, W.; Gruca, P.; Papp, M.; Nowak, G. Antidepressant-like activity of magnesium in the chronic mild stress model in rats: Alterations in the NMDA receptor subunits. *Int. J. Neuropsychopharmacol.* **2014**, *17*, 393–405. [CrossRef]

111. Vink, R. Magnesium in the CNS: Recent advances and developments. *Magnes. Res.* **2016**, *29*, 95–101. [CrossRef] [PubMed]

112. Zheltova, A.A.; Kharitonova, M.V.; Iezhitsa, I.N.; Spasov, A.A. Magnesium deficiency and oxidative stress: An update. *Biomed. Taipei* **2016**, *6*, 20. [CrossRef] [PubMed]

113. Brosschot, J.F.; Verkuil, B.; Thayer, J.F. The default response to uncertainty and the importance of perceived safety in anxiety and stress: An evolution-theoretical perspective. *J. Anxiety. Disord.* **2016**, *41*, 22–34. [CrossRef] [PubMed]

114. Somjen, G.G.; Baskerville, E.N. Effect of Excess Magnesium on Vagal Inhibition and Acetylcholine Sensitivity of the Mammalian Heart in situ and in vitro. *Nature* **1968**, *217*, 679–680. [CrossRef]

115. Toda, N.; West, T. Interaction between Na, Ca, Mg, and vagal stimulation in the S-A node of the rabbit. *Am. J. Physiol. Leg. Content* **1967**, *212*, 424–430. [CrossRef]

116. Murasato, Y.; Harada, Y.; Ikeda, M.; Nakashima, Y.; Hayashida, Y. Effect of Magnesium Deficiency on Autonomic Circulatory Regulation in Conscious Rats. *Hypertension* **1999**, *34*, 247–252. [CrossRef]

117. Brosschot, J.F.; Verkuil, B.; Thayer, J.F. Generalized Unsafety Theory of Stress: Unsafe Environments and Conditions, and the Default Stress Response. *Int. J. Environ. Res. Public Health* **2018**, *15*, 464. [CrossRef]

118. Stoian, M.; Stoica, V. The role of distubances of phosphate metabolism in metabolic syndrome. *Maedica Buchar.* **2014**, *9*, 255–260. [CrossRef]

119. Brosschot, J.F. Ever at the ready for events that never happen. *Eur. J. Psychotraumatol.* **2017**, *8*, 1309934. [CrossRef]

120. Kirkland, A.E.; Sarlo, G.L.; Holton, K.F. The Role of Magnesium in Neurological Disorders. *Nutrients* **2018**, *10*, 730. [CrossRef]

121. Lopresti, A.L. The Effects of Psychological and Environmental Stress on Micronutrient Concentrations in the Body: A Review of the Evidence. *Adv. Nutr.* **2019**, *11*, 103–112. [CrossRef] [PubMed]

122. Classen, H.G.; Marquardt, P.; Späth, M.; Schumacher, K.A. Hypermagnesemia Following Exposure to Acute Stress. *Pharmacology* **1971**, *5*, 287–294. [CrossRef] [PubMed]

123. Ising, H.; Handrock, M.; Günther, T.; Fischer, R.; Dombrowski, M. Increased noise trauma in guinea pigs through magnesium deficiency. *Arch. Oto Rhino Laryngol.* **1982**, *236*, 139–146. [CrossRef] [PubMed]

124. Joachims, Z.; Babisch, W.; Ising, H.; Günther, T.; Handrock, M. Dependence of noise-induced hearing loss upon perilymph magnesium concentration. *J. Acoust. Soc. Am.* **1983**, *74*, 104–108. [CrossRef] [PubMed]

125. Ising, H. Interaction of noise-induced stress and Mg decrease. *Artery* **1981**, *9*, 205–211.
126. Ando, I.; Karasawa, K.; Yokota, S.; Shioya, T.; Matsuda, H.; Tanaka, A. Analysis of serum magnesium ions in dogs exposed to external stress: A pilot study. *Open Vet. J.* **2017**, *7*, 367–374. [CrossRef]
127. Yasmin, F.; Haleem, D.J.; Haleem, M.A. Effects of repeated restraint stress on serum electrolytes in ethanol-treated and water-treated rats. *Pak. J. Pharm. Sci.* **2007**, *20*, 51–55.
128. Heroux, O.; Peter, D.; Heggtveit, A. Long-term Effect of Suboptimal Dietary Magnesium on Magnesium and Calcium Contents of Organs, on Cold Tolerance and on Lifespan, and its Pathological Consequences in Rats. *J. Nutr.* **1977**, *107*, 1640–1652. [CrossRef]
129. Terashima, Y.; Tucker, R.E.; Deetz, L.E.; Degregorio, R.M.; Muntifering, R.B.; Mitchell, G.E., Jr. Plasma Magnesium Levels as Influenced by Cold Exposure in Fed or Fasted Sheep. *J. Nutr.* **1982**, *112*, 1914–1920. [CrossRef]
130. Whyte, K.F.; Addis, G.J.; Whitesmith, R.; Reid, J.L. Adrenergic control of plasma magnesium in man. *Clin. Sci. Lond.* **1987**, *72*, 135–138. [CrossRef]
131. Tanabe, K.; Osada, N.; Suzuki, N.; Nakayama, M.; Yokoyama, Y.; Yamamoto, A.; Oya, M.; Murabayashi, T.; Yamamoto, M.; Omiya, K.; et al. Erythrocyte magnesium and prostaglandin dynamics in chronic sleep deprivation. *Clin. Cardiol.* **1997**, *20*, 265–268. [CrossRef] [PubMed]
132. Takase, B.; Akima, T.; Uehata, A.; Ohsuzu, F.; Kurita, A. Effect of chronic stress and sleep deprivation on both flow-mediated dilation in the brachial artery and the intracellular magnesium level in humans. *Clin. Cardiol.* **2004**, *27*, 223–227. [CrossRef] [PubMed]
133. Mocci, F.; Canalis, P.; Tomasi, P.A.; Casu, F.; Pettinato, S. The effect of noise on serum and urinary magnesium and catecholamines in humans. *Occup. Med.* **2001**, *51*, 56–61. [CrossRef] [PubMed]
134. Ising, H.; Dienel, D.; Günther, T.; Markert, B. Health effects of traffic noise. *Int. Arch. Occup. Environ. Health* **1980**, *47*, 179–190. [CrossRef]
135. Joborn, H.; Akerström, G.; Ljunghall, S. Effects of exogenous catecholamines and exercise on plasma magnesium concentrations. *Clin. Endocrinol.* **1985**, *23*, 219–226. [CrossRef]
136. Caddell, J.; Kupiecki, R.; Proxmire, D.; Satoh, P.; Hutchinson, B. Plasma Catecholamines in Acute Magnesium Deficiency in Weanling Rats. *JN* **1986**, *116*, 1896–1901. [CrossRef]
137. Amyard, N.; Leyris, A.; Monier, C.; Francès, H.; Boulu, R.G.; Henrotte, J.G. Brain catecholamines, serotonin and their metabolites in mice selected for low (MGL) and high (MGH) blood magnesium levels. *Magnes. Res.* **1995**, *8*, 5–9.
138. Henrotte, J.G.; Franck, G.; Santarromana, M.; Frances, H.; Mouton, D.; Motta, R. Mice selected for low and high blood magnesium levels: A new model for stress studies. *Physiol. Behav.* **1997**, *61*, 653–658. [CrossRef]
139. Henrotte, J.G.; Aymard, N.; Allix, M.; Boulu, R.G. Effect of pyridoxine and magnesium on stress-induced gastric ulcers in mice selected for low or high blood magnesium levels. *Ann. Nutr. Metab.* **1995**, *39*, 285–290. [CrossRef]
140. Sartori, S.B.; Whittle, N.; Hetzenauer, A.; Singewald, N. Magnesium deficiency induces anxiety and HPA axis dysregulation: Modulation by therapeutic drug treatment. *Neuropharmacology* **2012**, *62*, 304–312. [CrossRef]
141. Bourin, M.; Hascoët, M. The mouse light/dark box test. *Eur. J. Pharmacol.* **2003**, *463*, 55–65. [CrossRef]
142. Spasov, A.A.; Iezhitsa, I.N.; Kharitonova, M.V.; Kravchenko, M.S. Depression-like and anxiety-related behaviour of rats fed with magnesium-deficient diet. *Zhurnal Vysshei Nervnoi Deiatelnosti Imeni IP Pavlova* **2008**, *58*, 476–485.
143. Iezhitsa, I.N.; Spasov, A.A.; Kharitonova, M.V.; Kravchenko, M.S. Effect of magnesium chloride on psychomotor activity, emotional status, and acute behavioural responses to clonidine, d-amphetamine, arecoline, nicotine, apomorphine, and L-5-hydroxytryptophan. *Nutr. Neurosci.* **2011**, *14*, 10–24. [CrossRef] [PubMed]
144. Akarachkova, E. The role of magnesium deficiency in the formation of clinical manifestation of stress in women. *Probl. Women Health* **2013**, *8*, 57.
145. Nielsen, F.H.; Johnson, L.K.; Zeng, H. Magnesium supplementation improves indicators of low magnesium status and inflammatory stress in adults older than 51 years with poor quality sleep. *Magnes. Res.* **2010**, *23*, 158–168. [CrossRef]
146. Hermes Sales, C.; Azevedo Nascimento, D.; Queiroz Medeiros, A.C.; Costa Lima, K.; Campos Pedrosa, L.F.; Colli, C. There is chronic latent magnesium deficiency in apparently healthy university students. *Nutr. Hosp.* **2014** *30*, 200–204. [CrossRef]

147. Eby, G.A.; Eby, K.L. Magnesium for treatment-resistant depression: A review and hypothesis. *Med. Hypotheses* **2010**, *74*, 649–660. [CrossRef]

148. Forsyth, A.K.; Williams, P.G.; Deane, F.P. Nutrition status of primary care patients with depression and anxiety. *Aust. J. Prim. Health* **2012**, *18*, 172–176. [CrossRef]

149. Abumaria, N.; Yin, B.; Zhang, L.; Li, X.Y.; Chen, T.; Descalzi, G.; Zhao, L.; Ahn, M.; Luo, L.; Ran, C.; et al. Effects of elevation of brain magnesium on fear conditioning, fear extinction, and synaptic plasticity in the infralimbic prefrontal cortex and lateral amygdala. *J. Neurosci.* **2011**, *31*, 14871–14881. [CrossRef]

150. Pochwat, B.; Sowa-Kucma, M.; Kotarska, K.; Misztak, P.; Nowak, G.; Szewczyk, B. Antidepressant-like activity of magnesium in the olfactory bulbectomy model is associated with the AMPA/BDNF pathway. *Psychopharmacology* **2015**, *232*, 355–367. [CrossRef]

151. Pilchova, I.; Klacanova, K.; Tatarkova, Z.; Kaplan, P.; Racay, P. The Involvement of Mg(2+) in Regulation of Cellular and Mitochondrial Functions. *Oxid Med. Cell Longev.* **2017**, *2017*, 6797460. [CrossRef] [PubMed]

152. Zogović, D.; Pesić, V.; Dmitrasinović, G.; Dajak, M.; Plećas, B.; Batinić, B.; Popović, D.; Ignjatović, S. Pituitary-gonadal, pituitary-adrenocortical hormonal and IL-6 levels following long-term magnesium supplementation in male students. *J. Med. Biochem.* **2014**, *33*, 291–298. [CrossRef]

153. Wienecke, E.; Nolden, C. Long-term HRV analysis shows stress reduction by magnesium intake. *MMW Fortschr. Med.* **2016**, *158*, 12–16. [CrossRef] [PubMed]

154. Pouteau, E.; Kabir-Ahmadi, M.; Noah, L.; Mazur, A.; Dye, L.; Hellhammer, J.; Pickering, G.; Dubray, C. Superiority of magnesium and vitamin B6 over magnesium alone on severe stress in healthy adults with low magnesemia: A randomized, single-blind clinical trial. *PLoS ONE* **2018**, *13*, e0208454. [CrossRef] [PubMed]

155. Eby, G.A.; Eby, K.L. Rapid recovery from major depression using magnesium treatment. *Med. Hypotheses* **2006**, *67*, 362–370. [CrossRef]

156. Boyle, N.B.; Lawton, C.; Dye, L. The Effects of Magnesium Supplementation on Subjective Anxiety and Stress-A Systematic Review. *Nutrients* **2017**, *9*, 429. [CrossRef]

Permissions

The contributors of this book come from diverse backgrounds, making this book a truly international effort. This book will bring forth new frontiers with its revolutionizing research information and detailed analysis of the nascent developments around the world.

We would like to thank all the contributing authors for lending their expertise to make the book truly unique. They have played a crucial role in the development of this book. Without their invaluable contributions this book wouldn't have been possible. They have made vital efforts to compile up to date information on the varied aspects of this subject to make this book a valuable addition to the collection of many professionals and students.

This book was conceptualized with the vision of imparting up-to-date information and advanced data in this field. To ensure the same, a matchless editorial board was set up. Every individual on the board went through rigorous rounds of assessment to prove their worth. After which they invested a large part of their time researching and compiling the most relevant data for our readers.

The editorial board has been involved in producing this book since its inception. They have spent rigorous hours researching and exploring the diverse topics which have resulted in the successful publishing of this book. They have passed on their knowledge of decades through this book. To expedite this challenging task, the publisher supported the team at every step. A small team of assistant editors was also appointed to further simplify the editing procedure and attain best results for the readers.

Apart from the editorial board, the designing team has also invested a significant amount of their time in understanding the subject and creating the most relevant covers. They scrutinized every image to scout for the most suitable representation of the subject and create an appropriate cover for the book.

The publishing team has been an ardent support to the editorial, designing and production team. Their endless efforts to recruit the best for this project, has resulted in the accomplishment of this book. They are a veteran in the field of academics and their pool of knowledge is as vast as their experience in printing. Their expertise and guidance has proved useful at every step. Their uncompromising quality standards have made this book an exceptional effort. Their encouragement from time to time has been an inspiration for everyone.

The publisher and the editorial board hope that this book will prove to be a valuable piece of knowledge for researchers, students, practitioners and scholars across the globe.

List of Contributors

Svetlana Orlova
Department of Dietetics and Clinical Nutritiology of Continuing Medical Education, Medical Institute, RUDN University, 119571 Moscow, Russia

Galina Dikke
Department of Obstetrics and Gynecology with a Course of Reproductive Medicine, The Academy of Medical Education F.I. Inozemtsev, 190013 Saint-Petersburg, Russia

Gisele Pickering
Department of Clinical Pharmacology, University Hospital and Inserm 1107 Fundamental and Clinical Pharmacology of Pain, Medical Faculty, F-63000 Clermont-Ferrand, France

Sofya Konchits, Kirill Starostin and Alina Bevz
Medical Affairs, Sanofi, 125009 Moscow, Russia

Gozewijn D. Laverman
Department of Internal Medicine/Nephrology, ZGT Hospital, 7609 PP Almelo, The Netherlands

Christina M. Gant
Department of Internal Medicine/Nephrology, ZGT Hospital, 7609 PP Almelo, The Netherlands
Department of Internal Medicine, Division of Nephrology, University of Groningen, University Medical Centre Groningen, 9713EZ Groningen, The Netherlands

S. Heleen Binnenmars, Stephan J. L. Bakker and Gerjan Navis
Department of Internal Medicine, Division of Nephrology, University of Groningen, University Medical Centre Groningen, 9713EZ Groningen, The Netherlands

Sabita S. Soedamah-Muthu
Centre of Research on Psychology in Somatic Diseases (CORPS), Department of Medical and Clinical Psychology, Tilburg University, 5037 AB Tilburg, The Netherlands
Institute for Food, Nutrition and Health, University of Reading, Reading RG1 5EX, UK

Francesca Luongo, Giuseppe Pietropaolo, Federica I. Wolf and Valentina Trapani
Istituto di Patologia Generale, Università Cattolica del Sacro Cuore, Fondazione Policlinico Universitario "Agostino Gemelli" IRCCS, I-00168 Rome, Italy

Mathieu Gautier, Isabelle Dhennin-Duthille and Halima Ouadid-Ahidouch
Laboratoire de Physiologie Cellulaire et Moléculaire-EA4667, UFR Sciences, Université de Picardie Jules Verne, F-80039 Amiens, France

Nuria Rosique-Esteban, Pablo Hernández-Alonso and Jordi Salas-Salvadó
Human Nutrition Unit, Department of Biochemistry and Biotechnology, Faculty of Medicine and Health Sciences, University Hospital of Sant Joan de Reus, Pere Virgili Institute for Health Research, Rovira i Virgili University, St/Sant Llorenç 21, 43201 Reus, Spain
CIBERobn Physiopathology of Obesity and Nutrition, Institute of Health Carlos III (ISCIII), 28029 Madrid, Spain

Marta Guasch-Ferré
Human Nutrition Unit, Department of Biochemistry and Biotechnology, Faculty of Medicine and Health Sciences, University Hospital of Sant Joan de Reus, Pere Virgili Institute for Health Research, Rovira i Virgili University, St/Sant Llorenç 21, 43201 Reus, Spain
CIBERobn Physiopathology of Obesity and Nutrition, Institute of Health Carlos III (ISCIII), 28029 Madrid, Spain
Department of Nutrition, Harvard T.H. Chan School of Public Health, Boston, MA 02115, USA

Serafi Cambray, Marcelino Bermudez-Lopez, Manuel Marti-Antonio, Milica Bozic, Elvira Fernandez and Jose M. Valdivielso
Vascular and Renal Translational Research Group, Institute for Biomedical Research Pifarré Foundation, IRBLleida Av. Rovira Roure 80, 25198 Lleida, Spain

Merce Ibarz
Indicators and Specifications of the Quality in the Clinical Laboratory Group, Institute for Biomedical Research Pifarré Foundation, IRBLleida, 25198 Lleida, Spain

Evertine Wesselink, Renate M. Winkels, Harm van Baar, Anne J. M. R. Geijsen, Moniek van Zutphen, Ellen Kampman and Dieuwertje E. G. Kok
Division of Human Nutrition, Wageningen University & Research, Stippeneng 4, 6708 WE Wageningen, The Netherlands

Henk K. van Halteren
Department of Internal Medicine, Admiraal de Ruyter Ziekenhuis, 's-Gravenpolderseweg 114, 4462 RA Goes, The Netherlands

Bibi M. E. Hansson
Department of Surgery, Canisius Wilhelmina Ziekenhuis, Weg door het Jonkerbos 100, 6532 SZ Nijmegen, The Netherlands

Sandra A. Radema
Department of Medical Oncology, Radboud University Medical Centre, Geert Grooteplein-Zuid 22, 6525 GA Nijmegen, The Netherlands

Johannes H. W. de Wilt
Department of Surgery, Radboud University Medical Centre, Geert Grooteplein-Zuid 22, 6525 GA Nijmegen, The Netherlands

Anne-Sophie Garnier, Agnès Duveau, Martin Planchais and Johnny Sayegh
LUNAM Université, 49180 Angers, France
Université Angers, CHU Angers, Service de Néphrologie-Dialyse-Transplantation, CHU d'Angers, 49933 Angers CEDEX 9, France

Jean-François Subra and Jean-François Augusto
LUNAM Université, 49180 Angers, France
Université Angers, CHU Angers, Service de Néphrologie-Dialyse-Transplantation, CHU d'Angers, 49933 Angers CEDEX 9, France
CRCINA, INSERM, Université de Nantes, Université d'Angers, LabEx IGO Immunotherapy, Graft, Oncology, 44007 Angers, France

Giuseppe Pietropaolo, Federica I. Wolf and Valentina Trapani
Sezione di Patologia Generale, Dipartimento di Medicina e Chirurgia Traslazionale, Fondazione Policlinico Universitario A. Gemelli IRCCS — Università Cattolica del Sacro Cuore, 00168 Rome, Italy

Daniela Pugliese, Alessandro Armuzzi, Luisa Guidi, Antonio Gasbarrini and Gian Lodovico Rapaccini
UOC Medicina Interna e Gastroenterologia, Dipartimento di Medicina e Chirurgia Traslazionale, Fondazione Policlinico Universitario A. Gemelli IRCCS — Università Cattolica del Sacro Cuore, 00168 Rome, Italy

Beata Ryszewska-Pokraśniewicz
Nowowiejski Hospital, 00-685 Warsaw, Poland

Anna Mach, Michał Skalski, Piotr Januszko and Maria Radziwoń-Zaleska
Department of Psychiatry, Medical University of Warsaw, 00-685 Warsaw, Poland

Zbigniew M. Wawrzyniak
Faculty of Electronics and Information Technology, Warsaw University of Technology, 00-685 Warsaw, Poland

Ewa Poleszak
Faculty of Pharmacy, Medical University of Lublin, 20-093 Lublin, Poland

Gabriel Nowak and Andrzej Pilc
Institute of Pharmacology, Polish Academy of Sciences, 31-343 Kraków, Poland

Pamela L. Lutsey and Melanie Jaeb
Division of Epidemiology & Community Health, School of Public Health, University of Minnesota, 1300 South 2nd Street, Suite 300, Minneapolis, MN 55454, USA

Lin Y. Chen
Cardiovascular Division, Department of Medicine, University of Minnesota, Minneapolis, MN 55455, USA

Anne Eaton, Kyle D. Rudser and James D. Neaton
Division of Biostatistics, School of Public Health, University of Minnesota, Minneapolis, MN 55455, USA

Alvaro Alonso
Department of Epidemiology, Rollins School of Public Health, Emory University, Atlanta, GA 30322, USA

Anna E. Kirkland and Gabrielle L. Sarlo
Department of Psychology, Behavior, Cognition and Neuroscience Program, American University, Washington, DC 20016, USA

Kathleen F. Holton
Department of Health Studies, American University, Washington, DC 20016, USA
Center for Behavioral Neuroscience, American University, Washington, DC 20016, USA

Justyna Malinowska
Students Scientific Group of Laboratory Medicine, Medical University of Warsaw, 02-097 Warsaw, Poland

Milena Małecka and Olga Ciepiela
Department of Laboratory Medicine, Medical University of Warsaw, 02-097 Warsaw, Poland

Kristien J. Ledeganck, Charlotte Anné, Amandine De Monie, Sarang Meybosch, Gert A. Verpooten, Marleen Vinckx, Annelies Van Eyck and Benedicte Y. De Winter
Laboratory of Experimental Medicine and Pediatrics, University of Antwerp, Universiteitsplein 1, T3.34, 2610 Antwerp, Belgium

Koen Van Hoeck and Dominique Trouet
Laboratory of Experimental Medicine and Pediatrics, University of Antwerp, Universiteitsplein 1, T3.34, 2610 Antwerp, Belgium
Department of Pediatric Nephrology, Antwerp University Hospital, Wilrijkstraat 10, 2650 Edegem, Belgium

Nora M. O'Brien
School of Food and Nutritional Sciences, University College Cork, T12 K8AF Cork, Ireland

Valeria D. Felice
Department of Pharmacology and Therapeutics and Department of Physiology, University College Cork, T12 K8AF Cork, Ireland
School of Food and Nutritional Sciences, University College Cork, T12 K8AF Cork, Ireland
APC Microbiome Ireland, University College Cork, T12 K8AF Cork, Ireland

Niall P. Hyland
Department of Pharmacology and Therapeutics and Department of Physiology, University College Cork, T12 K8AF Cork, Ireland
APC Microbiome Ireland, University College Cork, T12 K8AF Cork, Ireland

Yutaka Shindo and Kohji Hotta
Department of Bioscience and Informatics, Faculty of Science and Technology, Keio University, Yokohama, Kanagawa 223-8522, Japan

Ryu Yamanaka
Department of Bioscience and Informatics, Faculty of Science and Technology, Keio University, Yokohama, Kanagawa 223-8522, Japan
Faculty of Pharmaceutical Sciences, Sanyo-Onoda City University, Sanyo-Onoda, Yamaguchi 756-0884, Japan

Kotaro Oka
Department of Bioscience and Informatics, Faculty of Science and Technology, Keio University, Yokohama, Kanagawa 223-8522, Japan
Waseda Research Institute for Science and Engineering, Waseda University, Shinjuku, Tokyo 162-8480, Japan
Graduate Institute of Medicine, College of Medicine, Kaohsiung Medical University, Kaohsiung 80708, Taiwan

Nikolina Banjanin and Goran Belojevic
Institute of Hygiene and Medical Ecology, Faculty of Medicine, University of Belgrade, 11000 Belgrade, Serbia

Gisèle Pickering
Plateforme d'Investigation Clinique/CIC Inserm 1405, University Hospital CHU, 63000 Clermont-Ferrand, France

André Mazur
INRAE, UNH, Unité de Nutrition Humaine, Université Clermont Auvergne, 63001 Clermont-Ferrand, France

Denise M. O'Gorman
Marigot Ltd., P43 NN62 Cork, Ireland

Marion Trousselard
Independent Regulatory Board for Auditors (IRBA), 91220 Bretigny-sur-Orge, France

Przemyslaw Bienkowski
Department of Psychiatry, Warsaw Medical University, 02-091 Warsaw, Poland

Natalia Yaltsewa
Department of General Medicine, The Yaroslavl State Medical University Institute of Postgraduate Education, 150000 Yaroslavl, Russia

Mohamed Amessou, Lionel Noah and Etienne Pouteau
Medical Affairs Department, Consumer HealthCare, Sanofi, Gentilly, 94250 Paris, France

Index